Epilepsy - Advances in Diagnosis and Therapy

Edited by Isam Jaber Al-Zwaini
and Ban Adbul-Hameed Majeed Albadri

Published in London, United Kingdom

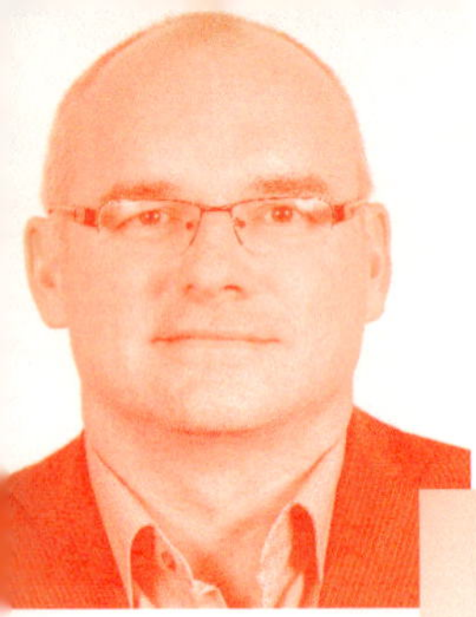
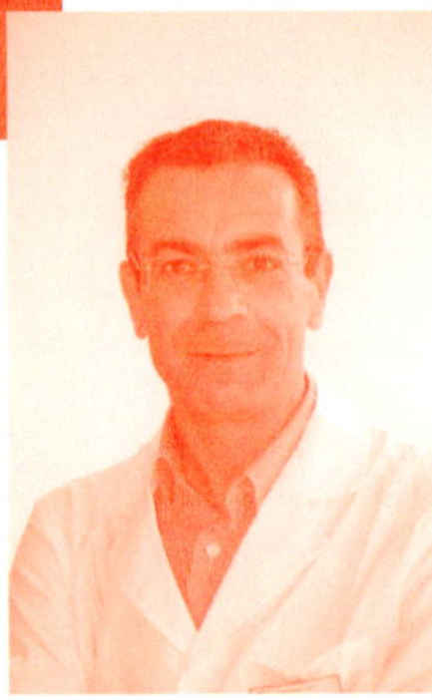
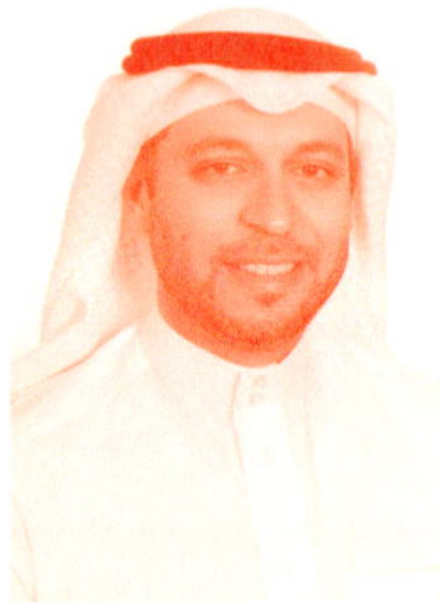
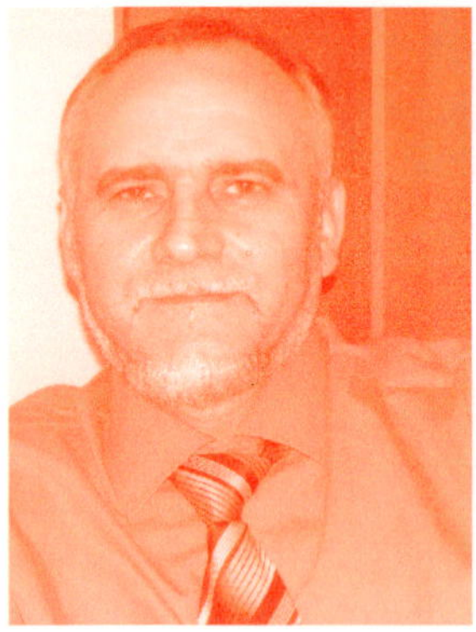
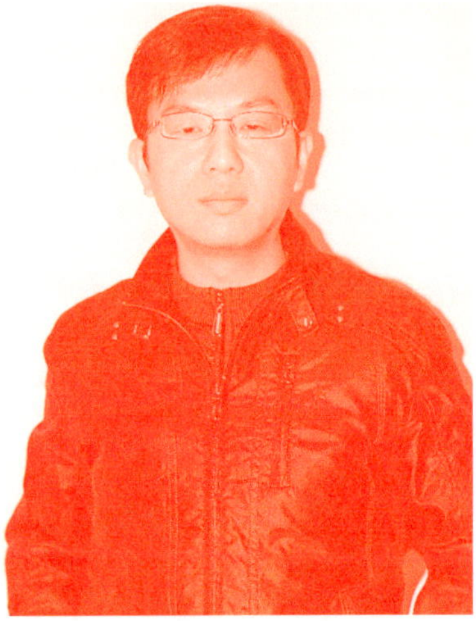
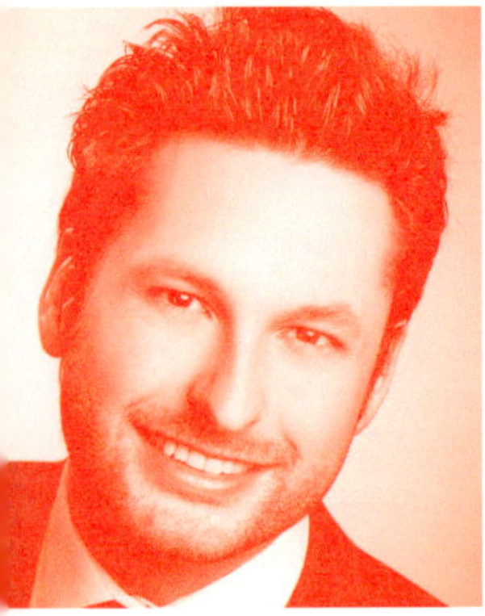
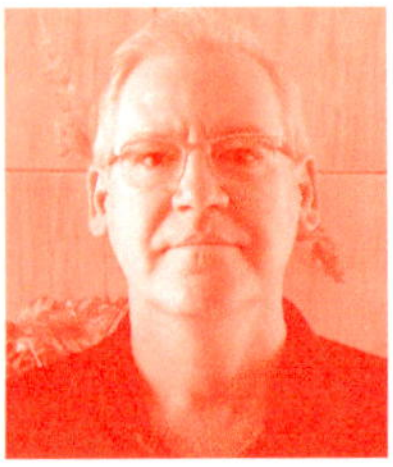

IntechOpen

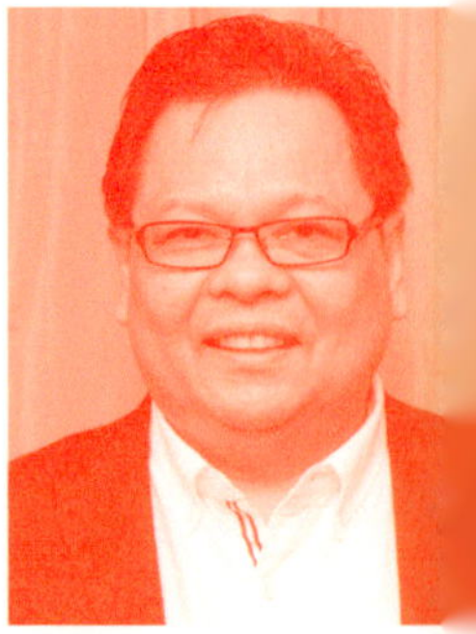
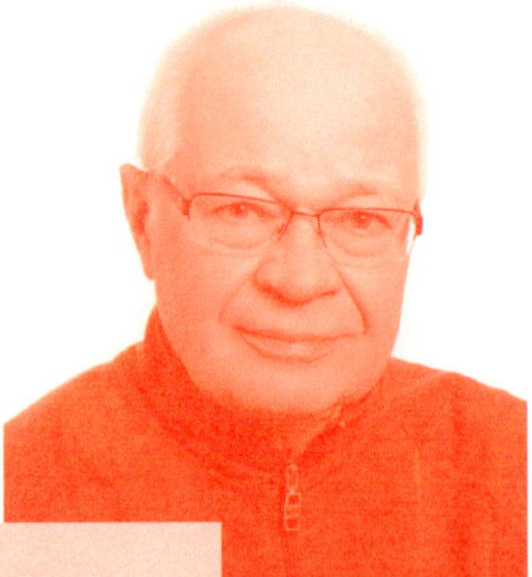
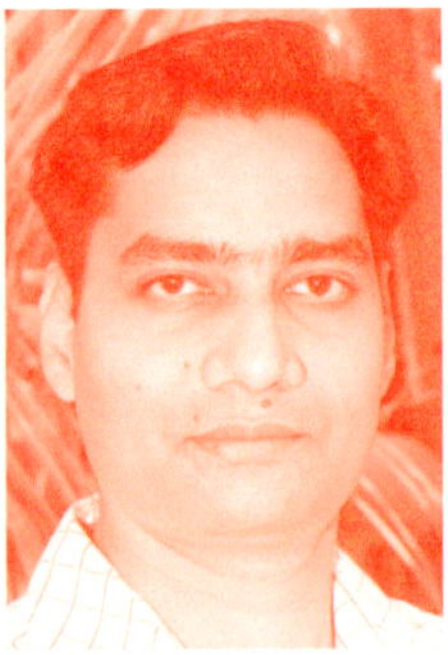
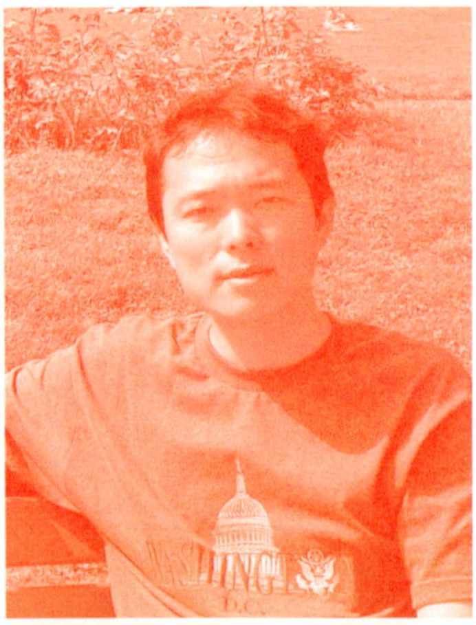
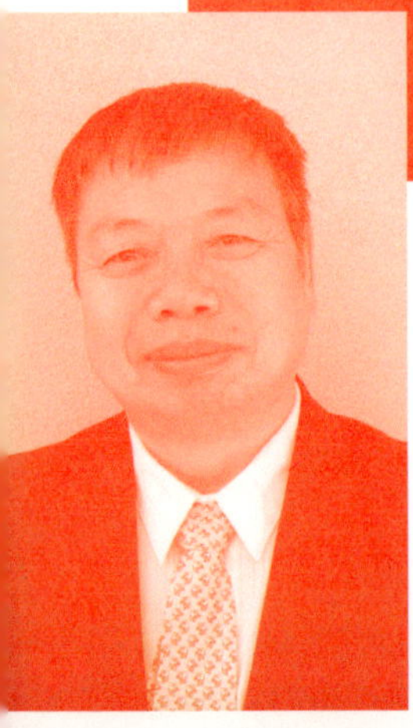
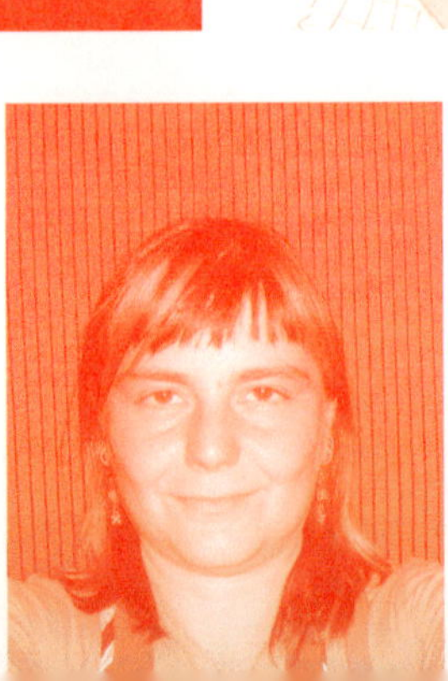

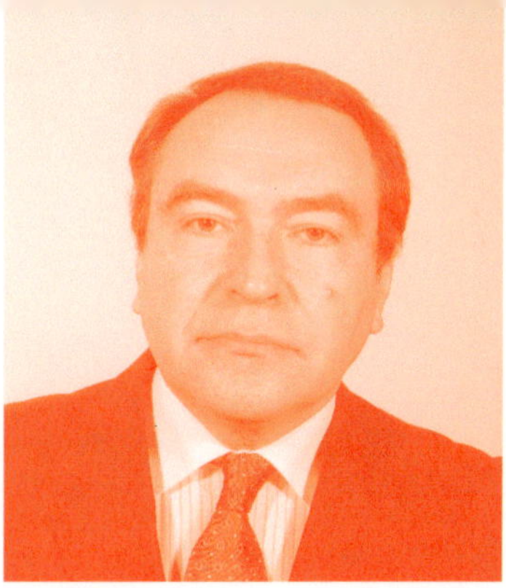
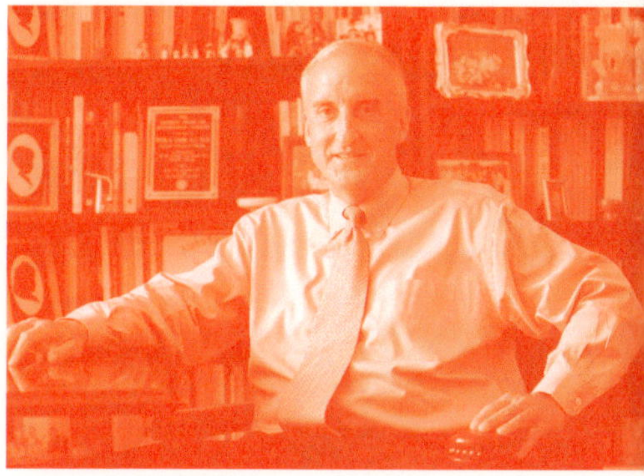
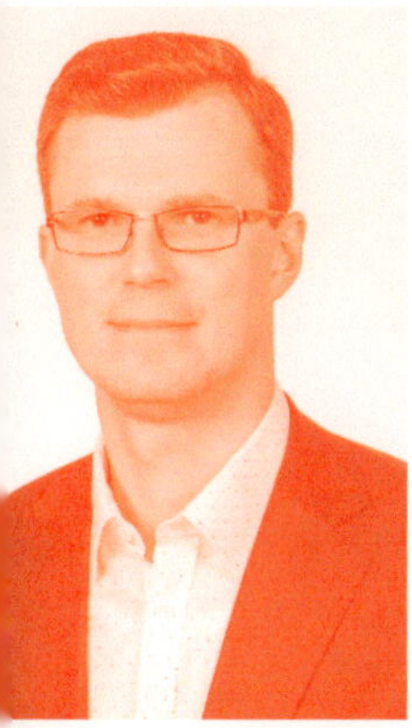
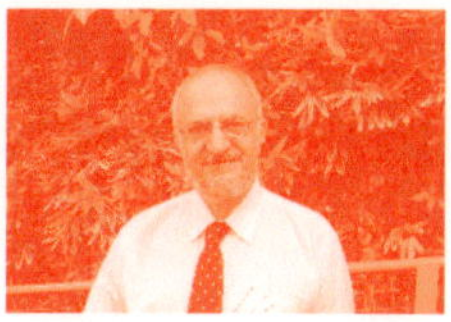
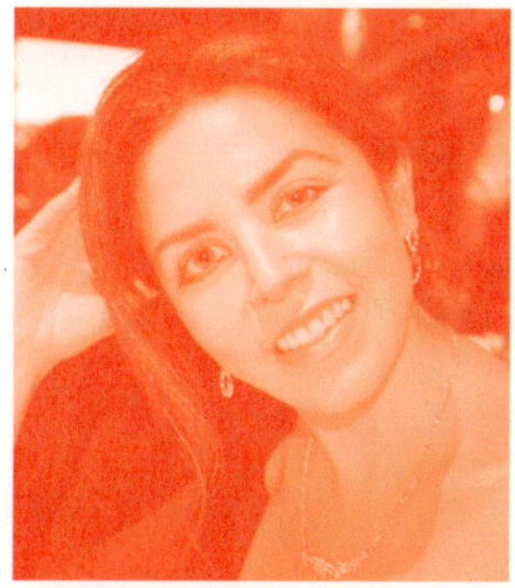

Supporting open minds since 2005

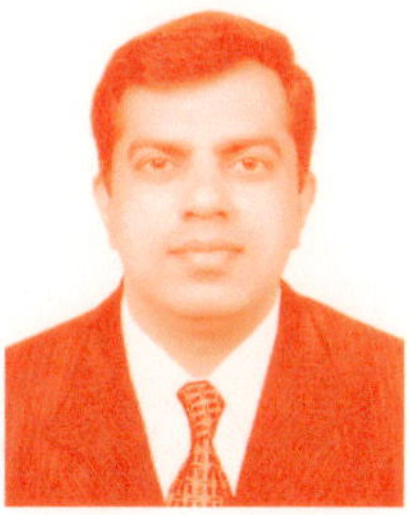
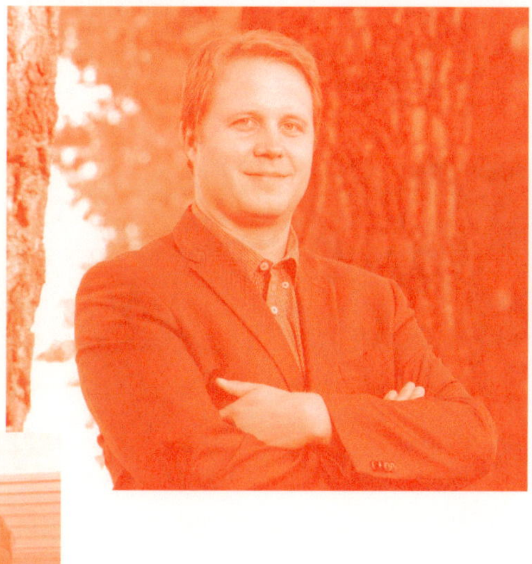
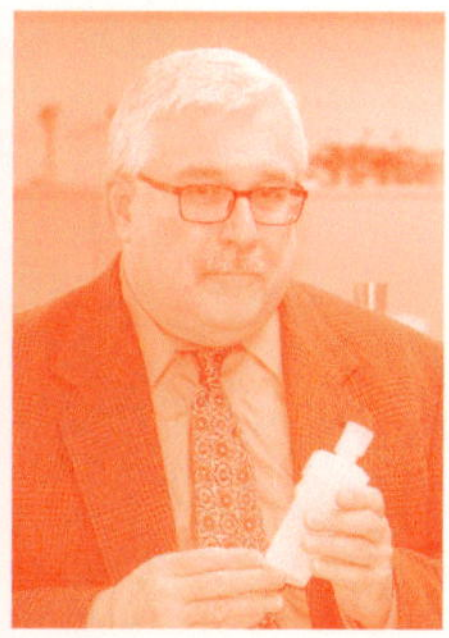
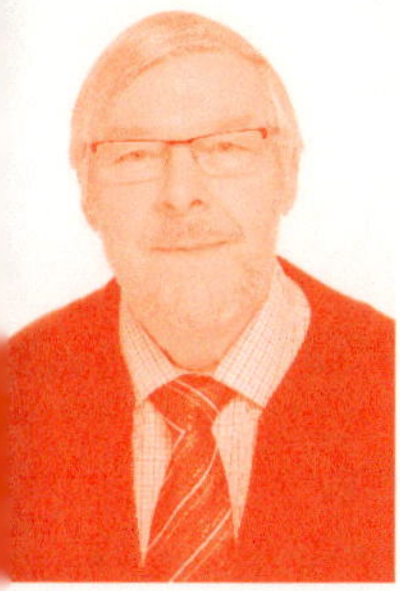
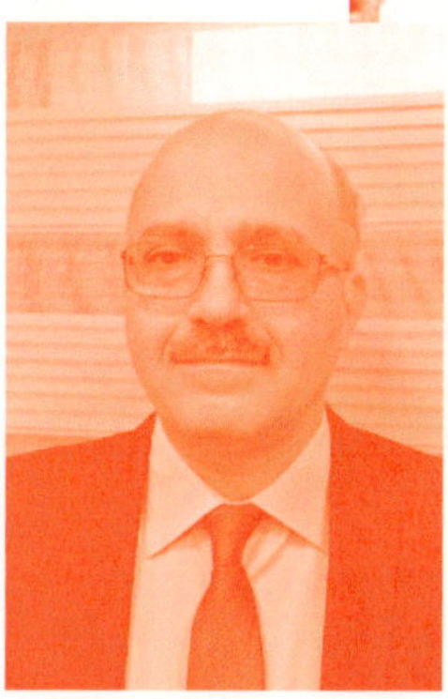
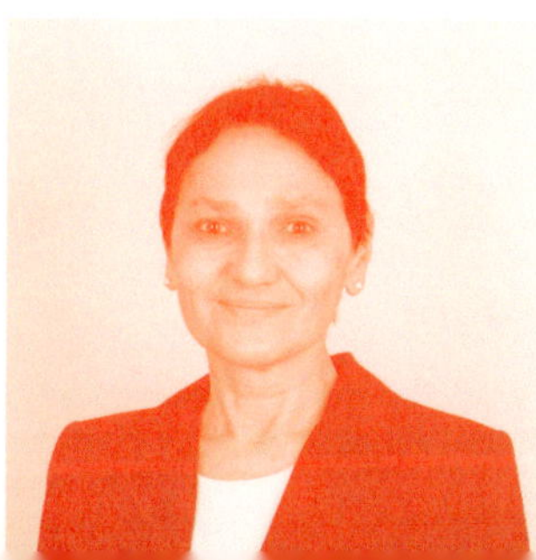
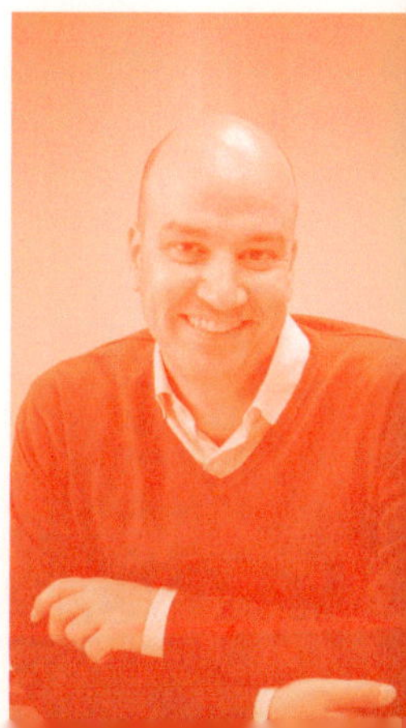

Epilepsy - Advances in Diagnosis and Therapy
http://dx.doi.org/10.5772/intechopen.77678
Edited by Isam Jaber Al-Zwaini and Ban Adbul-Hameed Majeed Albadri

Contributors
Boulenouar Mesraoua, Dirk Deleu, Hassan Al Hail, Gayane Melykian, Naim Haddad, Musab Ali, Lubna El Sheikh, Yasser Osman M Ali, Ali Alsadi Pooya, Peter Kaplan, Mohd Farooq Shaikh, Vanessa Lin Lin Lee, Suguna Nanthini, Alexey Kholin, Otman Fernandez-Concepcion, Melvin Lopez-Jimenez, Natalia Shnayder, Ekaterina Narodova, Valeriya Narodova, Andrey Narodov, Evgeniy Erakhtin, Halil Kocamaz, Sedat Isikay, Jie Tao, Shuzhang Zhang, Yudan Zhu, Jiwei Cheng, Laadraoui Jawad, Chait Abderrahman, Matthew Phillips, Isam Jaber Al-Zwaini

First published in London, United Kingdom, 2019 by IntechOpen
IntechOpen is the global imprint of INTECHOPEN LIMITED, registered in England and Wales, registration number: 11086078, 7th floor, 10 Lower Thames Street, London, EC3R 6AF, United Kingdom
Printed in Croatia

British Library Cataloguing-in-Publication Data
A catalogue record for this book is available from the British Library

Additional hard and PDF copies can be obtained from orders@intechopen.com

Epilepsy - Advances in Diagnosis and Therapy
Edited by Isam Jaber Al-Zwaini and Ban Adbul-Hameed Majeed Albadri
p. cm.
Print ISBN 978-1-78923-867-9
Online ISBN 978-1-78923-868-6
eBook (PDF) ISBN 978-1-83962-570-1

For EU product safety concerns:
IN TECH d.o.o., Prolaz Marije Krucifikse Kozulić 3, 51000 Rijeka, Croatia, info@intechopen.com or visit our website at intechopen.com.

Meet the editors

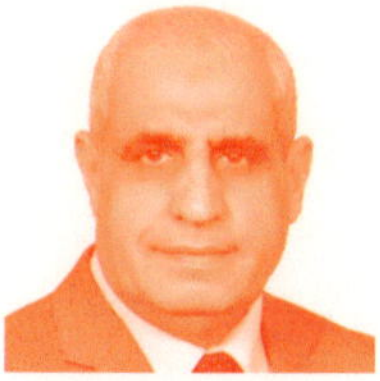

Prof. Isam Jaber AL-Zwaini was born on 4 January 1963 in Baghdad, Iraq. After graduation from the AL-Mustansiryia College of Medicine in 1987, he worked as a house officer in different hospitals in Baghdad for 15 months, followed by military service for 3 years. He started his pediatric study in 1991 and gained the Fellowship of Iraqi Commission for Medical Specializations in 1996. He started his work as a lecturer in the Department of Pediatrics, AL-Anbar Medical College from 1996 to 2001 when he was promoted to Assistant Professor. In 2005, he started working in the Department of Pediatrics, AL-Kindy Medical College, University of Baghdad and was promoted to Professor in 2008. He has an Associate Membership of the Royal College of Pediatrics and Child Health, UK since 2007. He became Head of the Pediatric Department in AL-Anbar and AL-Kindy Medical College for many years. He has published more than 30 scientific papers in different pediatric fields and he has a special interest in pediatric hematology, neurology, and nutrition.

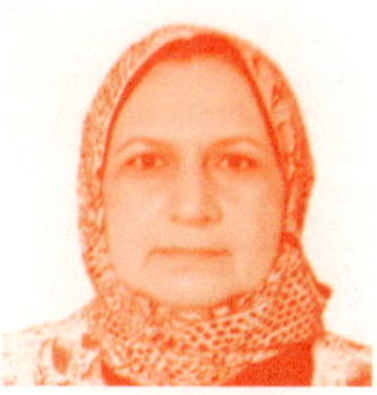

Assistant Prof. Ban Adbul-Hameed Majeed Albadri was born in 1962 in Baghdad, Iraq. After graduation from the AL-Mustansiryia College of Medicine in 1986, she worked as a house officer in different hospitals in Baghdad for one year. She started her pediatric study in 1991 and was awarded her Higher Diploma in Pediatrics from the Al-Mustansyria Medical College in October 1995. She gained the Fellowship of Iraqi Commission for Medical Specializations in March 1997. She started her work as a pediatrician in Tikrit General Teaching Hospital in April 1997. She applied to AL-Kindy General Hospital as a pediatrician in May 2003 and was appointed as a senior lecturer at AL-Kindy Medical College, Baghdad University in March 2005. She was promoted to Assistant Professor in 2010. She has published many scientific papers in different pediatric fields and she has a special interest in pediatric neurology and nutrition.

Contents

Preface

Epilepsy is the most common neurological disorder globally, affecting approximately 50 million people of all ages. It is one of the oldest diseases described in literature from remote ancient civilizations 2000–3000 years ago. Despite its long history and wide spread, epilepsy is still surrounded by myth and prejudice, which can only be overcome with great difficulty. The term *epilepsy* is derived from the Greek verb *epilambanein*, which by itself means to be seized and to be overwhelmed by surprise or attack. Therefore, epilepsy is a condition of getting over, seized, or attacked. The twelve very interesting chapters of this book cover various aspects of epileptology from the history and milestones of epilepsy as a disease entity to the most recent advances in understanding and diagnosing epilepsy.

The first chapter is an introductory chapter written by the editors. In this chapter, we trace the earliest records and the major milestones in the history of epilepsy since the early civilization in Mesopotamia (the ancient name of Iraq), almost 2000–3000 B.C. These early establishments include the Sumerian, Babylonian, Assyrian, and Akkadian civilizations. The first description of epilepsy was written in the Akkadian language in about 2000 B.C., in which the author described a condition similar to epileptic seizures in a patient. The contribution of the ancient Egyptian, old Chines, and Greek civilizations to the history of epilepsy is also described in this chapter. The father of medicine, Hippocrates, in his book "Sacred Disease" written in 400 B.C, raised the first dispute about the divine origin of epilepsy. He said "This disease is in my opinion no more divine than any other; it has the same nature as other diseases and the cause that gives rise to individual diseases. This chapter also follows the evolution of epilepsy as a disease entity and the discovery of anticonvulsant therapy throughout the middle ages and provides a short review about the misconceptions, incorrect beliefs, and myths surrounding epilepsy.

The second chapter by Vanessa Lin Lin Lee and Mohd. Farooq Shaikh, briefly discusses how neuroinflammation is involved in epileptogenesis as well as the status of inflammation in post-epileptic conditions; whether it is the cause or consequence of epilepsy, together with experimental evidence. The exact cause of epilepsy is still unknown, but there is mounting evidence showing that the development of epileptogenesis can be linked to a wide array of factors such as genetic predisposition, developmental disorders, and neurological insults. Neurological insults, which contribute to up to 60% of epilepsy cases, include traumatic brain injuries, cerebrovascular accidents, central nervous system infections, and strokes. Inflammation is one of the key features of epileptogenesis. However, the role of inflammation in epilepsy is still being actively studied, with various arguments on whether inflammation is the cause or consequence of epilepsy. The blood-brain barrier (BBB), which functions as a protector of the central nervous system, has an important role in regulating the transfer of blood constituents in the brain extracellular space. Increased BBB permeability or BBB leakage is said to be one of the earliest characteristics of the pathophysiology of epileptogenesis. BBB dysfunction may contribute to epileptogenesis via a cascade of events triggered by leakage of inflammatory mediators into the central nervous system (CNS), which causes neuroinflammation.

The third chapter is by Jawad Laadraoui and Abderrahman Chait in which they evaluate the convulsive effects of intracerebroventricular administration of cigarette smoke condensate in rats and compare the intensity of seizures with kainic acid induced-seizures as a model of epilepsy. They also evaluate the role of the cholinergic system using mAChRs antagonist in cigarette smoke condensate induced seizures. Tobacco smoke is a complex multi-component system, in which there are more than 4800 compounds, many of which are carcinogens. As a result, chronic obstructive pulmonary disease, chronic bronchitis, cardiovascular disease, emphysema, stroke, and many forms of cancer are directly related to smoking. The results of this study indicate that the central injection of cigarette condensate provides an epileptic behavior similar to that induced by kainic acid. However, pretreatment with atropine reduced seizures and all their parameters.

In the fourth chapter, Dr. Boulenouar Mesraoua et al describe non-convulsive status epilepticus (NCSE) in patients with altered mental status admitted to Hamad General Hospital, Doha, Qatar. The authors aim to update the current status of NCSE with particular emphasis on NCSE in the Middle Eastern and North African region, to find the prevalence of NCSE in patients with altered mental status, describing the clinical presentation, EEG findings, etiology, neuroimaging, treatment and outcome of NCSE in Qatar, and to discuss the time it takes to record NCSE in the intensive care unit using continuous EEG monitoring in patients with altered mental states. This study shows disappointing results regarding NCSE, which appears to be an emerging condition requiring rapid diagnosis and rapid treatment.

The fifth chapter, by Halil Kocamaz, is dedicated to gastrointestinal disorders associated with epilepsy. The gastrointestinal system communicates with the brain via the vagus nerve fibers and gut-brain axis. There is a well-known relationship between autoimmune diseases and epileptogenesis and this may explain why gut microbiota can interfere in the course of epilepsy. Many seizures that are described, depending on the severity and/or duration, as benign may have gastrointestinal origin. Epilepsy and related neurological symptoms may alert the clinician for additional life-threatening conditions and complications during the course of gastrointestinal-based chronic diseases such as inflammatory bowel disease and celiac disease. As the gut is the only exposed part of the inner body to environment gut-microbiota, novel therapeutic options that targets the gut may be promising in many diseases including epilepsy.

The sixth chapter, by Otman Fernandez-Concepcion and Melvin Lopez-Jimenez, reviews epileptic encephalopathies in infants and children. The concept of epileptic encephalopathies is based on the clinical descriptions of some epileptic syndromes during the last century. It represents a group of devastating epileptic disorders that appear early in life and are characterized by drug-resistant, generalized or focal seizures, persistent severe EEG abnormalities, and cognitive dysfunction or decline. In this review, the authors discuss the clinical and electroencephalographic characteristics, evaluation, and management of age-related epileptic encephalopathies, recognized by the International League Against Epilepsy. These include early infantile epileptic encephalopathy (Ohtahara syndrome), early myoclonic encephalopathy, epilepsy of infancy with migrating focal seizures, West syndrome, severe myoclonic epilepsy in infancy (Dravet syndrome), myoclonic–atonic epilepsy (Doose syndrome), Lennox-Gastaut syndrome, epileptic encephalopathy with continuous spike-and-wave during sleep, and Landau-Kleffner syndrome. Their etiologies, clinical features, treatment, and prognoses are presented and updated.

In the seventh chapter, Professor Alexey Kholin gives a description of malignant migrating partial seizures in infancy, also known as Coppola-Dulac syndrome. This syndrome is a rare and usually unrecognized epileptic syndrome of infancy. The first publication presented by G. Coppola and colleagues in 1995 and O. Dulac in 2005 summarized 24 patients' follow-up in the Saint Vincent de Paul Hospital in Paris. Clinical cases have demonstrated a new epileptic syndrome, different from previously described forms of epileptic encephalopathies of infancy. Seizure onset is before the age of 6 months. From the age of 1 to 10 months, seizures become very frequent and polymorphic, usually clustered in nature, with mental and motor retardation clear. Clinical manifestation of seizures may include head and eye deviation, lateralized clonic eyelids twitching, fixed gaze, tonic or clonic spasm of one limb or hemi spasms, axial tonic spasms, chewing or sucking movements, episodes of apnea, flushing, hypersalivation, and secondary generalized seizures. Video-EEG monitoring plays the most important role in the diagnosis. Ictal EEG patterns involve different areas of the cerebral cortex of both hemispheres, the initial zone of ictal patterns shifts from one region to another. It is a drug-resistant type of epilepsy with serious prognosis.

The eighth chapter is by Irma Khachidze and is about the dynamics of EEG characteristics in epileptic children during treatment with valproic acid. In this chapter, the author discusses the results of her original article aiming to investigate the alteration of different characteristics of interictal EEG in epileptic children during AED therapy. The analysis of the dynamics of background EEG reveals possible early predictors of the treatment's benefits or adverse effects. Determination of the efficacy of AED based on EEG criteria is very important for optimization of anti-epileptic therapy in individual patients. The result of this study concludes that reduction of high-amplitude low-frequency waves and suppression of epileptiform patterns simultaneously with clinical improvement at three to six months after treatment can serve as an indicator of effective therapy. Brain mapping reveals the essential prognostic or predicting value of morphology of the theta-waves and their distribution.

The ninth chapter is by Natalia Shnayder et al and it is about the role of non-drug treatment methods in epilepsy treatment in adult patients in Russia and abroad. An important problem of epileptology is ensuring the safety and acceptability of the treatment as well as prevention of adverse drug reactions of antiepileptic drugs. The emergence of ASEs can often decrease patients' life quality, thereby offsetting the positive effect of the treatment. Moreover, such adverse side effects as depression and anxiety may aggravate epileptic seizures. The authors conduct a literature review to reveal the basic non-drug epilepsy treatment options. However, not all of these options have a sufficient evidence base, and some of them are not safe. Particularly, methods with a low level of evidence include acupuncture and aromatherapy. One of the methods, which can influence the pathogenesis of epilepsy, is the physical activity for patients with epilepsy since epileptiform activity on the EEG was reported to disappear during exercise. The positive results of the application of art therapy (music therapy) is also described in modern literature.

Dr. Matthew C.L. Phillips, in the tenth chapter, discusses the influence of the ketogenic diet in the treatment of epilepsy in children and adults. Despite a wide array of anti-epileptic drugs and the option of surgery, one-third of children and adults with epilepsy continue to suffer from drug-resistant seizures. Many of these patients may benefit from a ketogenic diet, a non-pharmacologic therapy proven to improve seizure control through a variety of mechanisms that collectively stabilize synaptic function. There are many similarities concerning patient selection, patient preparation, and diet implementation in children compared to adults, but there are also important differences. The most conspicuous challenge to the more widespread use of ketogenic diets in children and adults with epilepsy is a lack of access to ketogenic services in many regions of the world. Moreover, the culinary and social restrictions associated with conventional ketogenic diets pose a significant barrier to the diet for adults.

Shuzhang Zhang et al, in the eleventh chapter, highlight recent discoveries on the mutations in voltage-gated ion channels (VGICs), genes, and dysfunction of VGICs in epilepsy, focusing on the pathophysiological and pharmacological properties. VGICs are extensively distributed in the central nervous system and are responsible for the generation as well as modulation of neuroexcitability and are considered to be vital players in the pathogenesis of human epilepsy, by regulating the shape and duration of action potentials. For instance, genetic alterations or abnormal expression of voltage-gated sodium channels, Kv channels, and voltage-gated calcium channels are proved to be associated with epileptogenesis. Understanding the role of epilepsy-associated VGICs might not only contribute to clarifying the mechanism of epileptogenesis and genetic modifiers but also provide potential targets for the precise treatment of epilepsy.

The last chapter, by Dr. B. Suguna Nanthini, discusses the interesting subject about the development of automated expert systems in order to perform difficult jobs. The author discusses the components of soft computing include machine learning, fuzzy logic, evolutionary computation, and probabilistic theory. These components have the cognitive ability to learn effectively. They deal with imprecision and have a good tolerance of uncertainty. Components of soft computing are needed for developing automated expert systems. These systems reduce human interventions in completing a task. The system has been trained and tested using soft computing techniques. These systems are required in all kinds of fields and are especially useful in medical diagnosis. From these analyses, this chapter concludes that there are a number of features of the system that will allow for better accuracy of classification. The classifier, with a suitable learning method, can perform well for the automated epileptic seizure detection system. Furthermore, the level of decomposition of the EEG signal at level 4 is sufficient for seizure detection.

Prof. Isam Al-Zwaini, PhD and Prof. Ban Adbul-Hameed Majeed Albadri
Department of Pediatrics,
AL-Kindy Medical College,
University of Baghdad,
Baghdad, Iraq

Section 1

Introduction

Chapter 1

Introductory Chapter: Epilepsy—The Long Journey of the Sacred Disease

Isam Jaber AL-Zwaini and
Ban Adbul-Hameed Majeed Albadri

1. Introduction

Epilepsy is the most common neurological disorder globally, affecting approximately 50 million people of all ages [1]. It is one of oldest diseases described in literature from remote ancient civilizations 2000–3000 years ago. Despite its old description and its wider spread, epilepsy is still surrounded by myth and prejudice which can be overcome only with great difficulties. These myths and prejudice might have its historical origin. The aim of this introductory chapter is to follow the origin of epilepsy in ancient cultures, highlight the myth and stigmatism associated with epilepsy, and follow the major milestone in its development as a disease entity. The term epilepsy is derived from the Greek verb epilambanein, which by itself means to be seized and to be overwhelmed by surprise or attack. Therefore, epilepsy means a condition of getting over, seized, or attacked [2].

2. The major milestones in the history of epilepsy

The history of epilepsy goes together with the history of humankind in the globe. The earliest recorded account of epilepsy can be traced to the earliest civilization developing in Mesopotamia (the old name of the country IRAQ) almost 2000–3000 BC. These earliest establishments include the Sumerian, Babylonian, Assyrian, and Akkadian civilizations. The first description of epilepsy was written in the Akkadian language about 2000 BC in which the author described a condition similar to epileptic seizures in a patient. He described a patient whose neck turns to the left side, with his hands and feet being tense, with his eyes widely opened, and with his mouth drooling froth without him knowing. The condition diagnosed as antasubbû translated as the hand of sin brought about by the god of the Moon [5].

In a tablet from the Babylonian series (1067–1046 BC) present in the Babylonian collection of the British Museum(47,753), we find a report containing a detailed description of the symptoms of the condition known today as epilepsy with the supernatural forces suggested as an etiology (**Figure 1**). This table is written in Neo-Babylonian script dated approximately at the middle of the first millennium BC [4]. In this tablet, epilepsy was called Sakikku miqtu ("falling disease"), and the author describes various signs for the diagnosis, treatment, and prognosis of epilepsy. The etiology of epilepsy was presumed to be the effect of demons, evil spirits, and ghosts, and features of generalized seizures, simple and complex partial seizures, gelastic seizures, nocturnal epilepsy, febrile seizures, status epilepticus,

IntechOpen

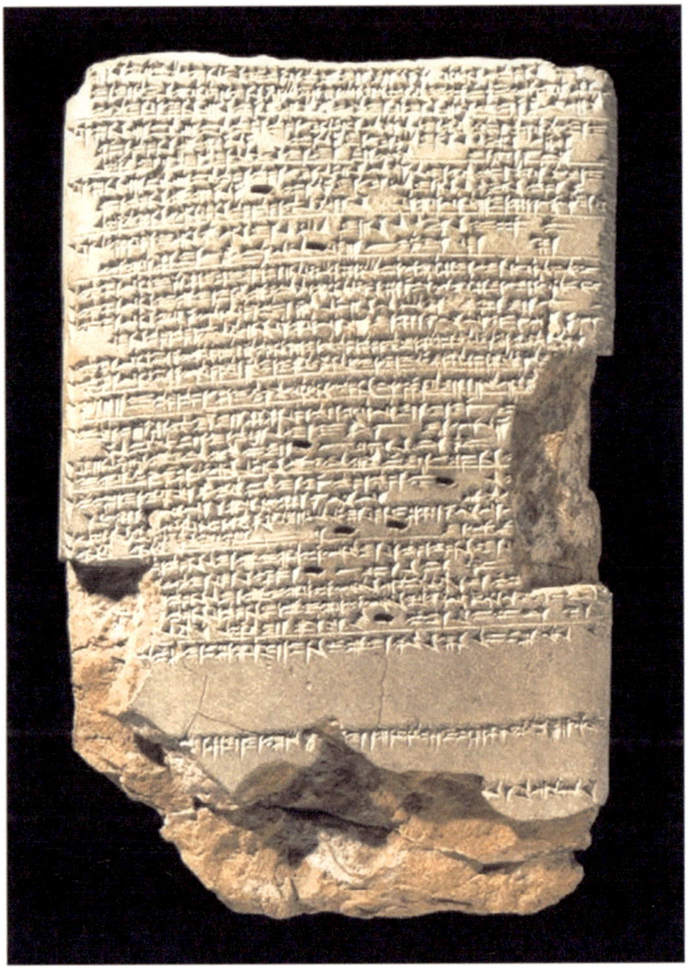

Figure 1.
British Museum Babylonian collection; Epilepsy tablet (47753) is an important Neo-Babylonian manuscript of Tablet 26 of the Diagnostic Handbook, the canonical Akkadian medical diagnostic series, composed of 40 tablets arranged into six chapters. This tablet gives symptoms of epilepsy and assigns disease names and etiologies to the various ways that the symptoms present themselves. Adopted by public domain at http://cdli.ox.ac.uk/wiki/doku.php?id=tablet_on_epilepsy.

chronic epilepsy, narcolepsy, and postictal states were described. This is by far the first written account of epilepsy [6, 7]. The king Hammurabi in his legislation (1790 BC) also refers to epilepsy (**Figure 2**). The legislation stated that a person with epilepsy could not marry, or testify in court, and a slave could be returned and the money refunded if bennu appeared within the month after the purchase. According to the researcher Marten Stol, bennu is another term for epilepsy [8].

The ancient Egyptian civilization medical reports (1700 BC) also contribute to the history of epilepsy by reporting five separate patients who shudder exceedingly. Probably these were the first reports of focal epilepsy following cortical irritation caused by examination or probing of wound or from an injury, e.g., gaping wound of the head. The last represents the earliest description of posttraumatic epilepsy [3].

In Greek civilization, epilepsy was referred to by many names including seliniasmos, sacred disease, Herculean disease, and demonism. These names related either to the etiology of the condition or to a figure. The scariness of the disease in Greek civilization may be related to the belief that epilepsy is vengeance of Mene,

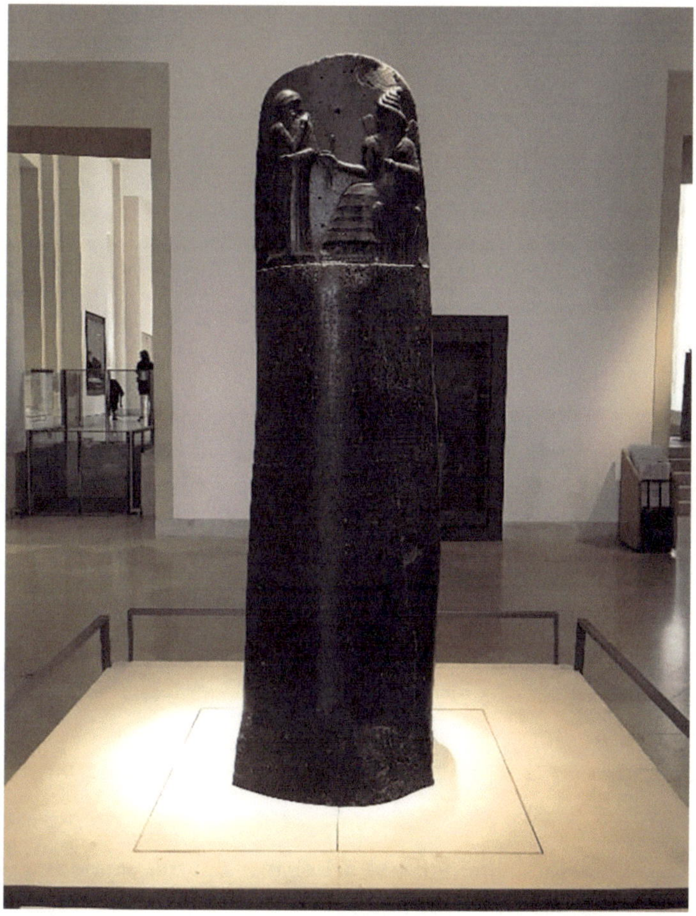

Figure 2.
The Hammurabi Obelisk containing his legislation (1790 B.C.). From the Louvre collection. Adopted by public domain at https://www.pinterest.com/pin/178173728990949335/.

Goddess of the Moon, on those with epilepsy and its cure could be of divine origin [3]. On the other hand, it might reflect the ambiguity of the disease, affecting body and mind, inspires, and has an Apollonian aspect. It is also considered as a disease of the genius since men like Persian King Cambyses II (522 BC), the Roman emperor Caesar, and the hero Hercules are said to have had epilepsy [3].

The father of the medicine, Hippocrates (**Figure 3**), in his book *On the Sacred Disease* (400 BC) (although still a controversy exists about the book authorship), who raised the first dispute about the divine origin of the epilepsy, had said "This disease is in my opinion no more divine than any other; it has the same nature as other diseases and the cause that gives rise to individual diseases." Hippocrates argued that epilepsy originates in the brain when an excess of phlegm enters the blood and is not of divine nature. He criticizes previous doctors who attribute epilepsy to divine intervention by stigmatizing them as magicians and charlatans [9]. Hippocrates was also the first to attempt a scientific approach toward the study of epilepsy by suggesting a possible etiology and therapy for the disease. He suggests brain dysfunction and heredity factors play a role in the etiology of epilepsy [10, 11].

By calling epilepsy as the great disease, he originates the term grand mal, and by linking convulsion to head injuries, he gives the base for the term posttraumatic epilepsy. He noticed that injury affecting the left side of the head could produce a right-sided convulsion. He describes the symptoms of focal seizures and suggests

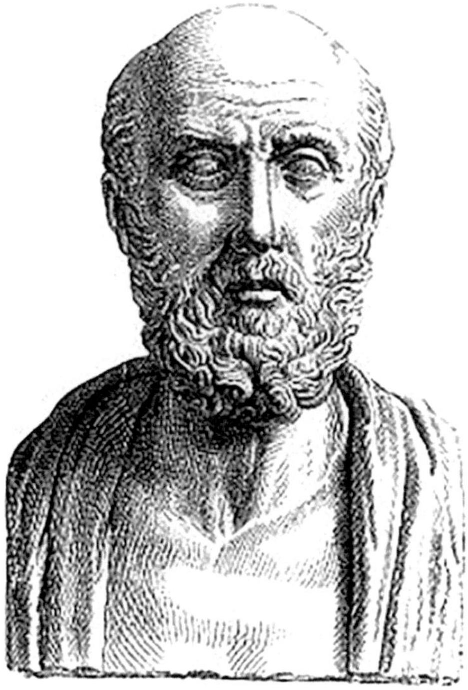

Figure 3.
Hippocrates wrote on the sacred disease 400 B.C. Adopted from the free domain https://en.wikipedia.org/wiki/Hippocrates.

many precipitating factors, among these are changes in the winds and temperature, exposure of the head to the sun, crying, and fear, and also he gives a prognostic clue by suggesting that disease manifesting at an early age has worse prognosis, and for older peoples, the prognosis is better. He considered epilepsy a curable disease unless if it is of long duration and ingrained as to be more powerful than the remedies that are applied [12]. Furthermore, Hippocrates in his book *On the Sacred Disease* described the first neurosurgical procedure, a craniotomy. He said craniotomy should be performed at the opposite side of the brain of the seizure in order to spare patients from "phlegmad" that caused the disease [13]. Many other famous Greek philosophers also wrote about epilepsy in their works like Plato (428–348 BC), who suggested in his laws a specific punishment for people selling slaves with epilepsy. Also Aristotle (384–322 BC), in his works *Problems*, *On Sleep and Waking*, and *Ethica Nicomachea*, presented his theories and views about epilepsy that had impressed many physicians in the post-Hippocratic and even Medieval era which had led the Catholic Church to validate his teaching and work and consider it as indisputable and beyond any criticism [3, 14–16]. The dominance of the Catholic Church during the era of the Middle Ages led to the continued existence of religious and magic beliefs about epilepsy.

In the old Chinese civilizations, also there are some references to the disease. Old Chinese physicians discuss a condition similar to generalized convulsions, T'ien-Hs'ien (770–221 BC). They thought that emotional shock bore by the mother during pregnancy is the cause for epilepsy in a child. Later on, Chinese scientist tries to classify seizures according to the age at onset, clinical symptoms, and the possible etiology. During the Tang dynasty (682 AD), two different classifications were proposed on the basis of the resemblance of noises a patient might utter during seizures to voices of animals and different organs as presumed sites of seizure origin [17, 18].

3. Epilepsy evolution as a disease entity

The first liberation of epilepsy from religious theories such as divine punishment or possession was made in the eighteenth and nineteenth centuries [19, 20]. In these centuries, a tremendous advance in the research on epilepsy with great emancipation from religious superstitions was made. At the beginning of the eighteenth century, epilepsy was regarded as idiopathic disease derived from brain and other internal organs. The work of William Culen (1710–1790) and Samuel A. Tissot (1728–1797) builds up the bases of the modern epileptology, and they described different types of epilepsies.

At the beginning of the nineteenth century, French physicians started to publish their research in the field of epileptology. Maisonneuve (1745–1826) [21], Calmeil (1798–1895) [22], and Jean-Etienne Dominique Esquirol (1772–1840) are among the famous physicians who work in this field. Maisonneuve stressed the importance of hospitalization of epileptic patients, categorized epilepsy into idiopathic and sympathetic, and described the so-called sensitive aura of sympathetic epilepsy. Esquirol distinguished between petit and grand mal and along with his pupils Bouchet and Cazauvieilh studied systematically insanity and epilepsy, conducting clinical and postmortem studies [19, 20]. In the second half of the nineteenth century, the etiology and pathophysiology of epilepsy and the topographic localization of epileptic seizures were stressed on. At that time important works were published by prestigious physicians such as Theodore Herpin (1799–1865) in 1852 and 1867, Louis François Delasiauve (1804–1893) in 1854, John Russell Reynolds (1828–1896) in 1861, and Sir William Richard Gowers (1845–1915) in 1881 [19].

The physiologist Fritsch (1838–1927) and the psychiatrist Hitzig (1838–1907) give the first proof that the brain was the origin of epilepsy. They presented experiments in which they provoked seizures by electric stimulation in the brain cortex of dogs [23]. An English neurologist, John Hughling Jackson (1835–1911), studied the pathological and anatomical bases of epilepsy extensively, and he set the scientific bases of epileptology. Jackson in 1873 defined epilepsy as the name given for occasional, sudden, excessive, rapid, and local discharges of gray matter. The presence of localized lesions on the cortex involved by epilepsy was the core of his studies on convulsions [19].

A Spanish pathologist, histologist, and neuroscientist, Santiago Ram'ony Cajal (1852–1934) at the beginning of the twentieth century, made an important advance in the field of the microscopic structure of the brain and nervous system. He was awarded with the Nobel Prize in 1906 for his advancement in the description of the structure of the neurons and synapses by employing the Golgi staining in the study of the nervous system. The famous book *The Borderlands of Epilepsy*, published by Sir William Richard Gowers in 1907, focuses on vagal and vasovagal attacks, faints, vertigo, migraine, and some sleep symptoms, especially narcolepsy.

Lennox (1884–1960) and Cobb (1887–1968) during the 1920s studied the effects of starvation, ketogenic diet, and altered cerebral oxygen in seizures. In their published monographs entitled "Epilepsy from the Standpoint of Physiology and Treatment" and "Epilepsy and Related Disorder" and their important paper summarizing their research entitled "The Relationship of Certain Physiochemical Processes to Epileptiform Seizures), they concentrate on the effects of various stimuli to the generation of epileptic convulsions. Most of these studied stimuli, as starvation, ketogenic diet, and lack of oxygen, give negative results. [24–26]. The relationship of behavioral changes to temporal lobe lesion was discovered during the 1940s by Klüver (1897–1979) and Bucy (1904–1992) who noticed this association on monkeys. Jasper (1906–1999) and Kershmann in 1941 proved that the temporal lobe is the site of origin of psychomotor seizures [27].

In 1969, James Kiffin Penry (1929–1996) published important treatises such as the series Basic Mechanisms of the Epilepsies and afterward Antiepileptic Drugs, Neurosurgical Management of the Epilepsies, Complex Partial Seizures, and their Treatment and Antiepileptic Drugs Mechanisms of Action and Advances in Epileptology. In the same year, Gastaut managed to organize a meeting in Marseilles attended by 120 members of the International League Against Epilepsy (ILAE), and preliminary classification of epilepsies was presented to a commission on the terminology of epilepsy. The General Assembly of the ILAE accepted the first publication of clinical and electroencephalographic classifications of epileptic seizures [28–30].

A great milestone in the understanding of epilepsy was by recording abnormal electrical discharge associated with seizures. The first scientist who notices electric changes in the brain during experimentally induced seizures, associating epileptic attacks with abnormal electric discharges, was a Russian physiologist, Kaufman (1877–1951), in 1912. In the same year, Pravdich-Neminsky (1879–1952), a Ukrainian physiologist, published the first animal EEG and the evoked potential of the mammalian (dog) [31]. The theories of the association of electric stimuli and brain activity inducing seizures dated back to the nineteenth century from the work of Fritch (1838–1927) and Hitzig (1838–1907), Caton (1842–1926), and Adolf Beck (186–1942) who did their experiments by inducing seizure in dogs, rats, and rabbits, by applying electric stimuli on the animals' cortex [30].

Hans Berger (1873–1941), a German neurologist, reported the first record of human EEG in 1929 (**Figure 4**). In 1932, he reported sequential postictal EEG changes after a generalized tonic-clonic seizure, and in 1933, he published the first example of interictal changes and a minor epileptic seizure with 3/s rhythmic waves in the EEG [32, 33]. Initially, his work was confronted by controversies and suspicions within the scientific society, but later Adrian (1899–1977) and Matthews

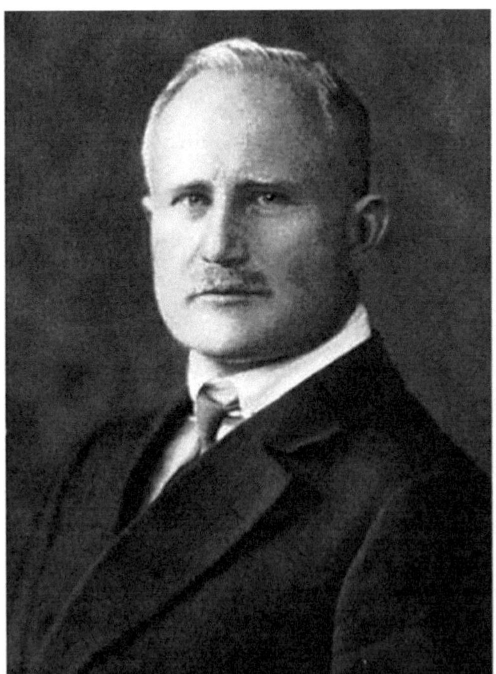

Figure 4.
Hans Berger, the first who record EEG in human. Adopted from the free domain https://neupsykey.com/historical-aspects-of-eeg/.

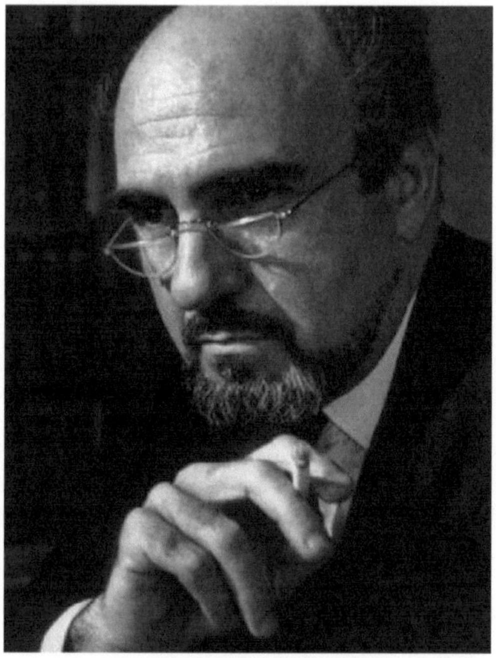

Figure 5.
Henri Jean Pascal Gastaut; the first who discover the photic stimulation as an EEG seizure activator and describe two syndromes adopted his name. Adopted from the free domain https://openi.nlm.nih.gov/detailedresult.php?img=PMC4158257 ERT2014-582039.002&req=4.

confirmed his results. The work of Berger on epileptic EEG was completed by an American neurologist Frederic Andrews Gibbs (1903–1992), and his wife and technician Erna Leonhardt-Gibbs (1904–1987), who is in collaboration with Lennox, establishes a correlation between EEG findings and epileptic seizures [34, 35]. In 1941, Gibbs and Lennox published the *Atlas of Electroencephalography* in which they included also mechanical and mathematical analyses of EEG [36].

Henri Jean Pascal Gastaut (1915–1995) did the great advance in the field of EEG in the 1950s (**Figure 5**). He discovered the photic stimulation as an EEG seizure activator and studied the role of thalamic reticular structures in the genesis of metrazol-induced generalized paroxysmal EEG discharges and developed the concept of centrencephalic seizures. Furthermore, he founded the International EEG Federation, and, in 1953, he became the head of the Marseilles Hospital Neurobiological Laboratories establishing a school of neurology that dominated for the next decades. He participated in the foundation of many education centers and research units. Also, he defined five major human EEG patterns (lambda waves, pi rhythm, mu rhythm, rolandic spikes, and posterior theta rhythm) and described two clinical syndromes that carried his name: Gastaut syndrome (a type of photosensitive epilepsy) and the Lennox-Gastaut syndrome (severe childhood encephalopathy) [37].

4. Evolution of anticonvulsant therapy

Herbal and chemical substances were the major therapy for epilepsy before the second half of the nineteenth century. In 1857, Sir Locock (1799–1875) discovered the anticonvulsant and sedative effect of potassium bromide, and he starts to treat his patients with this substance. Since that time, potassium bromide became the first drug of choice in the treatment of epilepsy, until the discovery of phenobarbital by a German physician, Hauptmann (1881–1948), in 1912. The drug company Bayer, under the brand name Luminal, introduced phenobarbital to the market. Hauptmann used phenobarbital as a sedative for his epileptic patient, and he discovered that their epileptic attacks were susceptible to the drug. The absence of the sedative effect of phenytoin, the next drug used as antiepileptic, leads to the delay of its use as anticonvulsant until 1938 despite its synthesis by Heinrich Biltz (1865–1943) in 1908. It was introduced as an anticonvulsant by Merritt (1902–1979) and Putnam (1894–1975) in 1938 under the name Dilantin. Phenytoin substitutes potassium bromide and phenobarbital as the first-line drug of choice for the prevention of partial and tonic seizures and for the treatment for acute cases of epilepsies and status epilepticus [38–42].

A new antiepileptic drug was introduced in 1946 under the name of trimethadione. Richards and Everett report the use of trimethadione to prevent pentylenetetrazol- induced seizures and for the treatment of absence seizures. In the 1950s, a set of new antiepileptic drugs were introduced: carbamazepine in 1953, primidone in 1954, ethosuximide in 1958, and sodium valproate in 1963 [43]. Serum level of antiepileptic drugs was first introduced in 1960 by Buchtal and Svenmark [44]. Other antiepileptic drugs were introduced in the 1970s, including clobazam, clonazepam, and piracetam. The last decade of the twentieth century and the early years of the twenty-first century mark the beginning of the use of new antiepileptic drugs. Among these drugs are vigabatrin (1989), lamotrigine (1990), gabapentin (1993), felbamate (1993), topiramate (1995), tiagabine (1998), zonisamide (1989 in Japan and 2000 in the USA), levetiracetam(2000), pregabalin (2004), rufinamide (2004), lacosamide (2008), eslicarbazepine (2009), and perampanel (2012). The field of anticonvulsant drugs is dynamic and in the last two decades a new generation of antiepileptic drugs introduced to the market, and there are a number of very new antiepileptic drugs which are under various stages of drug development such as brivaracetam and retigabine. The aim of the researches in this field is to improve tolerance and effectiveness of the drugs and to improve the quality of the life of the patient through improvement in the pharmacokinetics, safety, and efficacy of these drugs.

The role of diet in the management of epilepsy dated back to the era of Hippocratic were fasting and other types of diet used for the treatment of epilepsy [13]. The use of ketogenic diet (diet full with fat and low in protein and carbohydrates) for the treatment of epilepsy started in 1911 by two French physicians, Guelpa and Marie, who reported a decrease in the number of seizures in 20 children and adults with epilepsy when treated with ketogenic diet [45]. In 1922, an American physician, Hugh Conklin, stresses the importance of the ketogenic diet in the management of epilepsy since he believed that epilepsy caused by toxins damages the brain cell. He had a personal interest in ketogenic diet and tried to treat his nephew, who suffered from drug-resistant epilepsy, by this method. By using ketogenic diet, he had encouraging results. Since that time, many authors published many papers, but none explained the anticonvulsive mechanisms of ketogenic diets [46, 47].

In 1831, the first neurosurgical operation for an epileptic patient with brain abscess was done by Heyman [30]. Posttraumatic epilepsy was the most common indication for the operations done at that time. At the beginning of the twentieth century, a great advance in neurosurgical operations for epileptic patients is done, started by Dandy (1886–1946) who introduced hemispherectomy in 1923 and continued by Gibbs and Lennox in 1938 who introduced the notion of operating the epileptogenic focus [31, 48]. A further advance in the surgical procedure for epileptic patients was done by Penfield, Jasper, and Theodor Brown Rasmussen (1910–2002). They introduce the Foerster method for removing epileptogenic lesions in epileptic patients, invented Montreal procedure (using local anesthesia to remove part of the skull and expose brain), and published one the greatest classics in neurology, *Epilepsy and the Functional Anatomy of the Human Brain*, in 1954 [49, 50]. On the other hand, Van Wagenen and Herren (1897–1961) introduce the procedure of callosotomy, and Bailey (1892–1973) attempts temporal lobectomies for psychomotor seizures [51, 52].

The early introduction of EEG and the use of electrocorticography for intraoperative localization and later on the advent of modern diagnostic techniques such as MRI, PET, and SPECT was an important advance in the development of surgical techniques and approaches. Recently the application of microsurgery and the use of multiple transaction and gamma knife had revolutionized the neurosurgical operations for epileptic patients.

5. Misconception about epilepsy

Throughout the history of epilepsy, many misconceptions and wrong beliefs about the disease are conveyed. Some of these are referred to earlier in this chapter. These misconceptions and beliefs are variable in different parts of the world, from society to society and era to era, and it may lead to rejection, denial of education, and isolation in both developed and developing countries.

In the antiquity, one of the popular beliefs was that epilepsy is a contagious disease. People used to spit at a person with seizure and refuse to use the same dish. These beliefs continued in the Middle Ages where the clergy and synods of the early Christian church separated the possessed from the faithful because they thought that the possessed would desecrate the holy objects and would infect the sharing dishes and cups [53]. Berthold of Regensburg (1220–1272), a thirteenth-century-preacher, added breath as a rout of infection, and he warns people not to talk or bath with patients with seizures since the contagious nature of the infection is transmitted through the evil breath [4]. The beliefs that epilepsy is an infectious process continued until the eighteenth century [54].

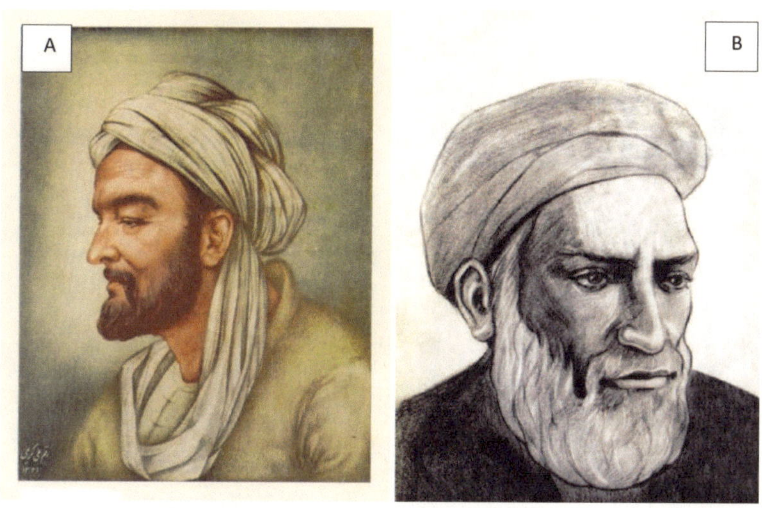

Figure 6.
Avicenna (Ibn Sina) (A) and Abubakr Muhammad ibn Zakariyya al-Razi (B) written manuscripts about epilepsy, which had great influences on the students and universities in Eastern and Western world till the 18 century. Adopted from the free Domain http://www.muslimphilosophy.com/sina/gal/IS-gal-16.htm and https://www.researchgate.net/figure/Portrait-of-Abubakr-Muhammad-ibn-Zakariyya-al-Razi-or-Rhazes-865-925-CE_fig1_236331515.

Other wrong beliefs were that people with epilepsy were demoniacs and that seizures caused by an unclean dumb and deaf spirit were common among priests in the old Christian world. These beliefs can be attributed to the biblical story of Jesus healing a boy with symptoms of an epileptic seizure. In the medieval Islamic era, we cannot find referring to epilepsy as caused by demons in any of the scientific texts of epilepsy written in that era. The two famous Islamic physicians, Avicenna and Mohammed Ibn Zakariya AL-Razi (**Figure 6**), had written manuscripts about epilepsy, which had great influences on the students and universities in Eastern and Western world till the eighteenth century [55]. Nowadays, still, misconceptions and wrong beliefs are prevalent and widely spread among societies from developing and developed countries throughout the world.

Author details

Isam Jaber AL-Zwaini* and Ban Adbul-Hameed Majeed Albadri
Department of pediatrics, AL-Kindy Medical College, University of Baghdad, Iraq

*Address all correspondence to: isamjaber@kmc.uobaghdad.edu.iq

References

[1] WHO. Epilepsy Fact Sheet. Available at: https://www.who.int/news-room/fact-sheets/detail/epilepsy

[2] Baloyannis SJ. Abstracts from the second international congress on epilepsy, brain and mind, Prague. Epilepsy & Behavior. 2012;**28**:303-332

[3] Magiorkinis E, Sidiropoulou K, Diamantis A. Hallmarks in the history of epilepsy: Epilepsy in antiquity. Epilepsy & Behavior. 2010;**17**:103-108

[4] Temkin O. The Falling Sickness. Baltimore: The Johns Hopkins University Press; 1945

[5] Labat R. Traité akkadien de diagnostics et pronostics médicaux. Paris/Leiden: Académie Internationale d'Histoire des Sciences/Brill; 1951. pp. 80-81, 188-199

[6] Wilson JVK, Reynolds EH. Texts and documents. Translation and analysis of a cuneiform text forming part of a Babylonian treatise on epilepsy. Medical History. 1990;**34**:185-198

[7] Reynolds EH, Wilson JVK. Psychoses of epilepsy in Babylon: The oldest account of the disorder. Epilepsia. 2008; **49**:1488-1490

[8] Stol M. Epilepsy in Babylonia. Amsterdam: Brill; 1993. pp. 5-7

[9] Hippocrate. De la maladie sacrée, livre 6. In: Littré E, editor. Oeuvres Completes d' Hippocrate. Paris: Baillière; 1849. p. 364

[10] Hippocrate. De la maladie sacrée, livre 6. In: Littré E, editor. Oeuvres Completes d' Hippocrate. Paris: Baillière; 1849. p. 354

[11] Hippocrate. De la maladie sacrée, livre 6. In: Littré E, editor. Oeuvres Completes d' Hippocrate. Paris: Baillière; 1849. p. 366

[12] Hippocrate. Sixième livre des épidémies, livre 5. In: Littré E, editor. Oeuvres Complètes d' Hippocrate. Paris: Baillière; 1849. p. 324

[13] Hippocrates. The Sacred Disease. Vol. 2. London, UK: Loeb Classical Library and Harvard University Press; 1965. translated by Jones WHS

[14] Aristotle. Problems, 30, 1. Vol. 2. London: Loeb; 1936. p. 154

[15] Aristotle. On sleep and waking. In: Hett WS, editor. On the Soul, Parva Naturalia, on Breath. Vol. 457A. London: Loeb; 1957. pp. 8-9

[16] Aristotle. Ethica nicomachea. In: Ross WD, editor. The Works of Aristotle, Vol. IX. Oxford: Oxford Univ. Press; 1925. 8, 1150B. pp. 32-35

[17] Lai CW, Lai YH. History of epilepsy in Chinese traditional medicine. Epilepsia. 1991;**32**:299-302

[18] Chaudhary UJ, Duncan JS, Lemieux L. A dialogue with historical concepts of epilepsy from the Babylonians to Hughlings Jackson: Persistent beliefs. Epilepsy & Behavior. 2011;**21**:109-114

[19] Sidiropoulou K, Diamantis A, Magiorkinis E. Hallmarks in 18th- and 19th-century epilepsy research. Epilepsy and Behavior. 2010;**18**(3):151-161

[20] Diamantis A, Sidiropoulou K, Magiorkinis E. Epilepsy during the middle ages, the renaissance and the enlightenment. Journal of Neurology. 2010;**257**(5):691-698

[21] Maisonneuve JGF. Recherches et observations sur l'épilepsie, presentées a

L' École de médecine de Paris, Paris, France. 1803

[22] Calmeil LF. De l' epilepsie etudiee sous le rapport de son siege et de son influence sur la production de l' alienation mentale [Thesis]. Paris, France: Imprimerie de Didot le jeune. 1824

[23] Fritsch G, Hitzig E. Ueber die elektrische Erregbarkeit des Grosshirns. Archiv für Anatomie, Physiologie und Wissenschaftliche Medicin. 1870;**37**: 300-332

[24] Lennox W, Cobb S. Epilepsy from the Standpoint of Physiology and Treatment. Medicine Monograph XIV. Baltimore, Maryland, USA: Williams and Wilkins; 1928

[25] Lennox W, Cobb S. Epilepsy. Baltimore, Md, USA: Wiiliams & Wilkins; 1928

[26] Lennox W, Cobb S. The relation of certain physicochemical processes to epileptiform seizures. The American Journal of Psychiatry. 1929;**85**:837-847

[27] Jasper H, Kershmann J. Electroencepahlografic classification of the epilepsies. Archives of Neurology and Psychiatry. 1941;**45**(6):903-943

[28] Gastaut H. Classification of the epilepsies. Proposal for an international classification. Epilepsia. 1969;**10**:14-21

[29] Gastaut H. Clinical and electroencephalographical classification of epileptic seizures. Epilepsia. 1969;**10**: 2-13

[30] Magiorkinis E, Diamantis A, Sidiropoulou K, Panteliadis C. Highlights in the history of epilepsy: The last 200 years. Epilepsy Research and Treatment. 2014;**2014**:582039

[31] Hermann BP, Stone JL. Ahistorical review of the epilepsy surgery program at the University of Illinois Medical Center: The contributions of Bailey, Gibbs, and collaborators to the refinement of anterior temporal lobectomy. Journal of Epilepsy. 1989; **2**(3):155-163

[32] Berger H. Uber das Elektroenzephalogram des Menschen. Archiv für Psychiatrie und Nervenkrankheiten. 1932;**97**:6-26

[33] Berger H. Uber das Elektroenzephalogram des Menschen. Archiv für Psychiatrie und Nervenkrankheiten. 1933;**100**:301-320

[34] Gibbs F, Davis H, Lennox W. The electroencephalogram in epilepsy and in conditions of impaired consciousness. Archives of Neurology and Psychiatry. 1935;**34**(6):1133-1148

[35] Gibbs FA, Gibbs EL, Lennox WG. Epilepsy: A paroxysmal cerebral dysrhythmia. Brain. 1937;**60**(4):377-388

[36] Gibbs FA, Gibbs E. Atlas of Electroencephalography. Oxford, UK: Boston City Hospital; 1941

[37] Cereghino JJ. The major advances in epilepsy in the 20th century and what we can expect (hope for) in the future. Epilepsia. 2009;**50**(3):351-357

[38] Locock C. Analysis of fifty-two cases of epilepsy observed by the author. The Lancet. 1857;**70**:527-529

[39] Hauptmann A. Luminal bei Epilepsie. Münchener medizinische Wochenschrift. 1912;**59**: 1907-1909

[40] Merrit H, Putnam T. A new series of anticonvulsant drugs tested by experiments in animals. Archives of Neurology and Psychiatry. 1938;**39**(5): 1003-1015

[41] Merrit H, Putnam T. Sodium diphenyl hydantoinate in the treatment

of convulsive disorders. JAMA. *1938*;**111**(12):1068-1073

[42] Pravdich-Neminsky V. Ein Versuch der Registrierung der elektrischen Gehirnerscheinungen. Zentralblatt für Physiologie. 1913;**27**:951-960

[43] Meunier H, Carraz G, Meunier Y, et al. Propri'et'es pharmacodynamiques de l'acide n-dipropylacetique. Thérapie. 1963;**18**:435-438

[44] Buchtal F, Svensmark O. Aspects of the pharmacology of phenytoin (dilantin) and phenobarbital relevant to their dosage in the treatment of epilepsy. Epilepsia. 1960;**1**:373-384

[45] Guelpa G, Marie A. La lutte contrel epilepsie parlade's intoxication et par la reeducation alimentaire. Revue de Thérapeutique Médico-Chirurgicale. 1911;**18**:8-13

[46] Peterman MG. The ketogenic diet in epilepsy. The Journal of the American Medical Association. 1925;**84**(26):1979-1983

[47] Huttenlocher PR, Wilbourn AJ, Signore JM. Mediumchain triglycerides as a therapy for intractable childhood epilepsy. Neurology. 1971;**21**(11):1097-1103

[48] Dandy WE. Removal of right cerebral hemisphere for certain tumors with hemiplegia. The Journal of the American Medical Association. 1928;**90**:823-825

[49] Penfield W, Jasper HH. Highest level seizures. Research Publications - Association for Research in Nervous and Mental Disease. 1947;**26**:252

[50] Penfield W, Jasper H. Epilepsy and the Functional Anatomy of the Human Brain. Boston, Mass, USA: Little, Brown; 1954

[51] Van Wagenen WP, Herren RY. Surgical division of commissural pathways in the corpus callosum. Relation to spread of an epileptic attack. Archives of Neurology and Psychiatry. 1940;**44**:740-759

[52] Bailey P, Gibbs FA. The surgical treatment of psychomotor epilepsy. The Journal of the American Medical Association. 1951;**145**(6):365-370

[53] International league against epilepsy. The history and stigma of epilepsy. Epilepsia. 2003;**44**(suppl. 6):12-14

[54] De Boer HM. Epilepsy and society. Epilepsia. 1995;**36**:S8-S11

[55] Vanzan A, Paladin F. Epilepsy and Persian culture: An overview. Epilepsia. 1992;**33**:1057-1064

Section 2

Epilepsy - Etiological and Pathophysiological Aspect

Chapter 2

Inflammation: Cause or Consequence of Epilepsy?

Vanessa Lin Lin Lee and Mohd. Farooq Shaikh

Abstract

Epilepsy is the third most common neurological disorder, affecting about 70 million people worldwide. It is defined as a central nervous system disorder which affects the neuronal activity in the brain, causing unprovoked seizures and other behavioral changes. Unfortunately, one-third of epilepsy patients are unresponsive to available therapies and patients who respond to antiepileptic drugs often complain of debilitating side effects. In the effort of devising a suitable therapy for epilepsy treatment, researchers delved into the origin of seizures and the epileptogenic process and found an association between epilepsy and inflammation. Here, we discuss the involvement of inflammatory mediators in the development and progression of seizures and epileptogenesis, supported by clinical shreds of evidence. Subsequently, we discuss the role of inflammation in the generation of seizures, as it is debatable whether inflammation is the cause or consequence of epilepsy, along with experimental models in inflammation and epilepsy research.

Keywords: inflammation, inflammatory mediators, seizures, epilepsy, animal models

1. Introduction

Epilepsy is a brain disorder denoted by the predisposition to generate seizures accompanied by emotional and cognitive dysfunction [1]. Currently, there are estimated to be 50–70 million people worldwide suffering from epilepsy but only about 70% of them respond well to existing antiepileptic drugs [2, 3]. Furthermore, epileptic patients suffer deteriorating quality of life as they face limitations on their physical activities and daily life as well as being subjected to prejudice due to their seizures [4]. This calls for more research to seek for novel and effective therapies for the management and treatment of epilepsy, by first understanding the basis for the onset and progression of seizures.

The exact cause of epilepsy is still unknown, but there are mounting evidence showing that the development of epileptogenesis can be linked to a wide array of factors such as genetic predisposition, developmental disorders and neurological insults [5]. Neurological insults, which contribute towards up to 60% of epilepsy cases, include traumatic brain injuries (TBI), cerebrovascular accidents (CVA), central nervous system (CNS) infections and strokes, where inflammation is one of the key features of epileptogenesis [6]. However, the role of inflammation in epilepsy is still being actively studied, with various arguments on whether inflammation is the cause or consequence of epilepsy [7]. The blood-brain barrier (BBB), which functions as a protector of the central nervous system, has an important role in regulating the transfer of blood constituents in the brain extracellular space [8]. Increased BBB permeability or BBB leakage is said to be one of the earliest characteristics of the pathophysiology of epileptogenesis [9, 10]. BBB dysfunction may contribute to epileptogenesis via a cascade of events triggered by leakage of inflammatory mediators into the CNS which causes neuroinflammation [11, 12]. Here, we discuss briefly how neuroinflammation is involved in epileptogenesis as well as the status of inflammation in post-epileptic conditions; whether it is the cause or consequence of epilepsy, together with experimental evidences.

2. Inflammatory response in epilepsy

Considering inflammation as one of the culprits of epileptogenesis, neuroinflammation occurs as a result of a cascade of inflammatory pathways. This involves inflammatory and anti-inflammatory molecules as a response to noxious stimuli or immune stimulation; targeted to defend against pathogenic threats. The activation of inflammatory mediators such as interleukins (ILs), interferons (IFNs), cyclooxygenase (COX)-2 and nuclear factor kappa B (NF-κB), and the surplus of downstream inflammatory mediators including IL-1β, IL-6, tumor necrosis factor (TNF)-α and prostaglandin E2 (PGE2) contribute to seizure progression [13, 14]. Inflammatory mediators are produced by the glia, neurons, endothelial cells of the BBB and peripheral immune cells. In the presence of noxious stimuli, cytokines are secreted by immunocompetent and endothelial cells as well as glial and neuronal cells in the CNS. In the presence of noxious stimuli, cytokines are released which enable effective communication between effector and target cells [7, 15].

Both innate and adaptive immunity is known to contribute in the generation of inflammation in the brain via the microglia, astrocytes and neurons [7]. In a non-epileptic condition, innate immunity activation occurs during infection and is instrumental for pathogen recognition as well as removal via homeostatic-type tissue inflammation [16]. In epileptic condition where pathogens are absent, innate immunity signaling is activated by damage-associated molecular patterns (DAMPs) which are secreted by injured or activated neurons, bringing about a phenomenon called 'sterile inflammation' [17]. The microglia and astrocytes recognize proteins such as high mobility group box 1 (HMGB1), S100 proteins, adenosine triphosphate (ATP), migration inhibitory factor-related protein 8 (MRP8), which makes are DAMPs, extracellular matrix degradation products and IL-1β to induce inflammation [17, 18]. On top of that, the inflammatory signaling disrupts the BBB integrity by inducing up-regulation of adhesion molecules as well as leukocyte recruitment. These processes reduces seizure threshold and contribute to epileptogenesis and seizure recurrence in epilepsy models [19, 20].

Clinically, it is observed that patients with autoimmune diseases such as systemic lupus erythematosus (SLE), Hashimoto's encephalopathy, Behcet's disease, and Sjogren's syndrome have an increased risk of developing epilepsy [5]. Another example of an autoimmune disease associated with a predisposition to seizures is Rasmussen encephalitis (RE), a rare inflammatory brain disease causing cerebral hemiatrophy, which progressively leads to severe seizures [21]. Patients of RE have higher levels of astrocytosis, proinflammatory mediators as well as lymphocytes and activated microglial cells in the brain [22, 23]. In these cases, usually, immunotherapies are more effective as compared to antiepileptic drugs in the management of epilepsy [24].

Moreover, a number of reports suggest that the onset and perpetuation of epilepsy can be driven by inflammation and is not caused by the autoimmune process.

Upregulation of proinflammatory markers and inflammation-related microRNAs are found in patients of generalized seizures and temporal lobe epilepsy (TLE) [25, 26]. Butler, Li [27] reported a significantly greater inflammation intensity and spatial extent using positron emission tomography (PET) scan in post-seizure patients [27].

3. Experimental models

Moving forward with the understanding on the clinical association of inflammation with epileptogenesis, researchers sought to decipher the role of inflammation and associated pathways in the genesis of a seizure in the brain. Experimental models of inflammation have been instrumental in understanding the role of inflammation in epilepsy. It is still an ongoing debate as there are two field of thoughts; (1) inflammation acts as the cause of seizures and (2) inflammation is the consequence of seizures [7]. Here, we discuss the different types of experimental models and the outcomes of the experimental work, summarized in **Table 1**.

3.1 Inflammation increases seizure susceptibility

3.1.1 Hyperthermia-induced seizures

Febrile seizures (FS) are common in children aged between 6 months and 5 years and occur in response to fever but without infection of the CNS. Fever is the elevation of the body temperature set point within the hypothalamus which results in an elevation of core temperature and is generated by inflammatory mediators such as cytokines and prostaglandins which then invokes a systemic inflammatory response [28, 29]. A widely used hyperthermia-induced seizure model for studying FS is one in which hyperthermia is induced using a regulated stream of mildly heated air to increase the body temperature of neonatal rats aged 10–13 days [30–32]. The brain development of rats between 10 and 15 postnatal days best corresponds to the development of brain in human infants when they are most susceptible to FS [30]. The 'ideal' increase of core temperature in the pups is around 2.9°C, which is reported to be parallel with the temperature increment observed in children experiencing FS [33].

In this model, seizures can be confirmed using electroencephalogram (EEG) [30]. The behaviors exhibited by the pups, such as biting tonic stiffening, and falling over, are similar to those observed after administration of convulsants. Generalized tonic seizures are rarely observed, however [30, 32]. In addition to biochemical analysis, behavioral tests such as the balance beam test and footprint test provide information on the severity and progression of seizures. Research has also shown that in this hyperthermic model, there is a remarkably high release of cytokines within the brain, specifically IL-1β within the hippocampus, and activation of astrocytes, which elevates the brain temperature. This finding is similar to those seen in children suffering from FS [31].

3.1.2 Systemic inflammation

Systemic inflammation is believed to have several CNS manifestations, such as fever, locomotor activity reduction and behaviors that are associated with brain hyperactivity during peripheral inflammation [34]. In other words, the inflammatory response which can be observed during the manifestation of peripheral inflammatory diseases is similar to the inflammatory response generated in the

Types of animal model	Dose/method	Outcome	References
Hyperthermic-induced seizure	Using a regulated stream of mildly heated air to increase core temperature.	• Mimics febrile seizures in children. • Core body temperature increase by around 2.9°C. • Marked release of cytokines within the brain and activation of astrocytes.	[28–31]
Inflammatory bowel disease model	Intracolonic administration of 2,4,6-trinitobenzene sulfonic acid (TNBS) at a dose of 50 mg/ml, 50mL per rat.	• Induces significant inflammatory response within the hippocampus. • Activation of microglial. • Increases levels of TNFα. • Increases susceptibility to PTZ-induced seizures.	[32–35]
Escherichia coli LPS injection	Intraperitoneal injection of 5 mg/kg or peritoneal infusion of 2.5 mg/kg/day for 7 days.	• Increases plasma levels of IL-1β, IL-6 and TNF-α. • Increases body temperature slightly (by 0.9°C). • Increases seizure susceptibility.	[36–38]
Kainic acid injection	Intraperitoneal injection of 2 mg/kg in rat neonates, 15 mg/kg in adult rats and 20 mg/kg in mice, 6 mg/kg in zebrafish.	• Induces limbic seizures characterized by a seizure scale devised by Racine. • Seizures induced resemble human temporal lobe epilepsy. • Leads to neuronal cell death and induction of proinflammatory gene expression.	[39–44]
Pilocarpine injection	Subcutaneous or intraperitoneal injection of 340–350 mg/kg in rats, 30 mM in zebrafish larvae.	• Induces status epilepticus, followed by recurrent spontaneous seizures. • Causes extensive neuronal cell loss, astrogliosis, and mossy fiber sprouting in hippocampus. • Developmental exposure to pilocarpine shows very little effect to startle response.	[45–50]
Serum albumin injection	Intracerebroventricular injection of 1.9 mM in rats.	• Mimics BBB breakdown following seizures. • Increased IL-1β immunoreactivity. • Astrocyte dysfunction. • Significant increase in interictal spikes and neuronal excitability. • Reduction in seizure threshold.	[51]

Table 1.
Animal models in epilepsy studies.

periphery [35]. It is important to note that systemic inflammation alone is insufficient to induce seizures, and therefore, a double-hit with a proconvulsant is usually adopted in experiments to show that the first hit of existing inflammation predisposes the subject to increased seizure susceptibility in response to a second hit. We discuss two models of systemic inflammation which have been used for the study of epilepsy and seizures.

The first one is a model of inflammatory bowel disease [36–38]. Inflammatory colitis is induced in adult male rats by intracolonic administration of 2,4,6-trinitobenzene sulfonic acid (TNBS) to initiate a T helper-1 cell-mediated model of inflammatory bowel disease. A dose of 50 mg/mL, 50 mL per rat, invoked an acute form of localized inflammatory colitis. To study the susceptibility to seizures, a convulsant, pentylenetetrazole (PTZ) was given through intravenous infusion to induce seizures. In this study by Riazi et al. [38], they found that TNBS-treated rats express increased susceptibility to PTZ-induced seizures that strongly correlates with the severity and progression of intestinal inflammation. The TNBS-treated rats present a prominent and reversible inflammatory response within the hippocampus along with microglial activation and TNF-α level elevation [38]. The inflammatory colitis model is also used by Rao, Medhi [39] to establish the correlation between systemic inflammation and seizures. They induced colitis using a method described by MacPherson and Pfeiffer [40], which is the application of acetic acid on the colonic lumen of adult rats. They too found that systemic inflammation can be associated with a decreased threshold to PTZ-induced seizures [39].

The second model of systemic inflammation is bacterial lipopolysaccharide (LPS) injection. In adult rats, an intraperitoneal injection of LPS results in an increase in body temperature elicited by an inflammatory response, which mimics febrile seizures, though a second-hit with a pro-convulsant drug, usually kainic acid, is usually required to generate febrile convulsions. LPS increases rat's body temperature by 1–1.5°C, which mimics fever and amplifies the convulsant actions of KA [41]. Single intraperitoneal injection of *Escherichia coli* LPS at 5 mg/kg or infusion of at a dose of 2.5 mg/kg/day into the peritoneal cavity of adult rats for 7 days via an osmotic mini-pump is sufficient to induce peripheral inflammation [42, 43]. In mice, a single dose of 1 mg/kg of LPS i.p. is sufficient to elicit effects on body temperature and seizure susceptibility [44]. Seizure susceptibility is then tested using an intraperitoneal injection of KA (10 mg/kg) or PTZ (10 mg/mL) after 2 hours [43, 44]. LPS infusion is reported to increase plasma levels of IL-1β, IL-6 and TNF-α. This means that the systemic inflammation induced by LPS infusion brings about the activation of microglia, enhancement of pro-inflammatory cytokines production and tissue oxidative stress in the hippocampus [43, 45]. As a result, LPS administration increases body temperature slightly and reduces PTZ-induced seizure susceptibility in a dose-dependent and time-dependent manner. Recent studies have shown that LPS acts as an activator for Toll-like receptor 4 (TLR 4) and induces seizures. The probable mechanism in explanation to this is that LPS mimics the actions stressed or damaged neurons which releases endogenous 'danger signals' via a protein called HMGB1. After being released from neurons, HMGB1 communicates with TLR4 to induce seizures, which activates a positive feedback cycle, by stimulating activated astrocytes and microglia for additional release of HMGB1.

3.2 Inflammation as a consequence of seizures

3.2.1 Kainic acid (KA) injection

KA is an agonist for α-amino-3-hydroxy-5-methylisoxazole-4-propionic acid (AMPA) and KA receptor. AMPA is a subtype of ionotropic glutamate receptor. Systemic and intracerebral injections of KA induce progressive limbic seizures, which resemble human temporal lobe epilepsy, in rats [46]. These peak in status epilepticus (SE) where, in limbic structures (i.e. hippocampal CA1 and CA3, and the hilus of dentate gyrus) of the brain, reactive oxygen species (ROS) production and mitochondrial dysfunction lead to neuronal cell death [47]. Moreover, the delayed release of proinflammatory gene expressions, such as TNF-α, IL-1β, IL-6, inducible nitric oxide synthase (iNOS) and cyclooxygenase-2 (COX-2), is believed to promote prolonged neurodegeneration [48]. For these reasons, KA is used for various studies into neurological disorders including inflammation and epilepsy.

Kainic acid injection into hippocampus of rats increases the number of IL-1ß, IL-6 and TNF-α positive cells in the hippocampus, indicating inflammatory response [49, 50]. There is also a higher number of GFAP-positive cells which shows that kainic acid promotes gliosis, also an indicator of neuroinflammation. Chen, Zhu [49] found that kainic acid administration causes swelling and deformities of endothelial cells and their nuclei in cerebromicrovessels. The BBB integrity is also destroyed following kainic acid injection with signs of vacuolation, perivascular edema and membrane damage [49].

KA is widely used in epilepsy studies and models include rodents as well as zebrafish. In rodents, KA works to induce seizures and SE in neonatal and adult rat and mice. In rat neonates, 2 mg/kg of KA injected intraperitoneally was found to induce seizures without mortality while 4 mg/kg of KA was shown to induce mortality in 60% of pups [51]. For adult rats and mice, a single dose of KA at15mg/kg for rats and 20 mg/kg for mice can be used for inducing seizures [52].

In rat neonates, the phases of convulsions that are generated by KA are automatism (forelimb/hind-limb scratching) and continuous generalized tonic-clonic seizures, with loss of righting reflex, indicating tonic extension and SE. In this model, SE is defined as continuous clonic seizures involving both forelimbs and hind-limbs and continual loss of the righting reflex [51].

In adult rats and mice, seizures are characterized by a seizure scoring scale devised by Racine as follows:

Stage 1: Wet dog shakes, facial clonus and staring.

Stage 2: Head nodding.

Stage 3: Forelimb clonus.

Stage 4: Forelimb clonus with rearing.

Stage 5: Rearing, jumping, falling and SE.

Despite being a relatively new model, zebrafish is acknowledged to be a fairly popular animal model in pre-clinical researches and as a suitable alternative to rodents and other animal models in epilepsy research [53]. KA is used to induce seizures in zebrafish at a dose of 6 mg/kg, injected intraperitoneally. The seizures induced by KA are characterized as follows [54]:

Stage 1: Immobility and hyperventilation.

Stage 2: Whirlpool-like swimming behavior.

Stage 3: Rapid left-to-right movements.

Stage 4: Abnormal and spasmodic muscular contractions.

Stage 5: Rapid, whole-body, clonus-like convulsions.

Stage 6: Death.

SE is represented by seizure scores fluctuating between 4 and 6 for a period of 30 minutes or more [55].

3.2.2 Pilocarpine injection

Pilocarpine is a cholinergic (muscarinic) agonist which induces SE, followed by recurrent spontaneous seizures (RSS), in animal models and is widely used to study the mechanisms of SE. It acts on the endothelial muscarinic receptors which compromises the integrity of the BBB [56]. It subsequently causes the influx of proinflammatory cytokines into the brain, which results in neuroinflammation [35]. The hippocampus is notably more vulnerable to pilocarpine-induced neuronal injury because it possesses numerous distinct neuronal circuits which are involved in the generation of seizures [57]. Pilocarpine causes extensive neuronal cell loss in CA1 and CA3 pyramidal cell layers, astrogliosis, and mossy fiber sprouting in the hippocampus [57, 58].

Upon administration of pilocarpine into rats, the levels of inflammatory biomarkers, IL-1β, TNF-α, NF-κβ and COX-2, are elevated in the hippocampus, indicating the presence of neuroinflammation [59]. During pilocarpine-induced seizures, ROS formation increases and glutathione (GSH) redox status becomes impaired in the hippocampus [60, 61]. The overproduction of ROS leads to an increase in oxidative stress which contributes to cell apoptosis in the brain [62]. Ali, Mahdy [59] reported that pilocarpine injection induces a significant elevation of hippocampal cytochrome c and caspase 3 levels which contributes to apoptosis. This apoptotic cell death is a key feature of hippocampal cell loss induced by SE [59]. Furthermore, apoptosis related proteins such as Bax, Bcl-2 family and caspase-3 can modify the neurotransmission pathways that are independent of cell death in the CNS and have significant contribution in epileptogenesis [63, 64].

Seizures can be induced in adult mice or rats with a subcutaneous or intraperitoneal injection of 340–350 mg/kg of pilocarpine hydrochloride [58, 65]. Pilocarpine treatment sequentially induces the following behavioral changes: akinesia, facial automatisms, forelimb clonus with rearing, salivation, masticatory jaw movements and falling [65, 66]. These behaviors build up progressively into motor limbic seizures that recur repeatedly and rapidly develop into SE, similar to that described in patients of temporal lobe epilepsy (TLE). EEG findings showed a significant surge of theta rhythms and isolated spikes in the hippocampus, synchronization of the hippocampal and cortical activities, isolated electrographic seizures and SE [65]. The electroencephalographical, behavioral, as well as anatomical alterations and characteristics of human TLE are emulated by this model [58].

Besides the rodent models, pilocarpine is also used to induce seizures in zebrafish larvae for anticonvulsant studies. A final concentration of 30 mM of pilocarpine is used with a 1-minute incubation before quantification of larval locomotor activity. Exposure to pilocarpine results in a more subtle convulsive behavior compared to PTZ, such as lurching/head banging, head-to-tail undulations, increased mouth movements, tremor, body contortions and loss of posture [67]. Eddins, Cerutti [68] reported the use of pilocarpine to induce seizures in zebrafish embryos to compare its effects on early exposure to developmental exposure to toxicants. Zebrafish embryos (2-hours post-fertilization) exposed to 100 μM pilocarpine exhibit very little to zero dose–response relationship of developmental pilocarpine exposure with regard to the startle response [68].

3.2.3 Albumin injection

Extravasation of serum albumin into the brain provokes prominent BBB dysfunction through the activation of transforming growth factor beta (TGF-β) receptor (RII) signaling. This causes the astrocytes to fail in buffering extracellular K^+ which causes BBB dysfunction [69–71]. BBB dysfunction is a commonly found following seizures or epileptogenic brain injuries [7].

Frigerio et al. [72] described a model using albumin to provoke BBB breakdown, mimicking brain excitability after SE. They showed that a single intracerebroventricular injection of albumin to rats causes the diffusion of albumin into the hippocampus before conveyed into principal neurons. The extravasation of albumin by parenchymal cells at pathological concentration causes the following conditions: (1) down-regulation of Kir4.1 channels and neuroinflammation in glial fibrillary acidic protein(GFAP)-positive astrocytes; (2) brief neuronal hyperexcitability manifested as involuntary epileptic spikes, and amplified KA–induced epileptic activity; and (3) chronic reduction in seizure threshold without causing cell loss or spontaneous epileptic activity [72].

BBB disruption was induced using a single dose of intracerebroventricular injection of 1.9 mM rat albumin into deeply anesthetized adult rats. After the injection, GFAP-positive glial cells and IL-1β staining in the hippocampus were evaluated. It was found that albumin injection prominently increases IL-1β immunoreactivity in GFAP-positive astrocytes and the number of IL-1β immunopositive cells, indicating the presence of inflammation. Besides that, the production of rapid onset and transient spiking activity in the hippocampus can be found on the EEG analysis of rats injected with rat albumin. This means that the injection of albumin provokes the increase in neuronal excitability. Interestingly, rats presented a significant decline in seizure threshold 3 months after albumin injection. This suggests that acute tissue exposure to albumin induces a long-lasting increase in brain excitability [72].

In short, this model is able to show the pro-ictogenic effect of serum albumin in the brain, mimicking those attained after prolonged seizures and BBB dysfunction. Albumin induces the production of inflammatory molecules and together, they significantly increase brain excitability and seizure susceptibility although insufficient to trigger spontaneous seizures.

4. Conclusion

Inflammation plays an important role in the development of epilepsy and understanding this inflammatory process that happens during epileptogenesis could provide a strong basis for drug development and therapeutic approaches. We briefly highlighted the inflammatory response during epilepsy and some clinical correlation. Besides, we outlined the experimental findings in epilepsy research pertaining to inflammation and hope to clear the doubts as to whether inflammation is a cause or consequence of epilepsy. Evidently, inflammation can be both the cause as well as consequence of epilepsy. Inflammation due to hyperthermia or infection activates the release of inflammatory molecules which increases seizures susceptibility. On the other hand, BBB dysfunction and prolonged seizures cause an influx of inflammatory molecules which causes neuroinflammation to take place.

Anti-inflammatory drugs, such as acetaminophen, celecoxib or aspirin, along with other anti-inflammatory agents such as anti-MGB1 antibodies and COX-2 inhibitors have been shown to possess anti-convulsant properties [73]. Therefore, we suggest incorporating anti-inflammatory drugs into anti-epileptic treatments or therapy could be beneficial in the management of epilepsy and ameliorating comorbidities and side effects that could be exacerbated by neuroinflammation.

Acknowledgements

The authors would like to thank Mr. Brandon Choo Kar Meng for proofreading the manuscript.

Conflict of interest

Authors declare no conflict of interest.

Author details

Vanessa Lin Lin Lee and Mohd. Farooq Shaikh*
Neuropharmacology Research Laboratory, Jeffrey Cheah School of Medicine and Health Sciences, Monash University Malaysia, Bandar Sunway, Malaysia

*Address all correspondence to: farooq.shaikh@monash.edu

References

[1] Duncan JS, Sander JW, Sisodiya SM, Walker MC. Adult epilepsy. Lancet. 2006;**367**(9516):1087-1100

[2] Cunliffe VT, Baines RA, Giachello CN, Lin WH, Morgan A, Reuber M, et al. Epilepsy research methods update: Understanding the causes of epileptic seizures and identifying new treatments using non-mammalian model organisms. Seizure. 2015;**24**:44-51

[3] Thurman DJ, Begley CE, Carpio A, Helmers S, Hesdorffer DC, Mu J, et al. The primary prevention of epilepsy: A report of the prevention task force of the international league against epilepsy. Epilepsia. 2018;**59**(5):905-914

[4] Johan Arief MF, Choo BKM, Yap JL, Kumari Y, Shaikh MF. A systematic review on non-mammalian models in epilepsy research. Frontiers in Pharmacology. 2018;**9**:655

[5] Rana A, Musto AE. The role of inflammation in the development of epilepsy. Journal of Neuroinflammation. 2018;**15**(1):144

[6] Klein P, Dingledine R, Aronica E, Bernard C, Blümcke I, Boison D, et al. Commonalities in epileptogenic processes from different acute brain insults: Do they translate? Epilepsia. 2018;**59**(1):37-66

[7] Vezzani A, French J, Bartfai T, Baram TZ. The role of inflammation in epilepsy. Nature Reviews. Neurology. 2011;7(1):31-40

[8] Tomkins O, Feintuch A, Benifla M, Cohen A, Friedman A, Shelef I. Blood-brain barrier breakdown following traumatic brain injury: A possible role in posttraumatic epilepsy. Cardiovascular Psychiatry and Neurology. 2011;**2011**:765923

[9] Gorter JA, Van Vliet EA, Aronica E. Status epilepticus, blood-brain barrier disruption, inflammation, and epileptogenesis. Epilepsy & Behavior. 2015;**49**:13-16

[10] Van Vliet EA, Aronica E, Gorter JA. Blood–brain barrier dysfunction, seizures and epilepsy. In: Seminars in cell & Developmental biology. Academic Press. 2015;**38**:26-34

[11] Liebner S, Dijkhuizen RM, Reiss Y, Plate KH, Agalliu D, Constantin G. Functional morphology of the blood-brain barrier in health and disease. Acta Neuropathologica. 2018;**135**(3):1-26

[12] Maroso M, Balosso S, Ravizza T, Liu J, Aronica E, Iyer AM, et al. Toll-like receptor 4 and high-mobility group box-1 are involved in ictogenesis and can be targeted to reduce seizures. Nature Medicine. 2010;**16**(4):413

[13] Huang HL, Lin CC, Jeng KC, Yao PW, Chuang LT, Kuo SL, et al. Fresh green tea and gallic acid ameliorate oxidative stress in kainic acid-induced status epilepticus. Journal of Agricultural and Food Chemistry. 2012;**60**(9):2328-2336

[14] Teocchi MA, Ferreira AÉD, EPDL d O, Tedeschi H, D'Souza-Li L. Hippocampal gene expression dysregulation of Klotho, nuclear factor kappa B and tumor necrosis factor in temporal lobe epilepsy patients. Journal of Neuroinflammation. 2013;**10**(1):53

[15] Allan SM, Rothwell NJ. Cytokines and acute neurodegeneration. Nature Reviews. Neuroscience. 2001;**2**(10):734-744

[16] Ulevitch R, Tobias P. Receptor-dependent mechanisms of cell stimulation by bacterial endotoxin. Annual Review of Immunology. 1995;**13**(1):437-457

[17] Bianchi MEDAMP. PAMPs and alarmins: All we need to know about

danger. Journal of Leukocyte Biology. 2007;**81**(1):1-5

[18] Tsan MF, Gao B. Endogenous ligands of Toll-like receptors. Journal of Leukocyte Biology. 2004;**76**(3):514-519

[19] Vezzani A, Maroso M, Balosso S, Sanchez M-A, Bartfai T. IL-1 receptor/Toll-like receptor signaling in infection, inflammation, stress and neurodegeneration couples hyperexcitability and seizures. Brain, Behavior, and Immunity. 2011;**25**(7):1281-1289

[20] Vezzani A, Aronica E, Mazarati A, Pittman QJ. Epilepsy and brain inflammation. Experimental Neurology. 2013;**244**:11-21

[21] Bien CG, Tiemeier H, Sassen R, Kuczaty S, Urbach H, von Lehe M, et al. Rasmussen encephalitis: Incidence and course under randomized therapy with tacrolimus or intravenous immunoglobulins. Epilepsia. 2013;**54**(3):543-550

[22] Schneider-Hohendorf T, Mohan H, Bien CG, Breuer J, Becker A, Görlich D, et al. CD8+ T-cell pathogenicity in Rasmussen encephalitis elucidated by large-scale T-cell receptor sequencing. Nature Communications. 2016;**7**:11153

[23] Cepeda C, Chang JW, Owens GC, Huynh MN, Chen JY, Tran C, et al. In Rasmussen encephalitis, hemichannels associated with microglial activation are linked to cortical pyramidal neuron coupling: A possible mechanism for cellular hyperexcitability. CNS Neuroscience & Therapeutics. 2015;**21**(2):152-163

[24] Vincent A, Irani SR, Lang B. The growing recognition of immunotherapy-responsive seizure disorders with autoantibodies to specific neuronal proteins. Current Opinion in Neurology. 2010;**23**(2):144-150

[25] Alsharafi W, Xiao B. Dynamic expression of MicroRNAs (183, 135a, 125b, 128, 30c and 27a) in the rat Pilocarpine model and temporal lobe epilepsy patients. CNS & Neurological Disorders Drug Targets. 2015;**14**(8):1096-1102

[26] Ishikawa N, Kobayashi Y, Fujii Y, Kobayashi M. Increased interleukin-6 and high-sensitivity C-reactive protein levels in pediatric epilepsy patients with frequent, refractory generalized motor seizures. Seizure. 2015;**25**:136-140

[27] Butler T, Li Y, Tsui W, Friedman D, Maoz A, Wang X, et al. Transient and chronic seizure-induced inflammation in human focal epilepsy. Epilepsia. 2016;**57**(9):e191-e194

[28] Gatti S, Vezzani A, Bartfai T. Mechanisms of fever and febrile seizures: Putative role of the interleukin-1 system. In: Febrile Seizures. Massachusetts: Elsevier; 2002. pp. 169-188

[29] Zetterstrom M, Sundgren-Andersson AK, Ostlund P, Bartfai T. Delineation of the proinflammatory cytokine cascade in fever induction. Annals of the New York Academy of Sciences. 1998;**856**:48-52

[30] Baram TZ, Gerth A, Schultz L. Febrile seizures: An appropriate-aged model suitable for long-term studies. Developmental Brain Research. 1997;**98**(2):265-270

[31] Dube CM, Ravizza T, Hamamura M, Zha Q, Keebaugh A, Fok K, et al. Epileptogenesis provoked by prolonged experimental febrile seizures: Mechanisms and biomarkers. The Journal of Neuroscience. 2010;**30**(22):7484-7494

[32] Crespo M, DA L-N, Martin M. Cerebellar oxidative stress and fine motor impairment in adolescent rats exposed to hyperthermia-induced

seizures is prevented by maternal caffeine intake during gestation and lactation. European Journal of Pharmacology. 2018;**822**:186-198

[33] Dupuis N, Auvin S. Inflammation and epilepsy in the developing brain: Clinical and experimental evidence. CNS Neuroscience & Therapeutics. 2015;**21**(2):141-151

[34] Simard AR, Rivest S. Do pathogen exposure and innate immunity cause brain diseases? Neurological Research. 2005;**27**(7):717-725

[35] Riazi K, Galic MA, Pittman QJ. Contributions of peripheral inflammation to seizure susceptibility: Cytokines and brain excitability. Epilepsy Research. 2010;**89**(1):34-42

[36] Pol O, Ferrer I, Puig MM. Diarrhea associated with intestinal inflammation increases the potency of mu and delta opioids on the inhibition of gastrointestinal transit in mice. The Journal of Pharmacology and Experimental Therapeutics. 1994;**270**(1):386-391

[37] Puig MM, Pol O. Peripheral effects of opioids in a model of chronic intestinal inflammation in mice. The Journal of Pharmacology and Experimental Therapeutics. 1998;**287**(3):1068-1075

[38] Riazi K, Galic MA, Kuzmiski JB, Ho W, Sharkey KA, Pittman QJ. Microglial activation and TNFalpha production mediate altered CNS excitability following peripheral inflammation. Proceedings of the National Academy of Sciences of the United States of America. 2008;**105**(44):17151-17156

[39] Rao RS, Medhi B, Khanduja KL, Pandhi P. Correlation of seizures and biochemical parameters of oxidative stress in experimentally induced inflammatory rat models. Fundamental & Clinical Pharmacology. 2010;**24**(3):325-331

[40] MacPherson BR, Pfeiffer CJ. Experimental production of diffuse colitis in rats. Digestion. 1978;**17**(2):135-150

[41] Patterson KP, Baram TZ, Shinnar S. Origins of temporal lobe epilepsy: Febrile seizures and febrile status epilepticus. Neurotherapeutics. 2014;**11**(2):242-250

[42] Yamanaka D, Kawano T, Nishigaki A, Aoyama B, Tateiwa H, Shigematsu-Locatelli M, et al. Preventive effects of dexmedetomidine on the development of cognitive dysfunction following systemic inflammation in aged rats. Journal of Anesthesia. 2017;**31**(1):25-35

[43] Ho Y-H, Lin Y-T, Wu C-WJ, Chao Y-M, Chang AY, Chan JY. Peripheral inflammation increases seizure susceptibility via the induction of neuroinflammation and oxidative stress in the hippocampus. Journal of Biomedical Science. 2015;**22**(1):46

[44] Sayyah M, Javad-Pour M, Ghazi-Khansari M. The bacterial endotoxin lipopolysaccharide enhances seizure susceptibility in mice: Involvement of proinflammatory factors: Nitric oxide and prostaglandins. Neuroscience. 2003;**122**(4):1073-1080

[45] Eun BL, Abraham J, Mlsna L, Kim MJ, Koh S. Lipopolysaccharide potentiates hyperthermia-induced seizures. Brain and Behavior. 2015;**5**(8):e00348

[46] Ben-Ari Y, Cossart R. Kainate, a double agent that generates seizures: Two decades of progress. Trends in Neurosciences. 2000;**23**(11):580-587

[47] Ben-Ari Y. Limbic seizure and brain damage produced by kainic acid: Mechanisms and relevance to human temporal lobe epilepsy. Neuroscience. 1985;**14**(2):375-403

[48] Rizzi M, Perego C, Aliprandi M, Richichi C, Ravizza T, Colella D, et al. Glia activation and cytokine increase in rat hippocampus by kainic acid-induced status epilepticus during postnatal development. Neurobiology of Disease. 2003;**14**(3):494-503

[49] Chen Y-C, Zhu G-Y, Wang X, Shi L, Du T-T, Liu D-F, et al. Anterior thalamic nuclei deep brain stimulation reduces disruption of the blood-brain barrier, albumin extravasation, inflammation and apoptosis in kainic acid-induced epileptic rats. Neurological Research. 2017;**39**(12):1103-1113

[50] Wang Z-h, M-c M, Y-c Y, M-c Y. Asiatic acid and maslinic acid attenuated kainic acid-induced seizure through decreasing hippocampal inflammatory and oxidative stress. Epilepsy Research. 2018;**139**:28-34

[51] Dhir A, Chavda V. Pre-and post-exposure talampanel (GYKI 53773) against kainic acid seizures in neonatal rats. Pharmacological Reports. 2016;**68**(1):190-195

[52] Chiu KM, Wu CC, Wang MJ, Lee MY, Wang SJ. Protective effects of bupivacaine against kainic acid-induced seizure and neuronal cell death in the rat hippocampus. Biological and Pharmaceutical Bulletin. 2015;**38**(4):522-530

[53] Kundap UP, Kumari Y, Othman I, Shaikh M. Zebrafish as a model for epilepsy-induced cognitive dysfunction: A pharmacological, biochemical and behavioral approach. Frontiers in Pharmacology. 2017;**8**:515

[54] Mussulini BH, Vizuete AF, Braga M, Moro L, Baggio S, Santos E, Lazzarotto G, Zenki KC, Pettenuzzo L, da Rocha JB, de Oliveira DL. Forebrain glutamate uptake and behavioral parameters are altered in adult zebrafish after the induction of Status Epilepticus by kainic acid. Neurotoxicology. Apr 19, 2018

[55] Sierra S, Alfaro JM, Sanchez S, Burgos JS. Administration of docosahexaenoic acid before birth and until aging decreases kainate-induced seizures in adult zebrafish. Brain Research Bulletin. 2012;**88**(5):467-470

[56] Kharatishvili I, Shan ZY, She DT, Foong S, Kurniawan ND, Reutens DC. MRI changes and complement activation correlate with epileptogenicity in a mouse model of temporal lobe epilepsy. Brain Structure and Function. 2014;**219**(2):683-706

[57] Pestana RR, Kinjo ER, Hernandes MS, Britto LR. Reactive oxygen species generated by NADPH oxidase are involved in neurodegeneration in the pilocarpine model of temporal lobe epilepsy. Neuroscience Letters. 2010;**484**(3):187-191

[58] Hadera MG, Smeland OB, McDonald TS, Tan KN, Sonnewald U, Borges K. Triheptanoin partially restores levels of tricarboxylic acid cycle intermediates in the mouse pilocarpine model of epilepsy. Journal of Neurochemistry. 2014;**129**(1):107-119

[59] Ali AE, Mahdy HM, Elsherbiny DM, Azab SS. Rifampicin ameliorates lithium-pilocarpine-induced seizures, consequent hippocampal damage and memory deficit in rats: Impact on oxidative, inflammatory and apoptotic machineries. Biochemical Pharmacology. 2018;**156**:431-443

[60] Liu J, Wang A, Li L, Huang Y, Xue P, Hao A. Oxidative stress mediates hippocampal neuron death in rats after lithium–pilocarpine-induced status epilepticus. Seizure. 2010;**19**(3):165-172

[61] Liu Y-F, Gao F, Li X-W, Jia R-H, Meng X-D, Zhao R, et al. The anticonvulsant and neuroprotective effects of baicalin on pilocarpine-induced epileptic model in rats. Neurochemical Research. 2012;**37**(8):1670-1680

[62] Méndez-Armenta M, Nava-Ruíz C, Juárez-Rebollar D, Rodríguez-Martínez E, Yescas Gómez P. Oxidative stress associated with neuronal apoptosis in experimental models of epilepsy. Oxidative Medicine and Cellular Longevity. 2014;**2014**:12

[63] Jiao S, Li Z. Nonapoptotic function of BAD and BAX in long-term depression of synaptic transmission. Neuron. 2011;**70**(4):758-772

[64] Kudryashova I, Onufriev M, Kudryashov I, Gulyaeva N. Caspase-3 activity in hippocampal slices reflects changes in synaptic plasticity. Neuroscience and Behavioral Physiology. 2009;**39**(1):13

[65] Cavalheiro EA. The pilocarpine model of epilepsy. The Italian Journal of Neurological Sciences. 1995;**16**(1-2):33-37

[66] Brandt C, Töllner K, Klee R, Bröer S, Löscher W. Effective termination of status epilepticus by rational polypharmacy in the lithium–pilocarpine model in rats: Window of opportunity to prevent epilepsy and prediction of epilepsy by biomarkers. Neurobiology of Disease. 2015;**75**:78-90

[67] Vermoesen K, Serruys A-SK, Loyens E, Afrikanova T, Massie A, Schallier A, et al. Assessment of the convulsant liability of antidepressants using zebrafish and mouse seizure models. Epilepsy & Behavior. 2011;**22**(3):450-460

[68] Eddins D, Cerutti D, Williams P, Linney E, Levin ED. Zebrafish provide a sensitive model of persisting neurobehavioral effects of developmental chlorpyrifos exposure: Comparison with nicotine and pilocarpine effects and relationship to dopamine deficits. Neurotoxicology and Teratology. 2010;**32**(1):99-108

[69] Cacheaux LP, Ivens S, David Y, Lakhter AJ, Bar-Klein G, Shapira M, et al. Transcriptome profiling reveals TGF-β signaling involvement in epileptogenesis. Journal of Neuroscience. 2009;**29**(28):8927-8935

[70] David Y, Cacheaux LP, Ivens S, Lapilover E, Heinemann U, Kaufer D, et al. Astrocytic dysfunction in epileptogenesis: Consequence of altered potassium and glutamate homeostasis. Journal of Neuroscience. 2009;**29**(34):10588-10599

[71] Ivens S, Kaufer D, Flores LP, Bechmann I, Zumsteg D, Tomkins O, et al. TGF-β receptor-mediated albumin uptake into astrocytes is involved in neocortical epileptogenesis. Brain. 2006;**130**(2):535-547

[72] Frigerio F, Frasca A, Weissberg I, Parrella S, Friedman A, Vezzani A, et al. Long-lasting pro-ictogenic effects induced in vivo by rat brain exposure to serum albumin in the absence of concomitant pathology. Epilepsia. 2012;**53**(11):1887-1897

[73] Paudel YN, Shaikh MF, Shah S, Kumari Y, Othman I. Role of inflammation in epilepsy and neurobehavioral comorbidities: Implication for therapy. European Journal of Pharmacology. 2018;**837**:145-155

Chapter 3

Cerebroventricular Injection of Cigarette Smoke Condensate Produce Generalized Seizures Decreased by Muscarinic Receptor Antagonist in Rats

Jawad Laadraoui and Abderrahman Chait

Abstract

Tobacco smoke is a complex multicomponent system, in which more than 4800 compounds have been identified by chromatographic techniques; many of these compounds are carcinogenic. However, there is a great deal of research into the association between smoking and diseases such as heart attacks, strokes and cancers. Nevertheless rare are the studies on the association between smoking and epilepsy because the exact roles of smoking and nicotine use in epilepsy have not been well examined. In this study the authors evaluate the convulsive effects of intracerebroventricular administration of cigarette smoke condensate in rats and compare intensity of seizures with kainic acid-induced seizures as a model of epilepsy. The role of cholinergic system was also evaluated using mAChRs antagonist in cigarette smoke condensate (CSC) induced seizures. Results indicate that central injection of cigarette condensate provides an epileptic behavior similar to that induced by kainic acid. However a pretreatment with atropine reduced seizures and all their parameters.

Keywords: seizures, epilepsy, cigarette smoke condensate, intracerebroventricular, kainic acid

1. Introduction

In the world, about 1% of people suffer from epilepsy [1]. Modern anticonvulsants can prevent and decrease the intensity of these convulsions. However, about 30% of people with epilepsy have uncontrollable seizures although of drugs availability. It is also known that the therapy ineffectiveness and chronic toxicity of antiepileptic drugs drawbacks the treatment procedure for nearly 20% of the patients [2].

Tobacco smoke is a complex multicomponent system, in which more than 4800 compounds, many of which are known carcinogens. As a result, chronic obstructive pulmonary disease, chronic bronchitis, cardiovascular disease, emphysema, stroke and many forms of cancer are directly related to smoking [3].

In March 2012, the Food and Drug Administration established a long list containing 93 harmful and potentially harmful components (HPHCs) and an abbreviated list containing 18 HPHCs in tobacco products and tobacco smoke (**Table 1**).

However, seizure control in the majority of epileptic patients is achieved primarily through the pharmacotherapeutic action of drugs targeting membrane ion channels or glutamatergic or gabaergic neurotransmission [4], which is dependent on a wide variety of modifications., glutamate and GABA [5]. For example, a weak activation of the GABAergic system induces epilepsy [6]. Generally, the risk of epilepsy should be higher in chronic tobacco smokers; this behavior is due to toxic components of tobacco smoke that can lead to seizure behavior in humans and animals [7, 8].

Many components in tobacco smoke are associated with seizures or epilepsy (**Table 2**) [9]. For example, nicotine, when overdosed, caused seizures in human subjects. Nicotine, a parasympathomimetic alkaloid in tobacco when overdosed, caused seizures in human [10]. The carbon monoxide causes seizures that can be focal or generalized and may even present as a status of epilepticus [11, 12]. Ammonia, hexane, lead, cresol, arsenic, toluene and acetone are other chemicals found in tobacco smoke that can trigger seizures in humans or animals [13].

HPHCs in cigarette smoke	HPHCs in smokeless tobacco	HPHCs in roll-your-own tobacco[a] and cigarette filler
Acetaldehyde	Acetaldehyde	Ammonia
Acrolein	Arsenic	Arsenic
Acrylonitrile	Benzo[a]pyrene	Cadmium
4-Aminobiphenyl	Cadmium	Nicotine (total)
1-Aminonaphthalene	Crotonaldehyde	NNK*
2-Aminonaphthalene	Formaldehyde	NNN**
Ammonia	Nicotine (total and free)	
Benzene	NNK*	
Benzo[a]pyrene	NNN**	
1,3-Butadiene		
Carbon monoxide		
Crotonaldehyde		
Formaldehyde		
Isoprene		
Nicotine (total)		
NNK*		
NNN**		
Toluene		

See Ref. [4]. *4-(Methylnitrosamino)-1-(3-pyridyl)-1-butanone.*

** *N-Nitrosonornicotine.*

[a] *Roll-your-own tobacco is defined in section 900(15) of the FD&C Act to mean "any tobacco product which, because of its appearance, type, packaging, or labeling, is suitable for use and likely to be offered to, or purchased by, consumers as tobacco for making cigarettes." The term cigarette filler is not defined in the FD&C Act. For purposes of this draft guidance, we intend cigarette filler to mean the cut, ground, powdered, or leaf tobacco that is a component of a cigarette.*

Table 1.
Abbreviated list of harmful and potentially harmful constituents (HPHCs) in tobacco products.

Chemicals in tobacco smoke	Seizure-inducing	Potentiating seizures
Nicotine	Nicotine patch (H)[a]	
Carbon monoxide	(H)	
5% carbon dioxide		Low dose increased the severity of the electroshock-induced seizures (M)
Arsenic		
Ammonia	(H), (R)	
Hexane	(H)	
Lead acetate	High dose induced forelimb	Potentiated PTZ-induced convulsions (M)
Toluene	clonus (M)	Increased susceptibility to aminophylline-induced seizures (IP) (M)
Cresol	(H)	
Selenium		
Zinc		
Copper		
Nickel		
Acetone	High dose caused seizures (M)	

[a]*H: human; M: mouse; R: rat.*

Table 2.
Effects of chemicals in tobacco smoke on seizures or epilepsy.

Animals have been a useful tool for elucidating the association between tobacco smoking or nicotine use and seizures or epilepsy. Nicotine induced seizure models include cats, mice, and rats, and it was reported that animals received nicotine via injection develop seizures but not through the automatic smoking machine (ASM) [14, 15]. Other studies have shown that the activity of seizure-inducing chemicals such as pentylenetetrazole [16], kainic acid, pilocarpine, had been enhanced by prior pretreatment with nicotine [17].

In this study, we have investigated the convulsive effect of CSC as a crisis model compared to the intensity of the kainic acid model of epilepsy in rats. Thus examine the role of the cholinergic system in cigarette condensate seizures using a treatment with cholinergic muscarinic ligand.

2. Epileptic behavior induced by cerebral injection of cigarette smoke condensate

2.1 Methodology

The objective of the experiment was to demonstrate that a treatment with cigarette smoke condensate provides an epileptic behavior similar to this induced by a kainic acid, who reduced by a pretreatment with atropine.

The preparation of the cigarette smoke condensate was carried out by a cooling system consisting of a VP800 vacuum pump that generates and removes cigarette smoke to a tube and a balloon where the cigarette condensate is recovered [13]. Male

Sprague-Dawley rats (3–4 months old, 230–250 g weight) were used in this experiment, All animals were treated according to European decree, related to the ethical evaluation and authorization of projects using animals for experimental procedures, 1st February 2013, NOR: AGRG1238767A efforts were made to minimize the number and suffering of animals used. Before the experience all rats are anesthetized with an intraperitoneal injection of Hydrate chloral (400 mg/kg (6%)), before being placed in a Horsley-Clarke stereotactic frame. The head is secured with two bars that are inserted into the ear canal to the inner ears. The muzzle is well fixed by an oral part. After shaving the head, we made a median skin incision 1.5 cm long. The skin is spread laterally to clear the bone surface and highlight the coronal suture with the points, Bregma forward and Lambda back. The coordinates of the injection point with respect to the Bregma point are determined using the stereotaxic atlas of Paxinos and Watson [18]. The stereotaxic coordinates of the ventricle were as follows: the incisor bar −0.92 mm behind Bregma, ±1.5 mm laterally to the sagittal suture and 3.2 mm from the top of the skull. With a suitable milling machine, small openings are made in the cranial box for the placement (unilaterally) of the guide cannulas of approximately 23 gauge and the stainless steel anchor screws that will fix these cannulas. Stainless steel stylets (30 gauges) are placed in each guide cannula to prevent obstruction. These cannulas are then fixed by white dental cement. Then, with the help of pink dental cement, we put a crown in order to protect this preparation against any collision with the walls of the cage in which the animals were placed for 8 days to recover from surgery and eliminate anesthesia [13].

The animals were divided into four groups of six animals each. Control (saline 9%), kainic acid (1 μl/rat), CSC extract (2 μl/rat), atropine + CSC (Atr + CSC), a CSC was injected before 30 min of intraperitoneally injection of atropine (1 ml/kg).

For the KA and CSC infusion, the animals were gently retained by hand and the styles were removed from the guide cannulae and introduced 27 gauge injection needles. Injection was carried out using a Hamilton syringe (10 μl) which is connected to an injection cannula by a polyethylene catheter filled with distilled water. This was lowered into the guide cannula to a distance of 1.5 mm below its lower end to reach the target structure.

Total volume of 1 μl/rat for kainic acid and 2 μl/rat for CSC injected solutions were administered for a period of 60 s, and then the injection needles were left in the guide cannulae for a supplementary period of 60 s to facilitate drug delivery.

The animals were placed in the convulsion cage for 1 day before the beginning of the experiment to adapt the animals in the new environment.

A seizure was caused by intracerebroventricular injection of kainic acid and SCC. Immediately after the injection, each rat was placed in the center of the cage and its behavior was recorded and monitored within 90 min. The epileptic and mortality behaviors observed were classified as follows: latency of the seizure, latency of the tonic-clonic seizure, duration of the tonic-clonic seizure [13].

The scoring of seizures severity after KA injection was recorded during observation period (90 min) according to the scale:

0: normal activity; 1: immobility and/or staring; 2: rigidity, extension of the tail, swaying of the head; 3: repetitive movements, bilateral paws, breeding, tremor of hind limbs; 4: minor or flickering convulsions, jumps, falls; 5: tonic-clonic or multiple convulsions and/or appearance of score 4; 6: severe tonic-clonic seizure; 7: death [13].

The rats were randomly tested and to avoid the presence of odors that could lead to a change in behavior the convulsive cage was cleaned at the end of each test. Each rat has been subjected to a seizure test only once, and seizures have always occurred between 1:00 pm and 4:00 pm to minimize the confusional effects of the circadian rhythm [19].

2.2 Results

The results indicate that cigarette smoke condensate causes similar seizure behavior to this induced by kainic acid. However, the atropine-treated group showed a significant decrease in the convulsion score compared to the kainic acid group (**Figure 1**). There were no significant differences between the kainic acid and group treated with CSC concerning the time latency of seizures. However this parameter was significantly increased after treatment with atropine (**Figure 2**) [13].

Regarding to the latency of tonic-clonic seizures, the atropine-pretreated group showed a maximum value of score, which decreased significantly in the CSC group (**Figure 3**). However duration of tonic-clonic seizures was significantly decreased in the group pretreated with atropine compared to kainic acid and CSC groups. Nevertheless there is no significant deference between kainic acid and the CSC treated groups in the latency and duration of tonic-clonic seizures (**Figure 4**) [13].

2.3 Discussion

In this study, the authors explore the effects of intracerebroventricular pretreatment with tobacco smoke condensate on seizures and compare its severity to the administration of chemical-induced seizures, such as kainic acid as an important agent for the studying the function related to the excitatory transmission of amino acid-like neurotoxic powerful glutamate used in the rat [20]. The main finding of our study was that the central injections of CSC induce an epileptically behavior in rats. Furthermore, time latency of seizures; duration and latency of tonic-clonic seizures were significantly similar in the experimental groups. The modulation of the cholinergic system in the rat brain by activation or blockade of cholinergic receptors using atropine as a cholinergic antagonist has shown us the pathway and mechanism by which the preparation of SCC generates epileptic behavior. In this case, our results indicate that pretreatment with atropine reduced the intensity of seizures as well as other parameters recorded in the rat.

Nicotine is a major alkaloid in tobacco smoke, cigarette smoking has been the most famous method to intake nicotine [9]. Several laboratory studies were found that administration of low dose of nicotine produces behavioral effects

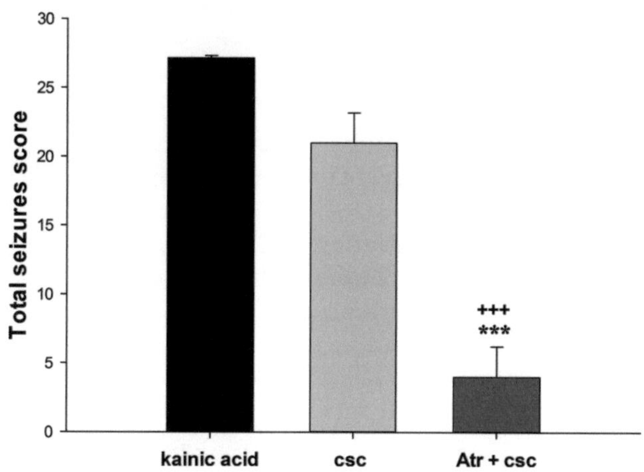

Figure 1.
Total seizure scores of all the groups. Rats received intracerebroventricularly administration of a cigarette smoke condensate (CSC), kainic acid and cigarette smoke condensate after intraperitoneally administration of atropine (atropine + CSC). Mean ± SEM: $^{***}P < 0.001$ *significantly different from the kainic acid group.* $^{+++}P < 0.001$ *significantly different from CSC extract.*

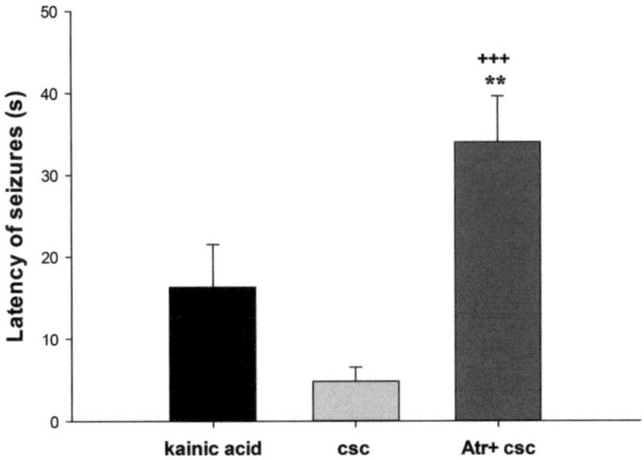

Figure 2.
*Effect of intracerebroventricularly administration of kainic acid and cigarette smoke condensate (CSC) on latency of seizures. Mean ± SEM: **P < 0.01 significantly different from the kainic acid group. +++P < 0.001 significantly different from CSC extract.*

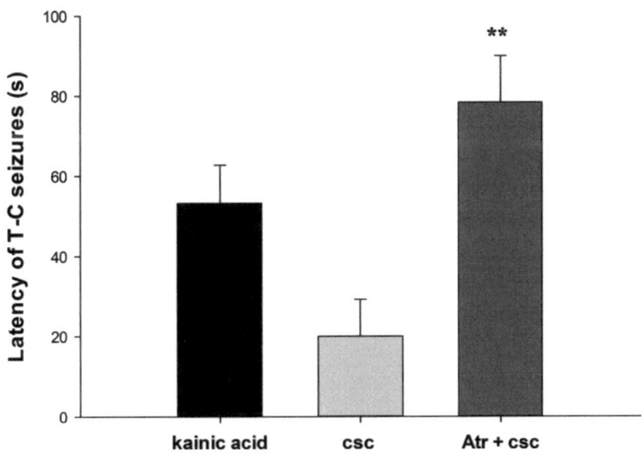

Figure 3.
*Total duration of seizures after intracerebroventricularly administration of kainic acid and cigarette smoke condensate (CSC), in a 90 min total time of epileptic behaviors recording. Mean ± SEM. **P < 0.01 significantly different from CSC extract.*

like nociception [21], locomotor activity [22], memory, learning, attention [23] and decrease or reduce anxiety [24], whereas high doses of nicotine cause seizures [25–27].

In our study, the central administration of CSC induces an epileptic behavior manifested by tonic-clonic seizures similar to this provoked by kainic acid. These results according to several electrophysiological studies indicated that intracerebroventricular administration of nicotine produces tonic-clonic seizures that have origin in the hippocampus structure [23, 25, 27].

Biochemical and pharmacological data have suggested that implicates the contribution of α4β2 and α7-containing nAChRs situated in GABAergic interneuron, in the generation of nicotine induced seizures [25, 28]. Conti-Tronconi et al. [29] had proposed that α7-nAChR subtype to underlie nicotine induced seizures for the reason that seizures sensibility is significantly correlates with quantity of α-bungarotoxin binding sites exists in the hippocampus. Several studies have examined to define the interrelationship between the nicotinic cholinergic system

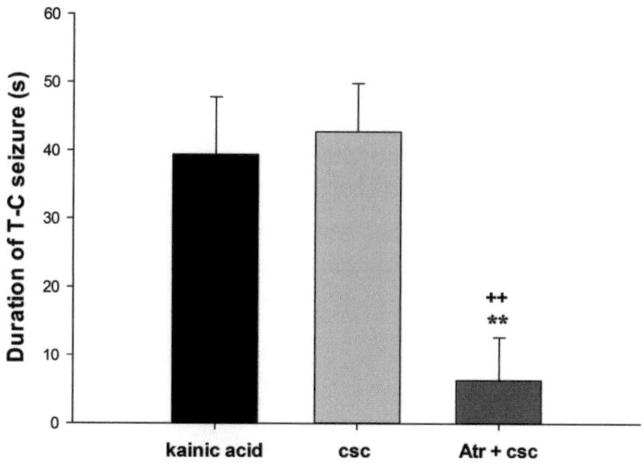

Figure 4.
*Duration of tonic-clonic seizure after intracerebroventricularly administration of kainic acid and cigarette smoke condensate (CSC). Mean ± SEM: **P < 0.01 significantly different from the kainic acid group. ++P < 0.01 significantly different from CSC extract.*

with the excitatory glutamatergic system and inhibitory gabaergic neurotransmitter in the brain. New study have reported that the α7-containing nAChRs receptors activation situated on glutamatergic nerve terminal conducing to synaptic liberation of glutamate which in turn stimulate *N*-methyl-D-Aspartate (NMDA) receptors located on pyramidal cells in of the hippocampus, are the most important mechanism that leads to nicotine seizures [25]. Though, other studies have demonstrated the contribution of α4β2 as well as α7-containing nAChRs receptors, localized in gabaergic interneurons in the creation of nicotine induced seizures [28, 30]. Contradictory to the glutamatergic hypothesis mentioned above, Dobelis et al. [28], proposed that nicotine-induced excitation was principally on relationship of pyramidal cells disinhibition in the hippocampus due to desensitization of α4β2 nAChR subtype situated on the cell bodies and dendritic terminals of pre-synaptic gabaergic interneurons.

Our results also indicate that pretreatment with atropine, a cholinergic blocking agent decreased score and latency of total seizures and tonic-clonic seizures of CSC-induced seizures; this experiment indicate that cholinergic circuit have an essential role in the mechanism underling the generation of seizures by cigarette smoke condensate. Supporting to this finding, numerous studies reporting that atropine acts as an anticonvulsant tool reducing the incidence and effectiveness of convulsions induced by an organophosphorus nerve agent [31]. A new study reporting that the anticonvulsant effects of atropine diminished with the seizures progression in a soman-induced seizures model in rats. This anticonvulsant action vanishes when the seizures had persisted for a period of 40 min [32]. Gholami et al. [33] reported a significant effect of cholinergic ligand in the pentylenetetrazole-induced epilepsy model in the rat hippocampus and they founded that cholinergic agonists leads to an augmentation of tonic-clonic seizures severity and rate mortality, however cholinergic antagonist decrease duration of tonic-clonic seizures, these data are in agreement with our study.

3. Conclusion

Data had revealed that the intracerebroventricular injection of CSC induces tonic and clonic seizures characterizing epieltical behavior similar to this triggered by acid kainic model of seizures and a significant modulatory effect of cholinergic antagonist ligands in the CSC induced seizures. In this epilepsy model, CSC led to an increment of time latency, duration and latency of tonic-clonic seizures; while pretreatment with cholinergic antagonist increased all parameters recorded. This finding provide supplementary support for data that tobacco and specially nicotine had convulsing actions and confirmation of novel CSC induced seizures model of epilepsy in rats.

Author details

Jawad Laadraoui* and Abderrahman Chait
Laboratory of Pharmacology, Neurobiology and Behavior, Semlalia Faculty of Sciences, Cadi Ayyad University, Marrakech, Morocco

*Address all correspondence to: jawad.laadraoui@edu.uca.ac.ma

References

[1] World Health Organization. The World Health Report 2001: Mental Health: New Understanding, New Hope. World Health Organization; 2001

[2] Engel J Jr. Surgery for seizures. The New England Journal of Medicine. 1996;**334**:647-653

[3] Eriksen M, Mackay J, Ross H. The Tobacco Atlas, Revised 4th ed. 2012. http://www.tobaccoatlas.org [Accessed: March 2014]

[4] https://www.fda.gov/Tobacco Products/Guidance Compliance Regulatory Information/ucm297752.htm

[5] Sander JW. The epidemiology of epilepsy revisited. Current Opinion in Neurology. 2003;**16**:165-170

[6] Cavalheiro EA, Fernandes MJ, Turski L, Naffah-Mazzacoratti MG. Spontaneous recurrent seizures in rats: Amino acid and monoamine determination in the hippocampus. Epilepsia. 1994;**35**:1-11

[7] Nagatomo K, Ueda Y, Doi T, Takaki M, Tsuru N. Functional role of GABA transporters for kindling development in GLAST KO mice. Neuroscience Research. 2007;**57**:319-321

[8] Ortel TL, Bedrosian CL, Simel DL. Arsenic poisoning and seizures. North Carolina Medical Journal. 1987;**48**:627-630

[9] Rong L, Frontera AT Jr, Benbadis SR. Tobacco smoking, epilepsy, and seizures. Epilepsy & Behavior. 2014;**31**:210-218

[10] Silva-Filho AR, Pires MLN, Shiotsuki N. Anticonvulsant and convulsant effects of organic solvents. Pharmacology, Biochemistry, and Behavior. 1992;**41**:79-82

[11] Woolf A, Burkhart K, Caraccio T, Litovitz T. Self-poisoning among adults using multiple transdermal nicotine patches. Journal of Toxicology. Clinical Toxicology. 1996;**34**:691-698

[12] Kurt F, Bektas Ö, Kalkan G, Öncel MY, Yakut HI, Kocabas CN. Does age affect presenting symptoms in children with carbon monoxide poisoning? Pediatric Emergency Care. 2013;**29**:916-921

[13] https://www.epilepsybehavior.com/article/S1525-5050(17)30705-9/fulltext

[14] Brown KL, Wilson RF, White MT. Carbon monoxide. Journal of Burn Care & Research. 2007;**28**:533-536

[15] Sood N, Hota D, Sahai AK, Chakrabarti A. Nicotine reversal of anticonvulsant action of topiramate in kainic acid-induced seizure model in mice. Nicotine & Tobacco Research. 2011:ntr138

[16] Tunock Y, Hieda Y, Keyler DE, Brown S, Ennifar S, Fattom A, et al. Inhibition of nicotine-induced seizures in rats by combining vaccination against nicotine with chronic nicotine infusion. Experimental and Clinical Psychopharmacology. 2001;**9**:228-228

[17] Sood N, Sahai AK, Medhi B, Chakrabarti A. Dose-finding study with nicotine as a proconvulsant agent in PTZ-induced seizure model in mice. Journal of Biomedical Science. 2008;**15**:755-765. DOI: 10.1007/s11373-008-9272-9

[18] Paxinos G, Watson C. The Rat Brain in Stereotaxic Coordinates/George Paxinos. Amsterdam: Charles Watson; 2007

[19] Löscher W, Fiedler M. The role of technical, biological and pharmacological factors in the

laboratory evaluation of anticonvulsant drugs. VI. Seasonal influences on maximal electroshock and pentylenetetrazol seizure thresholds. Epilepsy Research. 1996;**25**:3-10

[20] Sperk G. Kainic acid seizures in the rat. Progress in Neurobiology. 1994;**42**:1-32

[21] Damaj MI, Fei-Yin M, Dukat M, Glassco W, Glennon RA, Martin BR. Antinociceptive responses to nicotinic acetylcholine receptor ligands after systemic and intrathecal administration in mice. The Journal of Pharmacology and Experimental Therapeutics. 1998;**284**:1058-1065

[22] Whiteaker P, Garcha HS, Wonnacott S, Stolerman IP. Locomotor activation and dopamine release produced by nicotine and isoarecolone in rats. British Journal of Pharmacology. 1995;**116**:2097-2105

[23] Stitzel JA, Lu Y, Jimenez M, Tritto T, Collins AC. Genetic and pharmacological strategies identify a behavioral function of neuronal nicotinic receptors. Behavioural Brain Research. 2000;**113**:57-64

[24] Picciotto MR, Brunzell DH, Caldarone BJ. Effect of nicotine and nicotinic receptors on anxiety and depression. Neuroreport. 2002;**13**:1097-1106

[25] Damaj MI, Glassco W, Dukat M, Martin BR. Pharmacological characterization of nicotine-induced seizures in mice. The Journal of Pharmacology and Experimental Therapeutics. 1999;**291**:1284-1291

[26] Miner LL, Collins AC. Strain comparison of nicotine-induced seizure sensitivity and nicotinic receptors. Pharmacology, Biochemistry, and Behavior. 1989;**33**:469-475

[27] Cohen SL, Morley BJ, Snead OC. An EEG analysis of convulsive activity produced by cholinergic agents. Progress in Neuro-Psychopharmacology. 1981;**5**:383-388

[28] Dobelis P, Hutton S, Lu Y, Collins AC. GABAergic systems modulate nicotinic receptor-mediated seizures in mice. The Journal of Pharmacology and Experimental Therapeutics. 2003;**306**:1159-1166

[29] Conti-Tronconi BM, McLane KE, Raftery MA, Grando SA, Protti MP. The nicotinic acetylcholine receptor: Structure and autoimmune pathology. Critical Reviews in Biochemistry and Molecular Biology. 1994;**29**:69-123

[30] Franceschini D, Paylor R, Broide R, Salas R, Bassetto L, Gotti C, et al. Absence of α7-containing neuronal nicotinic acetylcholine receptors does not prevent nicotine-induced seizures. Molecular Brain Research. 2002;**98**:29-40

[31] Shih T-M, McDonough JH. Organophosphorus nerve agents-induced seizures and efficacy of atropine sulfate as anticonvulsant treatment. Pharmacology, Biochemistry, and Behavior. 1999;**64**:147-153

[32] Wang Y-A, Zhou W-X, Li J, Liu Y-Q, Yue Y-J, Zheng J-Q, et al. Anticonvulsant effects of phencynonate hydrochloride and other anticholinergic drugs in soman poisoning: Neurochemical mechanisms. Life Sciences. 2005;**78**:210-223

[33] Gholami M, Saboory E, Zare S, Roshan-Milani S, Hajizadeh-Moghaddam A. The effect of dorsal hippocampal administration of nicotinic and muscarinic cholinergic ligands on pentylenetetrazol-induced generalized seizures in rats. Epilepsy & Behavior. 2012;**25**:244-249. DOI: 10.1016/j.yebeh.2012.07.004

Section 3

Epilepsy - Clinical Presentation and Associated Problem

Chapter 4

Nonconvulsive Status Epilepticus in Patients with Altered Mental Status Admitted to Hamad General Hospital, Doha, Qatar

Boulenouar Mesraoua, Dirk Deleu, Hassan Al Hail, Musab Ali, Naim Haddad, Gayane Melykian, Yasser Osman M. Ali, Lubna El Sheikh, Ali A. Asadi-Pooya and Peter Kaplan

Abstract

This is a prospective, hospital-based study reporting an update and the prevalence of nonconvulsive status epilepticus (NCSE) in patients with altered mental status (AMS) in Qatar. Patients presenting with NCSE are compared to controls. Two-hundred and fifty patients with AMS are involved. Patients with NCSE are: 65 (12–79 years, m, 37, f, 28); controls: 185 (12–80 years, m, 101, f, 84). Occurrence of NCSE in patients with AMS was 26%. NCSE patients were younger than controls ($p < 0.001$). Deaths in the NCSE group occurred in 31% and 19% in controls ($p < 0.0007$). Hospitalization length was longer in NCSE proper and in comatose NCSE compared to controls ($p < 0.02$, $p < 0.03$). Recovery occurred in 40% of NCSE patients and 53% of controls ($p < 0.08$). About 31% of patients ($n = 21$) had refractory NCSE and 9 died. This is the first study reporting the prevalence of NCSE in Qatar. This prevalence (26%) is in the middle range. NCSE did not do better than the controls, result being disappointing regarding comatose NCSE. NCSE is an emerging condition requiring rapid diagnosis and rapid treatment. Regarding the optimal duration of continuous EGG (cEEG) monitoring to diagnose the majority of NCSE cases, 3 days of cEEG monitoring could accomplish this task.

Keywords: nonconvulsive seizures, nonconvulsive status epilepticus, epidemiology, treatment, antiseizure medications, outcome

1. Introduction

Nonconvulsive status epilepticus (NCSE) is accompanied with an altered mental status (AMS) without convulsive motor activity [1]. Because of the paucity of clinical symptoms, EEG is mandatory for the diagnosis of NCSE. In the intensive care unit (ICU), where the patient is often obtunded/comatose, cEEG monitoring is required to reveal NCSE. cEEG monitoring is important because of the difficulty distinguishing when AMS and coma are ictal and differentiating them from non-ictal

Lethargy and confusion attributed to a postictal state
Ictal confusion mistaken for metabolic encephalopathy
Unresponsiveness and catalepsy presumed to be psychogenic
Obtundation thought to be due to alcohol or drug intoxication
Hallucinations and agitation mistaken for psychosis or delirium
Lethargy presumed secondary to hypoglycemia
Mutism attributed to aphasia
Laughing and crying ascribed to emotional lability

Table 1.
Examples of delayed or missed NCSE diagnosis; from Kaplan [48].

symptoms associated with underlying pathology such as posthypoxic, metabolic or septic encephalopathies, and the effects of sedative drugs. Furthermore, the diagnosis of NCSE is frequently delayed, with patients in the ICU having often other serious medical conditions. To diagnose NCSE a high degree of suspicion is required [2], and consequently NCSE remains unrecognized. **Table 1** shows how frequently the diagnosis of NCSE could be missed in the emergency room.

In the United States, the estimated incidence of status epilepticus (SE) is 15–20/100,000 cases per year [3], and NCSE is representing 63% of all SE [4]. Both nonconvulsive seizures (NCS) and NCSE occur very frequently in the ICU and emergency department (ED): NCSs/NCSE is recorded in 8% to 48% in ICU patients [5–8], many of which are fatal [9–11].

Prevalence of NCSE is reported from different geographical areas of the world in patients with AMS [12–16]; However, to our knowledge, there is no study reporting the frequency of NCSE in the Middle East and North Africa (MENA) region; in this vast geographic area, the only NCSE incidence/prevalence is described from the MENA's neighboring countries like Pakistan, India, Turkey, and Israel [17–21]. There is a need for studies regarding the prevalence and morbidity of NCSE in MENA countries [22].

There is also a lack of consensus regarding the EEG monitoring duration when looking for NCSE in ICU patients with AMS; the authors dealing with this issue report a considerable variation in the duration of cEEG monitoring [23–26].

The aims of this chapter are multiple:

a. Know the rate of occurrence of NCSE in patients with AMS admitted to Hamad General Hospital (HGH) Doha, Qatar, using cEEG monitoring.

b. Describe the clinical and EEG findings, causes, head CT/MRI, as well as the treatment and outcomes of NCSE in patients with AMS, and compare the results to a matched control group with similar clinical presentations of AMS.

c. Highlight and discuss the lack of consensus in the literature regarding the duration of cEEG monitoring while looking for NCSs/NCSE in patients with AMS.

2. Methods

This clinical study was performed according to the Good Clinical Practice (GCP) guidelines. Approval was obtained from Hamad Medical Corporation Ethical Committee and Institutional Review Board (IRB). All subjects/relative(s) (caregivers) provided consent before participating.

2.1 Definition of NCSE and AMS

NCSE was defined as an AMS with diminished responsiveness, a positive EEG. and a response to anti-seizure drug (ASD) therapy; as a status, NCSE should be present for a minimum of 30 minutes of continuous nonconvulsive seizure activity or after repeated seizures without recovery of consciousness between events [1]; recently shorter durations have been reported.

Young's criteria [27] of electrographic SE and modified criteria of Chong and Hirsch [28] were used to diagnose NCSE; In addition, the International League against Epilepsy (ILAE) definition and classification of Status Epilepticus [29] and EEG Salzburg Consensus Criteria for NCSE [30] were used to recognize NCSE; NCSE was diagnosed in the presence of continuous generalized spike wave discharges with changes in intensity or frequency, epileptiform activity with ictal patterns that wax and wane, rhythmic and periodic discharges, and subtle and discrete electrographic seizures, when lasting for 30 minutes [10, 13, 15]. In comatose patients, epileptiform discharges faster than 2.5 Hz or generalized periodic discharges (GPDs), lateralized periodic discharges (LPDs) and continuous 2/s GPDs with triphasic morphology [31] of less than 2.5 Hz, as well as rhythmic discharges (RDs) faster than 0.5 Hz were also taken into consideration as NCSE if they responded to benzodiazepine treatment with improvement in the EEG or in patient mental status [13, 15, 29, 32].

Two EEG specialists agreed independently that the patient condition and EEG findings represent NCSE particularly when an EEG pattern did not meet above criteria; finally NCSE was considered if the EEG/or level of consciousness responded to an ASD trial.

Unexplained confusional state, change in behavior, mild to moderate obtundation, alteration in cognition and behavior from baseline, and unexplained decrease in level of consciousness including after convulsive status epilepticus treatment [2, 33] were considered AMS; in elderly patients, delirium (altered level of consciousness, with a fluctuating course, disorganized thinking, and inattention) was also included [15].

2.2 Patient selection for cEEG monitoring

All patients with AMS, from the Emergency Department and from ICUs, aged 12 years or above, had a cEEG monitoring [2, 33]. Not included were patients with open head injury, those whose relatives did not sign the consent form and patients with suspected brain death and an isoelectric EEG. In addition, patients treated for convulsive status epilepticus (CSE) who did not develop later NCSs/NCSE on cEEG monitoring were excluded.

2.3 Patients with NCSE and control group

Patients with AMS and those whose EEG was not compatible with NCSE during 3 days of cEEG monitoring recording were taken as controls. The NCSE and control groups were compared: this included the clinical presentation and medical condition, AMS etiology, neuroimaging, laboratory findings, length of stay, recovery, and outcome

2.4 cEEG monitoring and duration

2.4.1 cEEG recording

The following EEG recording system was used: international 10/20 system with 21 silver/silver chloride cup electrodes. Digital EEG signal stored electronically was filtered for display. High-pass filter and low-pass filter were 0.5–1 and 70 Hz. For extraneous electrical artifact, 50 Hz notch filter was used; impedance was 100 and 5000 ohms. cEEG was done by EEG technologists and monitored at least twice a day by an EEG specialist.

2.4.2 EEG duration

The duration of cEEG monitoring was determined by the response to treatment of NCSs/NCSE, the presence of other EEG features like rhythmic and periodic discharges, and their responses to treatment.

2.5 Laboratory investigations and Neuroimaging

The following investigations were performed in most NCSE cases and controls: complete blood count, electrolytes, liver and renal functions, brain MRI, and/or CT head; imaging was performed either before or after cEEG monitoring

2.6 NCSs/NCSE treatment

Benzodiazepines (lorazepam or diazepam) were used when NCSs/NCSE was suspected. If seizures persisted, European Federation of Neurological Sciences (EFNS) Guidelines and Glauser et al. report on NCSE treatment were followed: IV diazepam or lorazepam first and then second-line ASDs were initiated—valproic acid, phenytoin, or levetiracetam. If no results, continuous infusions of propofol, midazolam, and barbiturates were used [34, 35].

Many patients received more than one ASD. refractory NCSE was treated with anesthetic agents; same treatment protocol was followed in comatose NCSE. ASDs were not used in control group.

2.7 Outcome parameters

Seizure control and survival/death were considered as primary outcome parameters, while complete recovery and length of stay were secondary outcome parameters.

2.8 Statistical methods

Descriptive statistics (mean with standard deviation) for continuous variables, frequency, and percentages for categorical variables was used; differences between mean levels of NCSE and controls, outcome and morbidity, and Student's t-test were calculated; to detect associations between categorical variables and NCSE vs controls, outcome, and morbidity, chi-square tests or Fisher's exact tests were used. For independent variables at univariate analysis, NCSE logistic regressions were performed using a significance level of 0.05. A P value of 0.05 (two tailed) was considered a statistically significant level. For statistical analysis, an SPSS 22.0 statistical software was used.

3. Results

3.1 Occurrence of NCSE

Six patients suffered from CSE; only one of them who showed later NCSE EEG features and was included in the study. Twenty patients presented NCSs; 30% of them (n = 6) responded to ASDs and did not develop NCSE on cEEG monitoring;

they were also excluded from the study; the rest (70%, n=14) developed later NCSE during cEEG monitoring. These patients were included in the study.

NCSE group: 250 patients with AMS or coma underwent cEEG monitoring. Sixty-two patients were excluded (see reasons above and patient selection). In total, 65 patient responded to the criteria of NCSE (**Table 2**). The occurrence rate of NCSE was 65/250 (26%).

3.2 Characterization of NCSE and the control group

The control group consisted of 185 patients with AMS or coma in which cEEG monitoring did not show any features of NCSE. **Table 2** shows the demographic and clinical features of NCSE and control subjects. Only age and presence of subtle motor phenomena differed between the two groups; the NCSE patients were relatively younger and displayed subtle motor phenomena more often. As for etiology and comorbid states, a history of previous seizures and presence of cortical dysplasia were significantly more common in the NCSE group (**Table 3**). Other etiologies were not informative. Head injury, stroke, and status postcardiac arrest were frequently encountered in accident and emergency patients with NCSE; CT head done in 52

Variable	NCSE (n 65)	Controls (n 185)	P value
Age	45.7 ± 19	52.3 ± 15.8	0.001
Gender	M = 37/F = 28	M = 101/F = 84	0.75
Unresponsive/somnolent	11 (17%)	46 (25%)	0.19
Acute confusion	7 (11%)	18 (10%)	0.81
Severely decreased level of consciousness	20 (31%)	61 (33%)	0.74
Stupor/coma	27 (42%)	60 (32%)	0.23
Subtle motor phenomena	12 (18%)	8 (4%)	0.001

Note: P values are calculated using Chi-square tests and student t tests wherever appropriate.

Table 2.
Characteristics of patients with NCSE and controls.

Variable	NCSE (n 65)	Controls (n 185)	P value
Stroke (hemorrhagic, ischemic, subarachnoid hemorrhage)	16 (25%)	67 (36%)	0.09
Status post cardiac arrest	15 (23%)	35 (19%)	0.59
Head injury	8 (12%)	34 (18%)	0.34
Previous seizures (uncontrolled)	12 (18.4%)	4 (2%)	0.001
Cortical dysplasia	3 (4.6%)	0	0.02
Sepsis	3 (4.6%)	7 (3.8%)	1.00
Hepatic encephalopathy	1 (1.5%)	3 (1.6%)	1.00
End stage renal disease, post renal transplant	2 (3%)	11 (6%)	0.37
Intoxications	0	8 (4.3%)	0.12
Hypertensive encephalopathy	1 (1.5%)	6 (3.2%)	0.68
Personality disorder	1 (1.5%)	3 (1.6%)	1.0
Unknown	3 (4.6%)	7 (3.8%)	1.0

Note: P values are calculated using Chi-square tests or Fisher's exact test wherever appropriate.

Table 3.
Etiology of patients with NCSE and controls.

NCSE cases and in 101 of controls and MRI head done in 41 NCSE cases and in 97 of controls showed hippocampal sclerosis, malformations of cortical development, and encephalomalacia, which were more commonly seen in the NCSE group (**Table 4**).

Abnormal cholesterol and liver enzymes were more often abnormal in the NCSE group than controls (NCSE 15%, controls 4%, p 0.004).

3.3 Length of cEEG monitoring and time of occurrence of NCSs/NCSE

Twenty patients showed NCSs; 65% of them (n = 13) had NCSs during the first 40 minutes of recording, whereas 35% (n = 7) had their seizures later but within the first 48 hours of cEEG monitoring.

In the NCSE group (n = 65), NCSE EEG patterns were recorded during the first 3 hours in 66% (n = 43), later but within the first 48 hours in 22% (n = 14), and in the third day in 12% (n = 8). Among the 22 patients with late NCSE, 17 (77%) were comatose.

3.4 NCSE proper and comatose NCSE

The NCSE group was further subdivided into two: NCSE proper without coma (n = 39) and comatose NCSE (n = 26) [32, 36]; NCSE proper is defined as clinical symptoms suggestive of SE with mild impairment of consciousness (absence status or complex focal SE); NCSE with coma-lateralized epileptiform discharges, NCSE with coma-generalized epileptiform discharges is defined as deep coma of various etiology with characteristic epileptiform EEG pattern but with no clinical motor signs of SE; NCSE proper patients are significantly younger than the comatose NCSE ones (**Table 5**). NCSE in comatose patients was often recorded after the first day of cEEG monitoring: during the first 24 hours in only 54% (n = 14/26), later but within 48 hours in 35% (n = 9/26), and in the third day in 11% (n = 3/26) of the patients; comparatively, NCSE proper was recorded during the first day in 77% (n = 30/39), later but within 48 hours in 10% (n = 4/39), and during the third day in 13% (n = 5/39) of patients.

The 14 patients with early comatose NCSE (first 24 hs) suffered from head injury (n = 4), stroke (n = 4), and cardiac arrest (n = 3); and no etiology was found in three patients; comparatively, in the NCSE proper group (n = 30), 18 patients suffered from previous seizures, 5 from stroke, 3 from sepsis, 2 from head injury, and 2 from cardiac arrest.

Variable	CT (n pts)			MRI (n pts)		
	NCSE (n 52)	Controls (n 101)	P value	NCSE (n 41)	Controls (n 97)	P value
Abnormal	32 (62%)	49 (49%)	0.17	33 (80%)	53 (55%)	0.01
Ischemia, intracerebral hemorrhage, subarachnoid & subdural hemorrhage	14 (27%)	18 (18%)	0.21	16 (39%)	32 (33%)	0.56
Cortical atrophy	5 (10%)	10 (10%)	1.0	3 (7%)	6 (6%)	1.0
Polymicrogyria, cortical dysplasia, heterotopia				3 (7%)	0	0.02
Hippocampal sclerosis	3 (6%)	0	0.04	3 (7%)	1 (1%)	0.08
Encephalomalacia				3 (7%)	10 (10%)	0.04
Meningeal/cortical enhancement	1 (2%)	2 (2%)	1.0	1 (2%)	2 (2%)	1.0

Note: P values are calculated using Chi-square tests or Fisher's exact test wherever appropriate.

Table 4.
Head CT and MRI findings (some patients had both CT and MRI).

3.5 Antiseizure drug (ASD) treatment

Patients with NCSs (n = 20) were treated as follows: 18 with benzodiazepines, 10 with valproate IV, and 8 with levetiracetam plus valproate IV. The 65 NCSE patients received the following: lorazepam 4–8 mg IV or diazepam 10 mg IV (n = 45), levetiracetam IV or PO (n = 22), phenytoin IV (n = 21), valproate IV or PO (n = 18), topiramate PO (n = 5), phenobarbitone IV (n = 7), midazolam IV (n = 15), propofol (n = 5), fentanyl (n = 2), and thiopental (n = 3).

3.6 Outcome

3.6.1 Primary outcome

NCSE group (n = 65): 69% (n = 45, m 25, f 20) responded to treatment within 48 hours, whereas 31% (n = 20, m 12, f 8) died.

Control group (n = 185): 19% (n = 35, m 20, f 15) died. Thus, compared to the control group, death was more frequent in the NCSE group; there was additional statistical significance when NCSE proper was compared to comatose NCSE and when comatose NCSE was compared to controls (**Table 5**), with comatose patients exhibiting a more ominous outcome. The majority of patients with early occurrence of NCSs/NCSE = 65% (40 minutes to 3 hours) died (n = 13/20). Causes of death in NCSE (n = 20) group were distributed as follows: cardiac arrest (n = 6), hemorrhagic and ischemic strokes (n = 5), sepsis (n = 3), head injury (n = 4), subarachnoid hemorrhage (n = 1), and cerebral abscess (n = 1).

3.6.2 Secondary outcome

Compared to controls, NCSE achieved complete recovery in 40% (n = 26, m 15, f 11) compared to controls 53% (n = 98, m 55, f 43); **Table 5** shows that this achieved statistical significance when comatose NCSE was compared to controls; NCSE group (NCSE proper plus comatose NCSE) had a longer hospital stay than the controls.

Variable	NCSE (n 65)	NCSE proper (=without coma) (n 39)	NCSE with coma (n 26)	Control (n 185)	P value
Deaths	20 (31%)	8 (21%)*	12 (46%)*§	35 (19%)§	* 0.05, § 0.0007
Gender male	37 (57%)	23 (59%)	14 (54%)	101 (55%)	
Age (years)	45.7 ± 19§	36.9 ± 24&	51.3 ± 16.9&	52.3 ± 15.8 §	§ 0.001, & 0.006
Hospital stay (days)	15.2 ± 7.7#	14.6 ± 7.8	16.4 ± 7.7^	12.7 ± 5.5#^	# 0.02, ^0.03
Complete recovery	26 (40%)	18 (46%)	8 (31%)a	98 (53%)a	a 0.04

Note: P values are calculated using Chi-square tests, Fisher exact tests and Student t tests wherever appropriate.

** and § compare Death occuring respectively in NCSE without coma to NCSE with coma and also Death occurring in NCSE with coma to controls (respectively 0.05 and 0.0007).*

§ and & compare patients and controls 's age respectively in NCSE group to controls and also in NCSE without coma to NCSE with coma (respectively 0.001 and 0.006).

 # and ^ compare hospital stay respectively in NCSE group to controls and also in NCSE with coma to controls (respectively 0.02 and 0.03); symbol a compares complete recovery in NCSE with coma to controls (0.04)

Table 5.
Occurrence and comparison of the listed variables in the NCSE groups and control group.

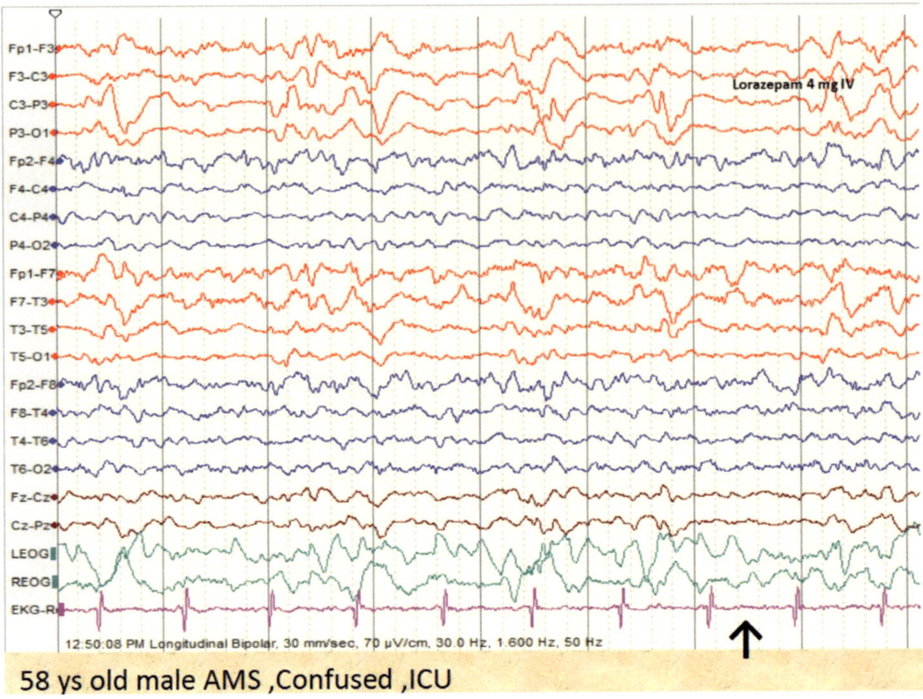

(a)

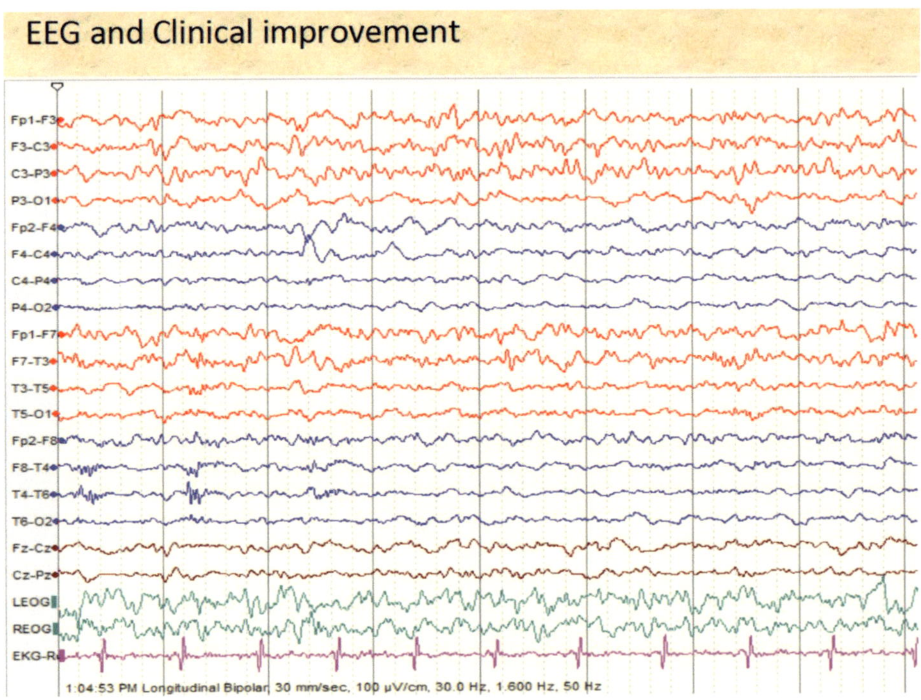

(b)

Figure 1.
(a) EEG shows left LPDs; patient received 4mg lorazepam IV and (b) EEG and clinical improvement following lorazepam IV.

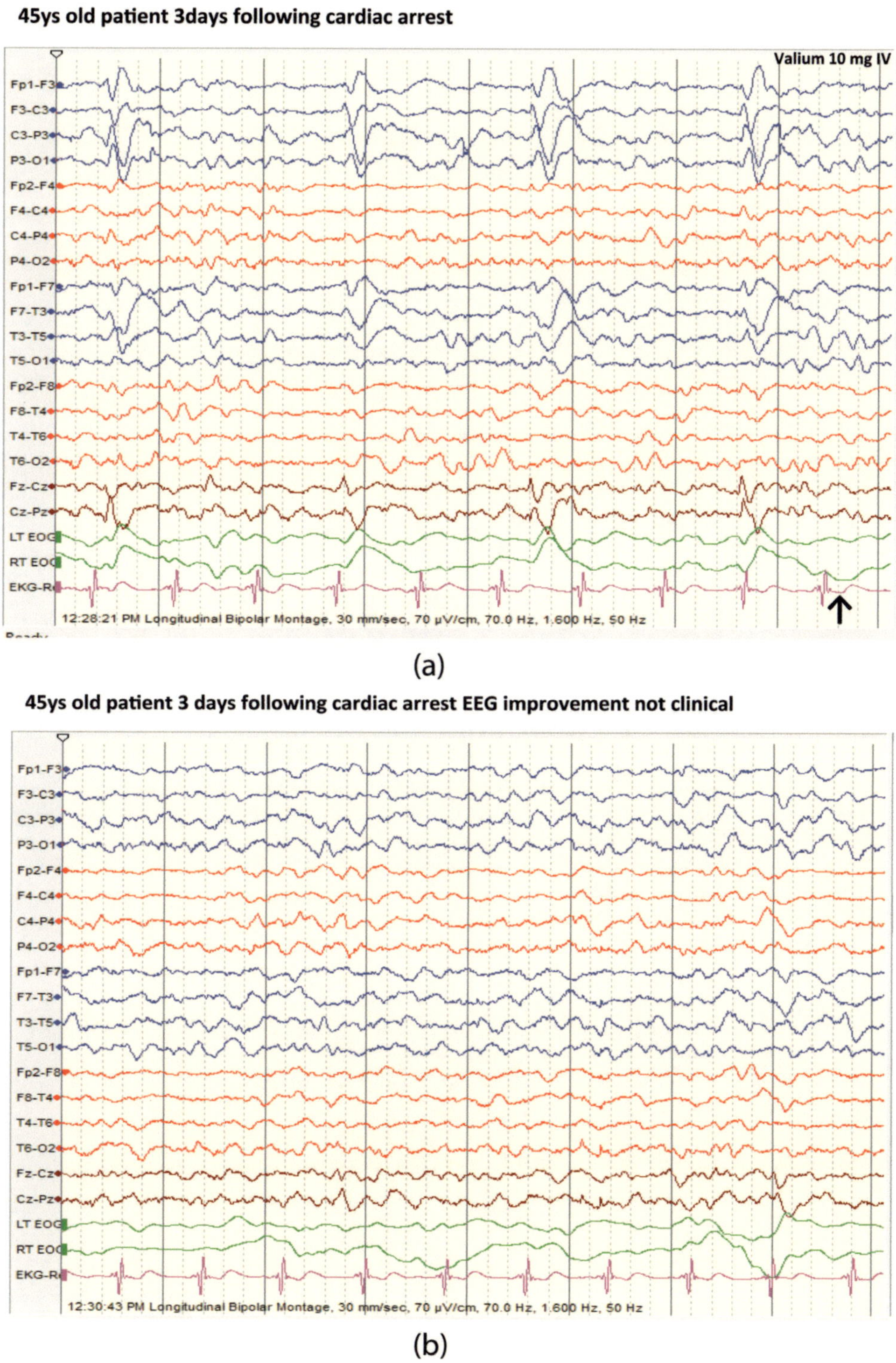

Figure 2.
(a) EEG shows left LPDs in a comatose patient following cardiac arrest; patient receives 10 mg Diazepam IV and (b) EEG shows dramatic improvement following Diazepam IV; however the patient remains comatose (possible NCSE ?).

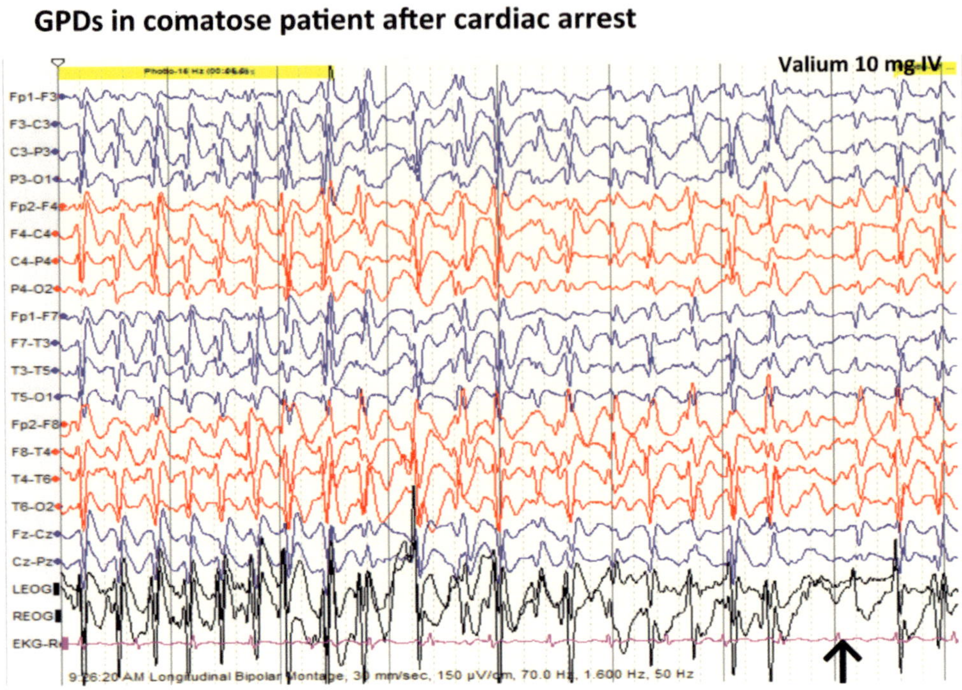

(a)

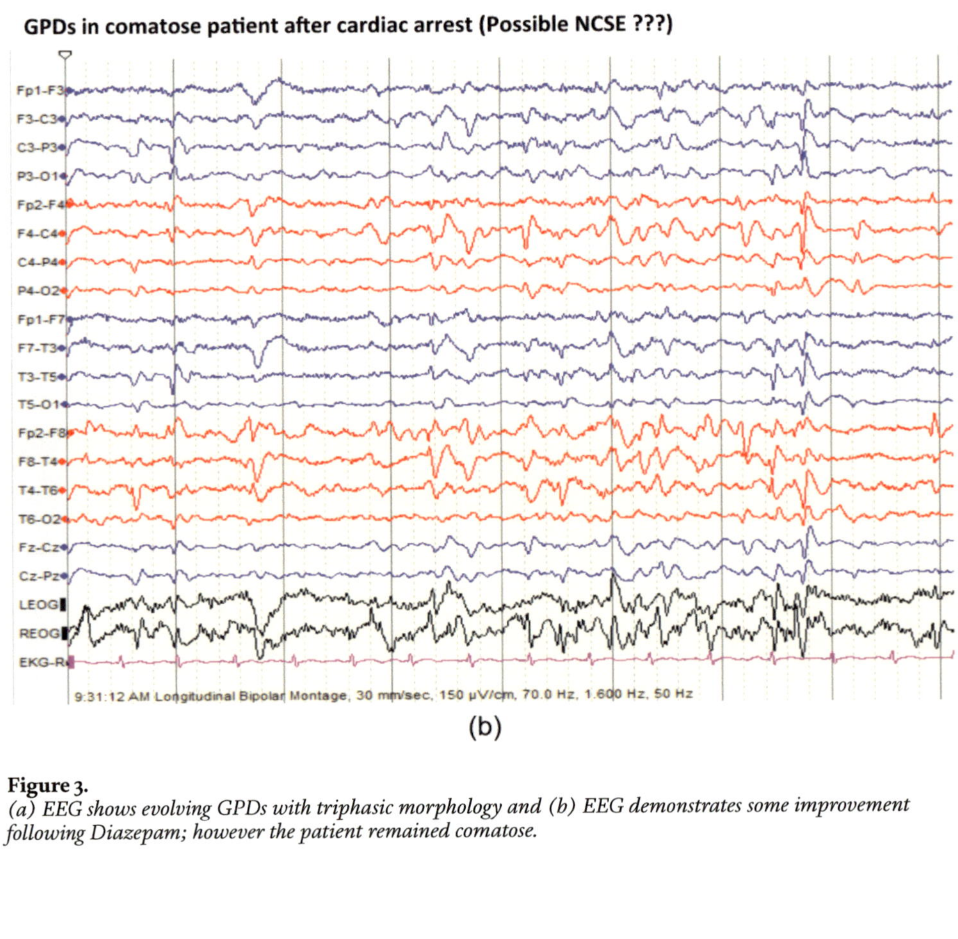

(b)

Figure 3.
(a) EEG shows evolving GPDs with triphasic morphology and (b) EEG demonstrates some improvement following Diazepam; however the patient remained comatose.

TWs patient with...

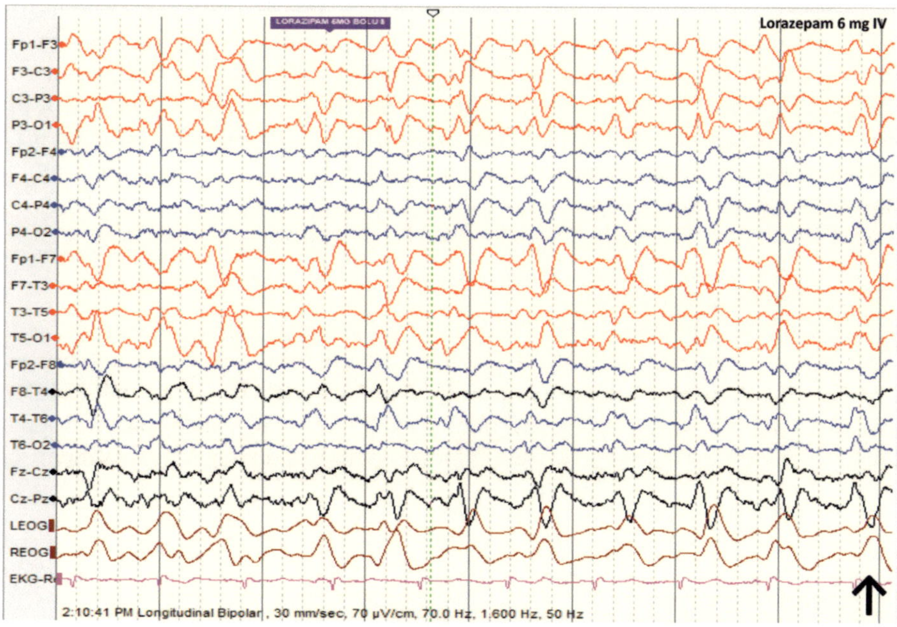

(a)

Dramatic improvement ...

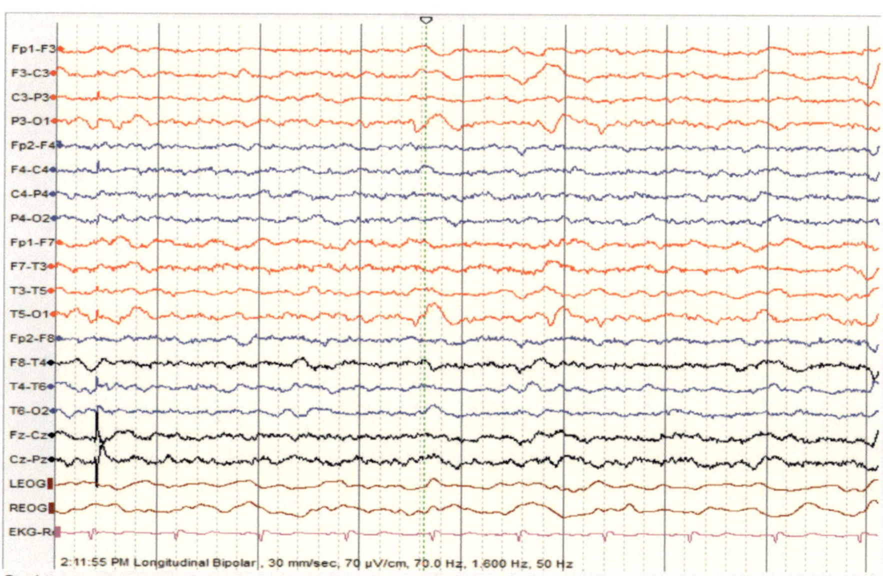

(b)

Figure 4.
(a) EEG shows predominantly left sided LPDs with triphasic morphology; 32 years old male given baclofen 30 mg for spasticity the first day of admission; 2 days later he presented an altered mental status with "akinetic mutism"; patient was given 6 mg lorazepam IV bolus. (b) Dramatic improvement in EEG and clinical status following IV lorazepam ; patient recovered completely, started talking and moving around normally; he was found to have a moderate to severe renal impairment (responsible for baclofen intoxication ?).

3.7 Refractory NCSE

Thirty-two percent of patients with NCSE (n = 21, m 13, f 8) suffered from refractory NCSE, defined as seizures lasting more than 60 minutes with failure of two ASDs [37]; they received the following treatment: midazolam IV (n = 10), propofol (n = 5), thiopental (n = 4), and fentanyl (n = 2). Fifty-seven percent (n = 12, m 8, f 4) survived; forty-three percent (n = 9, m 5, f 4) died with the following reasons: cardiac arrest (3), sepsis (3), ischemia (1), subarachnoid hemorrhage (1), and cerebral abscess (1). Only 33% (n = 7, m 4, f 3) recovered completely.

3.8 EEG patterns and location

EEG patterns recorded in the NCSE patients (n = 65): focal spike/sharp and wave >3/s in 43% (n = 28), generalized spike/sharp and wave >3/s in 28% (n = 18), GDPs, LPDs, continuous 2/s GPDs with triphasic morphology in 25% (n = 16), and multifocal spikes in 4% (n = 3); **Figures 1–5** show NCSE EEGs cases before and after ASD treatment.

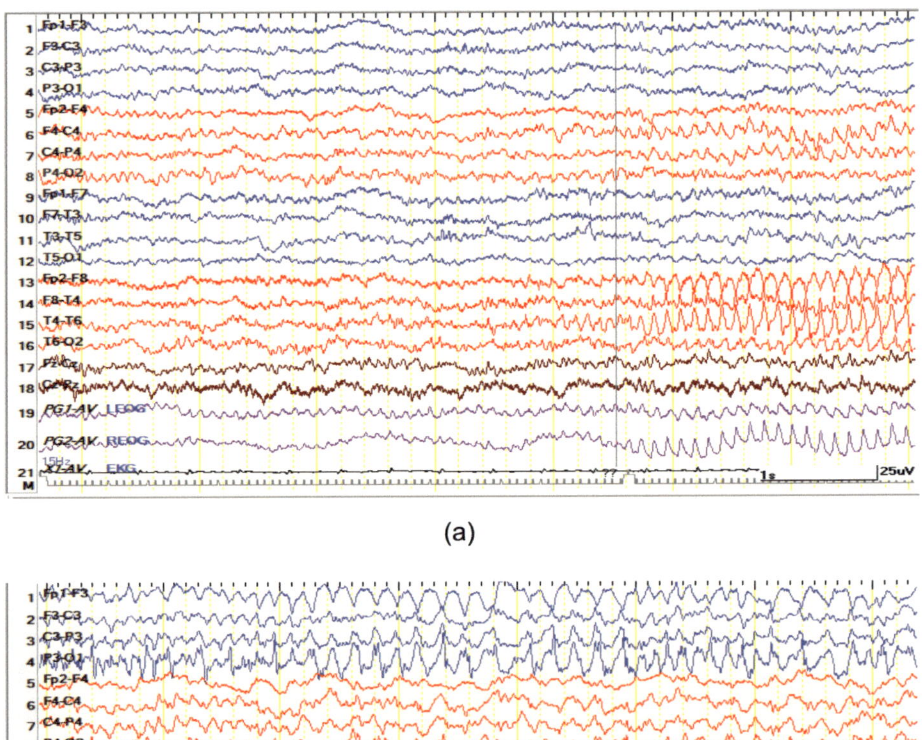

(a)

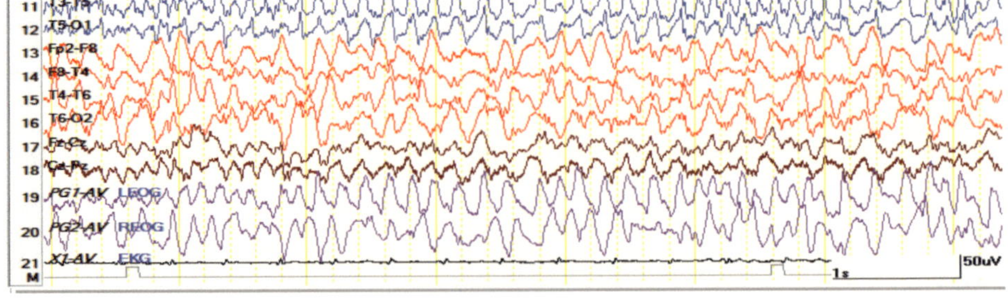

(b)

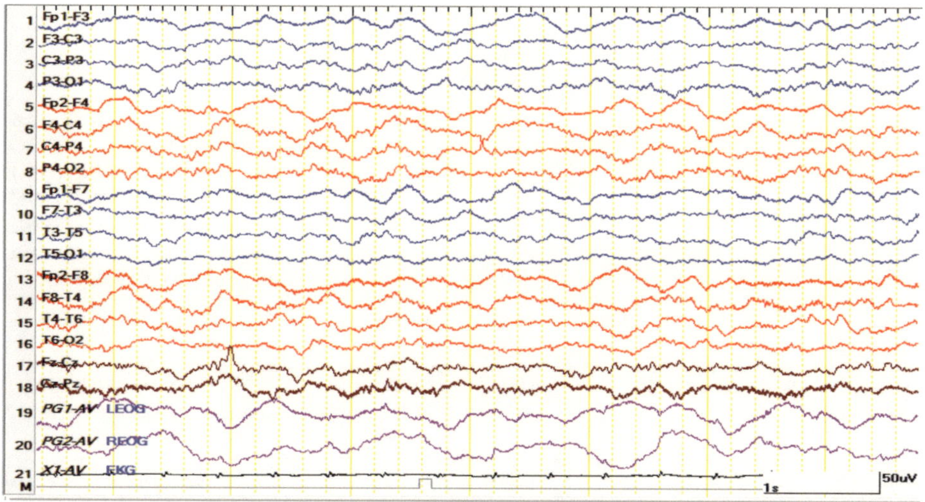

(c)

Figure 5.
(a) (Comatose focal NCSE) 67 years old male comatose, following head injury. EEG shows abnormal fast activity starting in right fronto-temporal leads accompanied by abnormal eye movements and facial twitching. (b) The ictal fast activity spreads to the contralateral fronto-temporal leads; patient shows same clinical manifestations (discrete twitching of the left face); the abnormal electrical activity was continuous for more than 30 mn. (c) 1 minute following 2 mg of lorazepam IV; patient remains comatose; EEG shows diffuse generalized slowing; no epileptiform activity; no clinical manifestations; survived with memory impairment and left hemiplegia.

EEG in NCSE patients who ultimately died (n = 20): 40% periodic patterns (n = 8), 30% continuous generalized spike/sharp and waves (n = 6), and 30% with focal spike/sharp and waves (n = 6). Fifty-two percent (n = 34) showed a continuous ictal pattern, and forty-three percent (n = 28) an intermittent/recurrent ictal pattern; five percent (n = 3) were not classified; forty-six percent (n = 30) showed a focal onset and 29% (n = 19) a generalized onset; twenty-five percent (n = 16) showed a periodic pattern; focal seizures originated from the temporal areas (55%) and from the frontal areas (31%). In the control group (n = 185), focal/generalized slowing was seen in 43% (n = 80) and slowing with some spike/sharp wave activity in 2% (n = 4).

4. Discussion

4.1 NCSE prevalence

In the current longitudinal prospective hospital-based study, we investigated the frequency of NCSE in patients with AMS admitted to Hamad Hospital, Doha, Qatar. The prevalence of NCSE among patients with AMS was 26% at our center that is compatible with previous similar studies (prevalence = 16–37%) (**Table 6**); these researchers used a similar design, with a parallel control group; however, most were retrospective, the cEEG recording duration often shorter or not mentioned. Five other authors from MENA' s neighboring countries (mentioned in Section 1) also reported the prevalence of NCSE in patients with AMS; however, they used different study designs, and therefore, those studies cannot be compared with our study.

4.2 NCSE outcome

NCSE is often associated with a poor outcome and a high mortality rate [9, 12, 13, 38]. In the current study, the mortality rate among patients with AMS and

Author (year)	Methods	Duration of EEG recording	Patients with AMS (n)	Patients with NCSE (n) (%)	Outcome
Mesraoua et al. (2017) Current study	Prospective	72 hs	(250)	65 (26)	Response to ASDs: NCSE 45/65 (69%); death: NCSE 20/65 (31%); death in controls: 35/185 (19%); complete recovery: NCSE 26/65 (40%); controls 98/185 (53%); NCSE longer hospital stay than controls $p < 0.02$ (**Table 5**)
Laccheo et al. [38] (2015)	Prospective	>24hs	(170)	36 (21)	Mortality 31% NCSE vs 14% in controls
Kurtz et al. [12] (2014)	Retrospective	?	(154)	NCSE/NCSs 24 (16), PEDs 45(29)	NCSs/NCSE independently associated with poor outcome 20% vs 3% controls, $p = 0.039$
Bottaro et al. [13] (2007)	Retrospective	20mn	(124)	22 (18)	NCSE significant association with mortality, longer hospitalization and poor outcome
Privitera et al. [9] (1994)	Prospective	30mn	(198)	74 (37)	Death was more common in NCSE (37%) compared to controls (23%)

Table 6.
Current and previous studies on NCSE prevalence and outcome.

Variable	OR	95% CI	P value
Age	1.16	1.0–1.34	0.05
Length of stay	2.03	1.29–3.20	0.002
Cardiac arrest	3.27	0.07–153	0.55
Stroke	35.0	0.33–3629	0.14
Head injury	30.1	0.02–56,392	0.38

Note: Variables significant at univariate analysis and having adequate numbers were used for multivariate analysis.

Table 7.
Multivariate logistic regression for mortality in NSCE.

NCSE was 31%, while the mortality rate among those with AMS and without NCSE was only 19%; NCSE carried a poor prognosis. Only one author reported similar outcome in NCSE and controls [9]; however death was more common in NCSE (37%) than in controls (23%). As previously reported by Young et al. [27], the length of stay and age were statistically significantly associated with mortality in the NCSE group (**Table 7**). In addition, in the current study, among patients with AMS and NCSE, head injury and stroke were associated with bad clinical outcomes with regard to recovery (**Table 8**). Also, we observed a longer hospitalization for NCSE group than that in the controls that is compatible with previous reports [13, 15].

We agree with Claassen [14] that most patients showing early NCSE EEG features (n = 13, =65%) did not achieve good outcome; we did not find any association between acute symptomatology and outcome as highlighted by Kang [39].

Patients with "periodic discharges" did not completely meet the EEG criteria for NCSE. In ICUs and cEEG monitoring units, these periodic EEG patterns are described as lying along an ictal–interictal continuum. There are convincing studies that these PDs, especially GPDs and LPDs, are strongly associated with NCSE and may be ictal [13, 15, 32, 40–45]; in fact, these EEG patterns have been found in patients with AMS,

Variable	OR	95% C.I.	P value
Age	1.0	0.96–1.05	0.74
Length of stay	1.10	0.90–1.34	0.36
Cardiac arrest	4.22	0.64–27.9	0.14
Stroke	26.30	3.24–213	0.03
Head injury	19.5	1.30–293	0.002

Note: Variables significant at univariate analysis and having adequate numbers were used for multivariate analysis.

Table 8.
Multivariate logistic regression for morbidity in NSCE.

some were evolving and some responded to benzodiazepines, as shown in **Figures 1–4**. Many studies reported that PDs carry a bad prognosis, and the final outcome depends mainly on the etiology of AMS [8, 18–20, 39]; in our study, 50% of patients with PDs died; they suffered from stroke, cardiac arrest, sepsis, or head injury. However, in multivariate logistic regression analysis, we did not find a correlation between these etiologies and mortality in patients with AMS and NCSE (**Table 7**). It seems that prognosis in NCSE depends on several factors (e.g., age, etiology, level of consciousness, etc.) and cannot be based on EEG or any one factor alone [20, 42].

Finally, the outcome of refractory NCSE was very poor in our study; 9 out of 21 patients (43%) with refractory NCSE died; this is much higher than that reported in a previous study (25%) [46]. However, in that study, 17% of refractory NCSE patients were in a vegetative state.

As reported previously, history of epilepsy/seizures could be a risk factor for NCSs/NCSE [12, 13, 38].

4.3 cEEG monitoring duration

The optimal length of cEEG monitoring in critically ill ICU patients with AMS is a controversial issue in the literature. In our study, majority (66%) of NCSE cases were detected during the first 3 hours of cEEG monitoring; this detection rate reached to 90% by 48 hours of monitoring. Various required cEEG monitoring durations have been suggested in the literature; 12–24 hours [8, 12, 19, 22], 72 hours [16, 18, 47], and finally 7–10 days [23]. A recent study reported that 1/5 of patients without early EEG epileptiform features develop them during 72 hours of cEEG monitoring [25]; Claassen et al. concluded that seizures are detected only in 87% of comatose patients compared to non-comatose patients (98%) in the first 48 hours of cEEG monitoring [14].

Based on the results from our study and review of the literature, and also considering the challenges and costs associated with cEEG monitoring, we suggest that 3 days of cEEG monitoring is optimal in ICUs and in patients with AMS to detect the majority of cases of NCSs/NCSE [14, 25].

5. Conclusion

To our knowledge, this is the first prospective study reporting the prevalence of NCSE in Qatar, a small country in the MENA region. This figure (26%) was in the middle range. Patients with NCSE did not do better than the controls, the result being disappointing regarding comatose NCSE. NCSE is an emerging condition requiring rapid diagnosis and rapid treatment. Regarding the duration of cEGG monitoring to diagnose the majority of NCSE cases, 3 days of cEEG monitoring could accomplish this task.

Author details

Boulenouar Mesraoua[1,2*], Dirk Deleu[1,2], Hassan Al Hail[1,2], Musab Ali[1], Naim Haddad[2], Gayane Melykian[1,2], Yasser Osman M. Ali[1,2], Lubna El Sheikh[1], Ali A. Asadi-Pooya[3,4] and Peter Kaplan[5]

1 Hamad General Hospital, Doha, Qatar

2 Weill Cornell Medical College-Qatar, Doha, Qatar

3 Jefferson Comprehensive Epilepsy Center, Thomas Jefferson University, Philadelphia, USA

4 Department of Neurology, Shiraz University of Medical Sciences, Shiraz, Iran

5 Johns Hopkins Bayview Medical Center, Baltimore, USA

*Address all correspondence to: boulenouar.mesraoua@wanadoo.fr

References

[1] Kinney MO, Craig JJ, Kaplan PW. Hidden in plain sight: Non-convulsive status epilepticus-Recognition and management. Acta Neurologica Scandinavica. 2017;**136**(4):280-292. DOI: 10.1111/ane.12732

[2] Kaplan PW. Nonconvulsive status epilepticus in the emergency room. Epilepsia. 1996;**37**(7):643-650

[3] Rüegg S. Non-convulsive status epilepticus in adults: An overview. Schweizer Archiv für Neurologie und Psychiatrie. 2008;**159**:53-83

[4] Knake S, Rosenow F, Vescovi M, et al. Incidence of status epilepticus in adults in Germany: A prospective, population-based study. Epilepsia. 2001;**42**:714-718

[5] Maganti R, Gerber P, Drees C, Chung S. Nonconvulsive status epilepticus. Epilepsy & Behavior. 2008;**12**:572-586

[6] Towne AR, Waterhouse EJ, Boggs JG, et al. Prevalence of nonconvulsive status epilepticus in comatose patients. Neurology. 2000;**54**:340-345

[7] Pandian JD, Cascino GD, So EL, Manno E, Fulgham JR. Digital video-electroencephalographic monitoring in the neurological–neurosurgical intensive care unit: Clinical features and outcome. Archives of Neurology. 2004;**61**:1090-1094

[8] Claassen J, Jetté N, Chum F, et al. Electrographic seizures and periodic discharges after intracerebral hemorrhage. Neurology. 2007;**69**:1356-1365

[9] Privitera M, Hoffman M, Moore JL, Jester D. EEG detection of nontonic–clonic status epilepticus in patients with altered consciousness. Epilepsy Research. 1994;**18**:155-166

[10] DeLorenzo RJ, Waterhouse EJ, Towne AR, et al. Persistent nonconvulsive status epilepticus after the control of convulsive status epilepticus. Epilepsia. 1998;**39**:833-840

[11] Kaplan PW. Nonconvulsive status epilepticus. Seminars in Neurology. 1996;**16**(1):33-40

[12] Kurtz P, Gaspard N, Wahl AS, et al. Continuous electroencephalography in a surgical intensive care unit. Intensive Care Medicine. 2014;**40**:228-234

[13] Bottaro FJ, Martinez OA, Pardal MM, Bruetman JE, Reisin RC. Nonconvulsive status epilepticus in the elderly: A case-control study. Epilepsia. 2007;**48**:966-972

[14] Claassen J, Mayer SA, Kowalski RG, Emerson RG, Hirsch LJ. Detection of electrographic seizures with continuous EEG monitoring in critically ill patients. Neurology. 2004;**62**:1743-1748

[15] Naeije G, Depondt C, Meeus C, Korpak K, Pepersack T, Legros B. EEG patterns compatible with nonconvulsive status epilepticus are common in elderly patients with delirium: A prospective study with continuous EEG monitoring. Epilepsy & Behavior. 2014;**36**:18-21

[16] Mehendale AM, Goldman MP, Mehendale RP, Rana K, Joppie K. Ambulatory electroencephalograms in neuropsychiatric practice: Opening Pandora's jar. World Journal of Neuroscience. 2014;**4**:125-132

[17] Siddiqui M, Jamil N, Malik A, Bano A, Khan FS, Siddiqui K. Frequency of non convulsive status epilepticus in patients with impaired level of consciousness. The Journal of the Pakistan Medical Association. 2009;**59**:296-298

[18] Rai V, Jetli S, Rai N, Padma MV, Tripathi M. Continuous EEG predictors

of outcome in patients with altered sensorium. Seizure. 2013;**22**:656-661

[19] Narayanan JT, Murthy JM. Nonconvulsive status epilepticus in a neurological intensive care unit: Profile in a developing country. Epilepsia. 2007;**48**:900-906

[20] Dericioglu N, Arsava EM, Topcuoglu MA. The clinical features and prognosis of patients with nonconvulsive status epilepticus in the neurological Intensive Care Unit of a tertiary referral center in Turkey. Clinical EEG and Neuroscience. 2014;**45**:293-298

[21] Shavit L, Grenader T, Galperin I. Nonconvulsive status epilepticus in elderly, a possible diagnostic pitfall. European Journal of Internal Medicine. 2012;**23**:701-704

[22] Mesraoua B, Deleu D, Wieser HG. Long term monitoring: An overview. In: Stevanovic D, editor. Epileptic Seizures. 1st ed. Intech; 2012. pp. 145-172

[23] Sutter R, Fuhr P, Grize L, Marsch S, Rüegg S. Continuous video EEG monitoring increases detection rate of NCSE. Epilepsia. 2011;**52**:453-457

[24] Vespa PM, Nuwer MR, Nenov V. Incidence of nonconvulsive and convulsive seizures in the ICU following traumatic brain injury: Increased incidence detected by continuous EEG monitoring. Critical Care Medicine. 1997;**25**(1 Suppl):A120

[25] Abend NS, Dlugos DJ, Hahn CD, Hirsch LJ, Herman ST. Use of EEG monitoring and management of non-convulsive seizures in critically ill patients: A survey of neurologists. Neurocritical Care. 2010;**12**:382-389

[26] Westover MB, Shafi MM, Bianchi MT, et al. The probability of seizures during EEG monitoring in critically ill adults. Clinical Neurophysiology. 2015;**126**:463-471

[27] Young GB, Jordan KG, Doig GS. An assessment of nonconvulsive seizures in the intensive care unit using continuous EEG monitoring: An investigation of variables associated with mortality. Neurology. 1996;**47**:83-89

[28] Chong DJ, Hirsch LJ. Which EEG patterns warrant treatment in the critically ill? Reviewing the evidence for treatment of periodic epileptiform discharges and related patterns. Journal of Clinical Neurophysiology. 2005;**22**:79-91

[29] Trinka E, Cock H, Hesdorffer D, et al. A definition and classification of status epilepticus—Report of the ILAE Task Force on Classification of Status Epilepticus. Epilepsia. 2015;**56**(10):1515-1523. DOI: 10.1111/epi.13121

[30] Leitinger M, Beniczky S, Rohracher A, Gardella E, Kalss G, Qerama E, et al. Salzburg consensus criteria for non-convulsive status epilepticus—Approach to clinical application. Epilepsy & Behavior. 2015;**49**:158-163

[31] Hirsch LJ, LaRoche SM, Gaspard N, Gerard E, Svoronos A, Herman ST, et al. American Clinical Neurophysiology Society's Standardized Critical Care EEG Terminology: 2012 version. Journal of Clinical Neurophysiology. 2013;**30**(1):1-27

[32] Bauer G, Trinka E. Nonconvulsive status epilepticus and coma. Epilepsia. 2010;**51**:177-190

[33] Hirsch LJ. Continuous EEG monitoring in the intensive care unit: An overview. Journal of Clinical Neurophysiology. 2004;**21**:332-340

[34] Meierkord H, Boon P, Engelsen B, et al. EFNS guideline on the management of status epilepticus in

adults. European Journal of Neurology. 2010;**17**:348-355

[35] Glauser T et al. Evidence-based guideline: Treatment of convulsive status epilepticus in children and adults: Report of the Guideline Committee of the American Epilepsy Society. Epilepsy Currents. 2016;**16**:48-61

[36] Fernández-Torre JL, Rebollo M, Gutiérrez A, López-Espadas F, Hernández-Hernández MA. Nonconvulsive status epilepticus in adults: Electroclinical differences between proper and comatose forms. Journal of Clinical Neurophysiology. 2012;**123**:244-251

[37] Liberalesso PB, Garzon E, Yacubian EM, Sakamoto AC. Refractory nonconvulsive status epilepticus in coma: Analysis of the evolution of ictal patterns. Arquivos de Neuro-Psiquiatria. 2012;**70**:501-505

[38] Laccheo I, Sonmezturk H, Bhatt AB, et al. Non-convulsive status epilepticus and non-convulsive seizures in neurological ICU patients. Neurocritical Care. 2015;**22**:202-211

[39] Kang BS, Jhang Y, Kim YS, et al. Etiology and prognosis of non-convulsive status epilepticus. Journal of Clinical Neuroscience. 2014;**21**:1915-1919

[40] Foreman B, Claassen J, Abou Khaled K, et al. Generalized periodic discharges in the critically ill: A case-control study of 200 patients. Neurology. 2012;**79**:1951-1960

[41] Trinka E, Leitinger M. Which EEG patterns in coma are nonconvulsive status epilepticus? Epilepsy & Behavior. 2015;**49**:203-222. DOI: 10.1016/j.yebeh.2015.05.005

[42] Sreedharan J et al. Falsely pessimistic prognosis by EEG in post-anoxic coma after cardiac arrest: The borderland of nonconvulsive status epilepticus. Epileptic Disorders. 2012;**14**(3):340-344

[43] Sivaraju A, Gilmore E. Understanding and managing the ictal interictal continuum in neurocritical care. Current Treatment Options in Neurology. 2016;**18**:1-13

[44] Braksick SA, Burkholder DB, Tsetsou S, et al. Associated factors and prognostic implications of stimulus-induced rhythmic, periodic, or ictal discharges. JAMA Neurology. 2016;**73**:585-590

[45] O'Rourke D, Chen PM, Gaspard N, et al. Response rates to anticonvulsant trials in patients with triphasic-wave EEG patterns of uncertain significance. Neurocritical Care. 2016;**24**:233-239

[46] Rohracher A, Höfler J, Kalss G, et al. Perampanel in patients with refractory and super-refractory status epilepticus in a neurological intensive care unit. Epilepsy & Behavior. 2015;**49**:354-358

[47] Altındağ et al. EEG patterns recorded by continuous EEG monitoring in neurological intensive care unit. Archives of Neuropsychiatry. 2017;**54**:168-174

[48] Kaplan PW. Behavioral manifestations of nonconvulsive status epilepticus. Epilepsy and Behavior. 2002 Apr;**3**:122-139

Chapter 5

Epilepsy and GI Disorders

Halil Kocamaz and Sedat Işıkay

Abstract

The gastrointestinal system communicates with the brain by way of vagus nerve fibers and the gut-brain axis. There is a well-known relationship between autoimmune diseases and epileptogenesis, and this may explain the involvement of gut microbiota in the course of epilepsy. Many seizures which are described, depending the severity and/or duration, as benign or epilepsy may be related and based on gastrointestinal origin. Epilepsy and related neurological symptoms may alert the clinician to additional life-threatening conditions and complications during the course of gastrointestinal system-based chronic disease such as inflammatory bowel disease and celiac disease. Since the gut is the only part of inner body exposed to environment, novel therapeutic options that target gut microbiata may be promising in many diseases including epilepsy.

Keywords: autoimmune, electrolyte, epilepsy, gastrointestinal, gut

1. Introduction

The enteric nervous system (ENS), located in the wall of the bowel, is also known as the "second brain." The ENS exhibits a wide similarity to the brain, both structurally and functionally. Its neuronal structure is not cemented by collagen and Schwann cells but by glial astrocytes of the central nervous system (CNS). It has similar complex functions to the brain and contains various neurotransmitters [1]. The gastrointestinal system communicates with the brain through vagus nerve fibers and the gut-brain axis. The interaction between the CNS and ENS is known as the gut-brain axis. This axis is mainly regulated by gut microbiota and related neurotransmitters such as 5-hydroxytryptamine (5-HT), also known as serotonin [2]. The common features in terms of function between the ENS and the CNS are reflected in the context of disorder, in that gastrointestinal dysfunction may be seen in neurological diseases, and neurological dysfunction may become evident in gastrointestinal disease processes [3]. Painful abdominal cramping, nausea, and cyclical vomiting syndrome are related to childhood epilepsy, and also in adults, abdominal symptoms are usually associated with idiopathic complex partial or secondary generalized seizures [4]. The ketogenic diet has beneficial effects on intractable seizures, and has been shown to affect the gut microbiota [5]. The gut microbiota and the immune system are interrelated [6]. Gut bacteria balance affects the development of autoimmune disorders. For instance, changing the balance of *Firmicutes* and *Bacteroidetes* in gut microbiota may promote autoimmune disorders such as type 1 diabetes mellitus [7]. The balance in the gut microbiota is also linked to the pro- and anti-inflammatory immune responses [8]. There is a well-known relationship between autoimmune diseases and epileptogenesis, and this may explain the involvement of gut microbiota in the course of epilepsy. The incidence of epilepsy differs between developed and developing countries, similarly to the differences observed in the gut microbiota [9]. Autoimmune diseases occur when the immune system exhibits redundant responses against the tissues of its own body. The etiology of autoimmune disease is still unclear, but some potential factors such as the environment, genetic predisposition, vaccines, an unbalanced diet, and immune disorders have been implicated [10, 11]. A large number of epilepsy cases have an autoimmune-related basis, and adjunctive immunotherapy has beneficial effects in such cases [12]. Some serum autoantibodies are also epileptogenic, and immunomodulatory therapy may attenuate the progression of some epilepsy syndromes [13]. In this context, gut microbiota-targeted therapy may be useful in the treatment of certain types of epilepsy syndromes by altering gut-related immunity and the gut-brain axis, which is also controlled by neurotransmitters. One case report stated that fecal microbiota transplantation cured refractory epilepsy in concomitant Crohn's disease [14].

2. GI disorders could be accompanied by epilepsy or seizures

Electrolyte imbalances resulting from acute or chronic vomiting and diarrhea may trigger severe seizures, especially in early childhood. Acute and profound electrolyte imbalances may lead to life-threatening neurological deterioration and intractable seizures [15]. Electrolyte imbalance and dehydration disrupt the regular voltage gradient across cellular membranes and lead to neuronal excitability following impaired neuronal discharge and epileptiform activities. Altered plasma osmolality is also substantially involved in the progression of abnormal neuronal discharge and disturbed brain metabolism. Electrolyte imbalance-related seizures are self-limited and do not commonly lead to morphological changes in the CNS if treated promptly and adequately. Epileptiform activities are commonly seen in patients with sodium abnormalities, hypocalcemia, and hypomagnesemia [16]. Seizures are related to electrolyte imbalance that usually presents as tonic-clonic type, although focal and other types may also be seen. Patients with electrolyte imbalance-related seizure frequently have a concomitant history of vomiting and diarrhea [17]. In order to identify the cause of seizures, prompt analyses of serum electrolytes and glucose levels should be performed in patients with first seizure at any age [18]. Hyponatremia is defined as a sodium level of less than 135 mEq/L. Acute hyponatremia (decreased sodium levels within a matter of hours) is mainly related to severe neurological deterioration including intractable seizures. Cerebral edema and cerebral herniation may be present as major life-threatening complications, particularly if serum sodium levels decrease to 120 mEq/L within a few hours [19]. Many clinical conditions and drugs may be responsible for hyponatremia, but antiepileptic drugs (AED) such as carbamazepine (CBZ), oxcarbazepine (OXC), and eslicarbazepine (ESL) should be remembered as causative drugs for developing hyponatremia due to inappropriate antidiuretic hormone syndrome [20]. Hyponatremia usually occurs as a non-specific wave slowing in EEG. Other EEG abnormalities include triphasic waves, high amplitude delta activity bursts, and central high amplitude delta waves with paroxysms. Interestingly, hypernatremia (when sodium levels exceed 145 mEq/L) may be seen as a consequence of tonic-clonic seizures. The pathological mechanism involved in hypernatremia after seizures depends on muscle contraction-related extracellular water depletion. Hypernatremia causes high intracellular osmolality of brain cells and shrinkage of the brain. The correction of hypernatremia should be gradual in order not to promote severe seizures. Hypocalcemia is defined as a plasma calcium level under 8.5 mg/dL, or an ionized calcium concentration less than 4 m/dL. Sodium and potassium abnormalities are more common in gastroenteritis, and hypocalcemia may also be seen during the course of gastroenteritis [21]. The clinical manifestations of hypocalcemia are related to the degree of hypocalcemia and the rate of decrease in serum calcium concentrations. The main clinical manifestation of hypocalcemia is neuromuscular excitability and tetany, although acute hypocalcemia may result in tonic-clonic, focal motor, and rarely absent seizures [22]. The major causes of hypocalcemia are vitamin D deficiency and drugs. Antiepileptic drugs (AEDs) such as phenobarbital, phenytoin, carbamazepine, and primidone may disrupt the absorption of intestinal calcium and lead to hypocalcemic symptoms, including seizures [23]. Hypocalcemia-related seizures can be easily treated with calcium therapy, and anticonvulsive therapy is not usually necessary [24].

Gastrointestinal infections are another cause of the development of epileptiform activities. There is a known relationship between diarrhea and seizures, especially in early childhood. Convulsion with mild gastroenteritis (CwG) was first reported in 1982 by the Japanese researcher Morooka, and is also known as "situation-related seizures" [25]. The diagnostic criteria for CwG were defined as follows [26]:

1. The child was previously healthy.
2. Nonfebrile convulsions accompanied by mild gastroenteritis, possible mild dehydration, absence of apparent acid intoxication, and electrolyte imbalance.
3. Convulsions mainly occurring during winter, and the gastroenteritis may persist for 1–5 days.
4. Convulsions may manifest as single or multiple episodes of generalized tonic-clonic seizure (GTCS).
5. Normal interictal electroencephalogram (EEG).
6. Normal serum electrolytes, serum glucose, and cerebrospinal fluid (CSF) with stool antigen test positive for rotavirus.
7. Favorable prognosis with rare relapse and unimpeded development.

CwG is primarily caused by rotavirus, norovirus, sapovirus, adenovirus, and coxsakie virus. Convulsions usually occur between the first and sixth day after the initial symptoms of gastroenteritis. The principal agent determined in cases of CwG is rotavirus. The mechanisms involved in CwG are still unknown [27]. Since CwG only appears in early childhood, it has been hypothesized to be related to the immature nervous system, similarly to febrile convulsions. Rotavirus can directly reach the central nervous system and cause cerebropathy, encephalitis, or convulsions [28]. Children with CwG do not require antiepileptic treatment. CWG has a short and benign course, with most episodes ending within 24 hours. Acute treatment with antiepileptic should be considered in patients with two or more convulsions [29]. Bacterial agents such as *Shigella* species are also related to neurological manifestations, including seizures. The pathophysiological mechanism of *Shigella*-related seizures has not been elucidated. Shiga toxin availability has been shown not to be essential for neurological complication [30]. Cytokines and host-immune responses are related to neurological complication during the course of disease [31]. Hyponatremia and hypoglycemia are also another factor for developing *Shigella*-related seizures and other neurological complications. *Shigella* infections are usually serious and life-threatening particularly in the case of extraintestinal and systemic involvement in developing countries. *Shigella* dysentery type 1 frequently leads to neurological complications. Appropriate treatment of *Shigella* infections with antibiotics will prevent recurrent seizures and neurological deterioration [32].

Abdominal epilepsy (*AE*) is characterized by a paroxysmal episode of abdominal pain, various abdominal symptoms, electroencephalogram (EEG) abnormalities, and favorable response to AEDs. AE is commonly seen in childhood although there have been reports of adults with AE [33]. Gastrointestinal symptoms associated with AE include abdominal pain, nausea, and vomiting, and patients may also have concomitant neurological symptoms, such as postictal lethargy, drowsiness, headache, blindness, paresthesia, and convulsions [34]. The pathophysiology of AE is not well understood, but several hypotheses have been suggested including the one which holds that abdominal epilepsy results from abnormal brain activity in the temporal lobe involving the amygdala. The amygdala then transmits activities to the gastrointestinal tract via direct projections to the dorsal motor nucleus of the vagus nerve through which gastrointestinal symptoms are felt to localized [35].

There are four diagnostic criteria for AE in the context of noninflammatory, neoplastic, metabolic, or anatomic abnormalities.

These are:

a. Otherwise unexplained, paroxysmal gastrointestinal complaints.

b. Symptoms arising from CNS disturbance.

c. An abnormal EEG with findings specific for a seizure disorder.

d. Improvement with anticonvulsant medication.

The most important differential for AE is abdominal migraine. In patients presenting with headache, it is very difficult to differentiate AE and abdominal migraine because symptoms usually overlap. Duration of the symptoms may be used to differentiate the two; being longer in migraine than in AE [36]. EEG is usually abnormal in AE and may confirm the diagnosis of AE. There is no recommended special AED therapy for abdominal epilepsy. Most of the patients may respond to single-drug therapy [37].

Inflammatory bowel disease: seizures may be seen as a clinical manifestation during the course of inflammatory bowel disease (IBD) particularly in severe cases. All types of seizures including status epilepticus have been reported. Thromboembolic events and various vitamin deficiencies such as thiamine and vitamin B12 are mostly responsible for seizures in IBD [38]. In case of seizure, a patient with IBD should be evaluated for a cranial thromboembolic event.

Celiac disease is characterized by malabsorption and gastrointestinal symptoms due to the intestinal villus injury. Approximately 10% of patients with celiac disease exhibit neurological manifestations including seizures [39]. The frequency of celiac disease in individuals with epilepsy ranges from 0.78 to 9.1% [40]. It has been suggested that vitamin deficiencies play an important role in the association between epilepsy and celiac disease because vitamins have neurotrophic and neuroprotective effects [41]. Immune mechanisms are also implicated in the pathogenesis of epileptic disorders in celiac disease. In support of this hypothesis, anti-Purkinje cell and anti-ganglioside antibodies have been determined in celiac disease patients with neurological dysfunction. Most of epileptic patients with celiac disease have been cured after adopting a gluten-free diet [42].

3. Gastrointestinal problems associated with antiepileptic drugs

AEDs have a relatively narrow therapeutic index, and their adverse effects can impact on any organ or system. Some 10–30% of patients with epilepsy discontinue their first prescribed AED due to adverse effects and intolerance [43]. Many AEDs cause gastrointestinal side effects. Multi-AEDs in particular may increase the potential side effects in intractable seizures. The most common AED-related side effects are vomiting and nausea [44]. Some important adverse gastrointestinal side effects of AEDs are mentioned below.

Valproic acid (*VA*) may cause gastrointestinal side effects such as nausea, diarrhea, abdominal pain, and vomiting. This problem may be seen particularly when the initial doses are taken. The meal time ingestion and slow release form of the drug will be tolerated by most patients [45]. Acute pancreatitis is also related to VA ingestion, and the clinician should suspect this in case of severe abdominal pain during VA therapy. Hepatotoxicity is a life-threatening condition related to VA therapy. Patients with organic brain disease, treated with several antiepileptic drugs, and younger than 2 years old have the highest risk for developing hepatotoxicity during VA treatment. Liver function tests, ammonia, and other tests are not reliable for assessing VA-related hepatotoxicity. However, clinical symptoms such as vomiting, nausea, anorexia, and lethargy may be an indicator of fatal hepatotoxicity [46].

Benzodiazepines are commonly prescribed drugs particularly in childhood epileptic syndromes. Although they exhibit sedation-related adverse effects, benzodiazepines are usually well tolerated in the gastrointestinal system and do not lead to hepatic damage unless combined with other AEDs [47].

Carbamazepine (*CBZ*) is well tolerated in the gastrointestinal system, but idiosyncratic reaction due to CBZ might be related to granulomatous hepatitis, fever, and rash [48].

Ethosuximide (*ESM*) has reversible, adverse gastrointestinal effects, such as abdominal discomfort, vomiting, diarrhea, and hiccups, but these can all be prevented if ESM is taken after meals [49].

Felbamate and *topiramate* (*TPM*) may cause anorexia, thus promoting weight loss, and there are reports of fatal hepatotoxicity due to felbamate [50, 51].

4. Conclusions

Gastrointestinal system manifestations may be a milestone of many neurological diseases, including epilepsy and benign seizures. Epilepsy and related neurological symptoms may alert the clinician to the presence of additional life-threatening conditions and complications during the course of gastrointestinal-based chronic disease such as inflammatory bowel disease and celiac disease. Since the gut is the only part of inner body exposed to environment, novel therapeutic options that target gut microbiata may be promising in many diseases including epilepsy.

Conflict of interest

The authors have no conflict of interest to report.

Author details

Halil Kocamaz[1*] and Sedat Işıkay[2]

1 Department of Pediatric Gastroenterology, Pamukkale University, Denizli, Turkey

2 Department of Pediatric Neurology, Hasan Kalyoncu University, Gaziantep, Turkey

*Address all correspondence to: drkocamaz@hotmail.com

References

[1] Gershon MD. The Enteric Nervous System: A Second Brain [Internet, cited: 23 January 2019]

[2] Mittal R, Debs LH, Patel AP, Nguyen D, Patel K, Hamed G, et al. Neurotransmitters: The critical modulators regulating gut-brain axis: HHS public access. Journal of Cellular Physiology. 2017;**232**(9):2359-2372 [cited 23 January 2019]

[3] Pfeiffer RF. Gastroenterology and neurology. Continuum: Lifelong Learning in Neurology. 2017;**23**(3, Neurology of Systemic Disease):744-761

[4] Shihabuddin BS, Harik SI. Episodic nausea and abdominal sensations as sole manifestations of simple partial seizures. Neurosciences (Riyadh, Saudi Arabia). 2007;**12**(4):327-329

[5] Xie G, Zhou Q, Qiu C-Z, Dai W-K, Wang H-P, Li Y-H, et al. Ketogenic diet poses a significant effect on imbalanced gut microbiota in infants with refractory epilepsy. World Journal of Gastroenterology. 2017;**23**(33):6164-6171

[6] Cerf-Bensussan N, Gaboriau-Routhiau V. The immune system and the gut microbiota: Friends or foes? Nature Reviews. Immunology. 2010;**10**(10):735-744

[7] Wen L, Ley RE, Volchkov PY, Stranges PB, Avanesyan L, Stonebraker AC, et al. Innate immunity and intestinal microbiota in the development of type 1 diabetes. Nature. 2008;**455**(7216):1109-1113

[8] Belkaid Y, Hand TW. Role of the microbiota in immunity and inflammation. Cell. 2014;**157**(1):121-141

[9] Heaney DC, MacDonald BK, Everitt A, Stevenson S, Leonardi GS, Wilkinson P, et al. Socioeconomic variation in incidence of epilepsy: Prospective community based study in south East England. BMJ. 2002;**325**(7371):1013-1016

[10] Cho JH, Gregersen PK. Genomics and the multifactorial nature of human autoimmune disease. The New England Journal of Medicine. 2011;**365**(17):1612-1623

[11] Molina V, Shoenfeld Y. Infection, vaccines and other environmental triggers of autoimmunity. Autoimmunity. 2005;**38**(3):235-245

[12] Palace J, Lang B. Epilepsy: An autoimmune disease? Journal of Neurology, Neurosurgery, and Psychiatry. 2000;**69**(6):711-714

[13] Peltola J, Kulmala P, Isojarvi J, Saiz A, Latvala K, Palmio J, et al. Autoantibodies to glutamic acid decarboxylase in patients with therapy-resistant epilepsy. Neurology. 2000;**55**(1):46-50

[14] He Z, Cui B-T, Zhang T, Li P, Long C-Y, Ji G-Z, et al. Fecal microbiota transplantation cured epilepsy in a case with Crohn's disease: The first report. World Journal of Gastroenterology. 2017;**23**(19):3565-3568

[15] Riggs JE. Neurologic manifestations of electrolyte disturbances. Neurologic Clinics. 2002;**20**(1):227-239, vii

[16] Castilla-Guerra L, del Carmen Fernandez-Moreno M, Lopez-Chozas JM, Fernandez-Bolanos R. Electrolytes disturbances and seizures. Epilepsia. 2006;**47**(12):1990-1998

[17] Beghi E, Carpio A, Forsgren L, Hesdorffer DC, Malmgren K, Sander JW, et al. Recommendation for a definition of acute symptomatic seizure. Epilepsia. 2010;**51**(4):671-675

[18] Schwartzkroin PA, Baraban SC, Hochman DW. Osmolarity, ionic flux, and changes in brain excitability. Epilepsy Research. 1998;**32**(1-2):275-285

[19] Bhardwaj A. Neurological impact of vasopressin dysregulation and hyponatremia. Annals of Neurology. 2006;**59**(2):229-236

[20] Van Amelsvoort T, Bakshi R, Devaux CB, Schwabe S. Hyponatremia associated with carbamazepine and oxcarbazepine therapy: A review. Epilepsia. 1994;**35**(1):181-188

[21] Devrajani B, Shah Z, Shaikh S, Shaikh S, Essa S. Hypocalcemia in acute gastroenteritis (a case-control study at Department of Internal Medicine). World Applied Sciences Journal. 2009;**7**(6):777-780

[22] Mrowka M, Knake S, Klinge H, Odin P, Rosenow F. Hypocalcemic generalised seizures as a manifestation of iatrogenic hypoparathyroidism months to years after thyroid surgery. Epileptic Disorders. 2004;**6**(2):85-87

[23] Fitzpatrick LA. Pathophysiology of bone loss in patients receiving anticonvulsant therapy. Epilepsy & Behavior. 2004;**5**(Suppl 2):S3-S15

[24] Modi S, Tripathi M, Saha S, Goswami R. Seizures in patients with idiopathic hypoparathyroidism: Effect of antiepileptic drug withdrawal on recurrence of seizures and serum calcium control. European Journal of Endocrinology. 2014;**170**(5):777-783

[25] Morooka K. Convulsions and mild diarrhea. Shonika (Tokyo). 1982;**23**:131-137

[26] Komori H, Wada M, Eto M, Oki H, Aida K, Fujimoto T. Benign convulsions with mild gastroenteritis: A report of 10 recent cases detailing clinical varieties. Brain and Development. 1995;**17**(5):334-337

[27] Li T, Hong S, Peng X, Cheng M, Jiang L. Benign infantile convulsions associated with mild gastroenteritis: An electroclinical study of 34 patients. Seizure. 2014;**23**(1):16-19

[28] Fischer TK, Ashley D, Kerin T, Reynolds-Hedmann E, Gentsch J, Widdowson M-A, et al. Rotavirus antigenemia in patients with acute gastroenteritis. The Journal of Infectious Diseases. 2005;**192**(5):913-919

[29] Ma X, Luan S, Zhao Y, Lv X, Zhang R. Clinical characteristics and follow-up of benign convulsions with mild gastroenteritis among children. Medicine (Baltimore). 2019;**98**(2):e14082

[30] Ashkenazi S, Cleary KR, Pickering LK, Murray BE, Cleary TG. The association of Shiga toxin and other cytotoxins with the neurologic manifestations of shigellosis. The Journal of Infectious Diseases. 1990;**161**(5):961-965

[31] Yuhas Y, Shulman L, Weizman A, Kaminsky E, Vanichkin A, Ashkenazi S. Involvement of tumor necrosis factor alpha and interleukin-1beta in enhancement of pentylenetetrazole-induced seizures caused by *Shigella dysenteriae*. Infection and Immunity. 1999;**67**(3):1455-1460

[32] Afroze F, Ahmed T, Sarmin M, Smsb Shahid A, Shahunja KM, Shahrin L, et al. Risk factors and outcome of *Shigella* encephalopathy in Bangladeshi children. PLoS Neglected Tropical Diseases. 2017;**11**(4):e0005561

[33] Kshirsagar VY, Nagarsenkar S, Ahmed M, Colaco S, C Wingkar K. Abdominal epilepsy in chronic recurrent abdominal pain. Journal of Pediatric Neurosciences. 2012;7:163-166

[34] Tiamkao S, Pratipanawatr T, Jitpimolmard S. Abdominal epilepsy: An uncommon of non-convulsive

status epilepticus. Journal of the Medical Association of Thailand. 2011;**94**(8):998-1001

[35] Siegel AM, Williamson PD, Roberts DW, Thadani VM, Darcey TM. Localized pain associated with seizures originating in the parietal lobe. Epilepsia. 1999;**40**(7):845-855

[36] Zinkin NT, Peppercorn MA. Abdominal epilepsy. Best Practice & Research. Clinical Gastroenterology. 2005;**19**(2):263-274

[37] Murai T, Tohyama T, Kinoshita M. Recurrent diarrhea as a manifestation of temporal lobe epilepsy. Epilepsy & Behavior Case Reports. 2014;**2**:57-59

[38] Casella G, Tontini GE, Bassotti G, Pastorelli L, Villanacci V, Spina L, et al. Neurological disorders and inflammatory bowel diseases. World Journal of Gastroenterology. 2014;**20**(27):8764-8782

[39] Işikay S, Kocamaz H. Prevalence of celiac disease in children with idiopathic epilepsy in Southeast Turkey. Pediatric Neurology. 2014;**50**(5):479-481

[40] Djuric Z, Nagorni A, Jocic-Jakubi B, Dimic M, Novak M, Milicevic R, et al. Celiac disease prevalence in epileptic children from Serbia. The Turkish Journal of Pediatrics. 2012;**54**(3):247

[41] Hadjivassiliou M, Gibson A, Davies-Jones GAB, Lobo AJ, Stephenson TJ, Milford-Ward A. Does cryptic gluten sensitivity play a part in neurological illness? Lancet. 1996;**347**(8998):369-371

[42] Pratesi R, Modelli IC, Martins RC, Almeida PL, Gandolfi L. Celiac disease and epilepsy: Favorable outcome in a child with difficult to control seizures. Acta Neurologica Scandinavica. 2003;**108**(4):290-293

[43] Wiebe S, Tellez-Zenteno JF, Shapiro M. An evidence-based approach to the first seizure. Epilepsia. 2008;**49**(Suppl 1):50-57

[44] Jahromi SR, Togha M, Fesharaki SH, Najafi M, Moghadam NB, Kheradmand JA, et al. Gastrointestinal adverse effects of antiepileptic drugs in intractable epileptic patients. Seizure. 2011;**20**(4):343-346

[45] Dreifuss FE, Langer DH. Side effects of valproate. The American Journal of Medicine. 1988 Jan;**84**(1A):34-41

[46] Powell-Jackson PR, Tredger JM, Williams R. Hepatotoxicity to sodium valproate: A review. Gut. 1984;**25**(6):673-681

[47] Czapinski P, Blaszczyk B, Czuczwar SJ. Mechanisms of action of antiepileptic drugs. Current Topics in Medicinal Chemistry. 2005;**5**(1):3-14

[48] Kristensen O, Klitgaard NA, Jönsson B, Sindrup S. Pharmacokinetics of 10-OH-carbamazepine, the main metabolite of the antiepileptic oxcarbazepine, from serum and saliva concentrations. Acta Neurologica Scandinavica. 1992;**85**(S138):145-150

[49] Pisani F, Perucca E, Bialer M. Ethosuximide: Chemistry, biotransformation P, and drug interactions. In: Levy RH, Mattson RH, Meldrum BS, Perrucca E, editors. Antiepileptic Drugs. 5th ed. Philadelphia, PA: Lippincott Williams & Wilkins; 2002. pp. 646-651

[50] O'Neil MG, Perdun CS, Wilson MB, McGown ST, Patel S. Felbamate-associated fatal acute hepatic necrosis. Neurology. 1996;**46**(5):1457-1459

[51] Ben-Menachem E, Axelsen M, Johanson EH, Stagge A, Smith U. Predictors of weight loss in adults with topiramate-treated epilepsy. Obesity Research. 2003;**11**(4):556-562

Section 4

Pediatric Epilepsy

Chapter 6

Epileptic Encephalopathies in Infants and Children

Otman Fernandez-Concepcion and Melvin Lopez-Jimenez

Abstract

Epileptic encephalopathies represent a group of devastating epileptic disorders that appear early in life. They are characterized by pharmacoresistant generalized or focal seizures, persistent severe EEG abnormalities, and cognitive dysfunction or decline. The ictal and interictal epileptic discharges are age-specific and either are the main cause or contribute to cognitive deterioration in the idiopathic or symptomatic group, respectively. Despite choosing the most appropriate antiepileptic drugs for the seizure type and syndrome, the results are often disappointing, and polytherapy and/or alternative therapy becomes unavoidable; in those cases, consideration should be given to the quality of life of the child and carers. In this chapter, we will discuss the clinical and electroencephalographic characteristics and evolution and management of age-related epileptic encephalopathies, recognized by the International League Against Epilepsy, as follows: early infantile epileptic encephalopathy (Ohtahara syndrome), early myoclonic encephalopathy, epilepsy of infancy with migrating focal seizures, infantile spasms (West syndrome), severe myoclonic epilepsy in infancy (Dravet syndrome), myoclonic-atonic epilepsy (Doose syndrome), Lennox-Gastaut syndrome, epileptic encephalopathy with continuous spike-and-wave during sleep, and Landau-Kleffner syndrome. Their clinical features, prognosis, etiologies, and treatment are presented and updated.

Keywords: electroclinical seizures, epileptic encephalopathy, pharmacoresistant epilepsy, epilepsy, electroencephalography

1. Introduction

The concept of epileptic encephalopathy (EE) is based on the clinical descriptions of some epileptic syndromes during the last century, such as West syndrome (WS) and Lennox-Gastaut syndrome (LGS). Delay in development in one, and intellectual disability in the other, was considered partly due to interictal epileptic discharges [1]. The idea that not only seizures but also apparently subclinical epileptic activity could affect cognitive functions was gaining strength in the scientific community related to epilepsy. According to this, the control of this epileptic activity could improve these deficits [1]. This notion was better profiled in the description of neuropsychological deficits related to continuous or sub-continuous paroxysmal activity during sleep, with the first description of the Landau-Kleffner syndrome (LKS) [2].

The definition of EE was better defined by Dulac in the 1990s and was incorporated into the proposed classification of the International League Against Epilepsy (ILAE) in 2001 [3]. In this proposal, the term EE was used for disorders in which "the epileptiform anomalies themselves are believed to contribute to the progressive disturbance of brain function." In 2006, Engel defined EE as disorders in which the evidence suggests the idea that neurological impairment depends on epilepsy and not on an underlying metabolic, degenerative, or encephalitic process, so that it excludes these progressive etiologies from the possible etiologies of EE [4]. Engel also emphasizes the importance of distinguishing between the deficits that are due to the cause of epilepsy, those that are due to pharmacotherapy, and those that are due to epilepsy itself.

The ILAE Working Group of 2010 pointed out the recognition achieved by the scientific community in relation to the EE [5]. The notion that epileptic activity itself may contribute to cognitive and behavioral deficiencies that exceed beyond what might be expected from causal pathology alone underlies the concept of EE. Deficits caused by epileptic discharges can be global or focal and can occur in a broad spectrum of severity.

In 2012, Capovilla proposed the term epileptogenic encephalopathy. They refer to progressive disorders of various etiologies that can cause deterioration and epilepsy, such as brain tumors, neurodegenerative or metabolic diseases, and presumed inflammatory or autoimmune conditions [1]. In epileptogenic encephalopathies, deterioration is independent of epilepsy, even if epilepsy could worsen the clinical picture; in some cases, the same etiology can produce encephalopathy without epilepsy. This distinction is important for the treatment; in the EE the treatment must be aggressive. On the other hand, if the deterioration is due to the etiology, there is a risk of unjustified excessive treatment. It is known that drugs, especially in polytherapy, can aggravate the neuropsychological deficits in these patients.

2. Neonatal epileptic encephalopathies: early infantile epileptic encephalopathy with suppression-burst pattern (Ohtahara syndrome) and early myoclonic encephalopathy (EME)

2.1 Overview

Early myoclonic epilepsy and early infantile epileptic encephalopathy (or Ohtahara syndrome) are age-dependent EEs that occur in the earliest stages of life. Although they share some clinical, electroencephalographic and prognostic characteristics, they are distinguished by their clinical presentations and different etiologies [6].

In 1976, Ohtahara et al. report an epileptic syndrome that affected very young babies with a typical electroencephalographic pattern, and they called it "early infant epileptic encephalopathy with suppression-burst" [7]. Ohtahara observed that this disorder progressed frequently to West syndrome (WS) and then to a Lennox-Gastaut syndrome (LGS) [8]. Ohtahara syndrome (OS), as it has been called since the 1980s, has also been known for other terms, such as myoclonic epilepsy with neonatal onset, neonatal epileptic encephalopathy with periodic electroencephalographic bursts, and early myoclonic epileptic encephalopathy.

In 2001, the ILAE Classification and Terminology Working Group included both OS and EME within EEs [3]. Both syndromes are similar in terms of age of onset, a characteristic of suppression-burst EEG, and the presence of several types of superimposed seizures; due to this, their differentiation is difficult and often impossible at the beginning of the disease [9]. On the other hand, motor manifestations at this age are difficult to classify.

2.2 Seizures: symptoms and semiology

In both syndromes, seizures begin almost after birth, usually during the first month of life [9]. In OS, the most typical seizures are epileptic spasms and tonic seizures, in groups or isolated [10]. In patients with hemispheric structural lesions, seizures can be unilateral or at least asymmetric. On the other hand, in the EME, myoclonic (axial, segmental, or erratic) seizures are more characteristic. The frequency of seizures is flexible and can be almost continuous. Erratic and segmental myoclonus usually occurs in the first days [11]. In erratic myoclonus, the jerking seems to change arbitrarily from one area of the body to another, mainly in the face and extremities, although axial myoclonus could also appear. Subtle focal or clonic seizures may continue to myoclonus. Additionally, the complex motor manifestations that are associated with bursts of paroxysmal activity on the EEG are difficult to classify as spasms or myoclonus. Both conditions can present focal seizures commonly; these can be with deviation of the eyes, tonic posture, or hemiconvulsions; subtle attacks can also occur with autonomic phenomena, such as flushing or apnea [9].

2.3 Electroencephalography features

2.3.1 Background

The EEG may be normal at the beginning of the EME, which is why successive EEGs must be repeated to define the diagnosis. When the clinical presentation is complete, there is no temporal or spatial organization or physiological characteristics in wakefulness or sleep [11].

2.3.2 Interictal abnormalities

The typical pattern is the suppression-burst (S-B); it consists of bursts of high-voltage asynchronous delta or theta waves, interspersed with spikes and polyspikes from 150 to 350 μV that last from 1 to 6 seconds and alternate with low voltage (<10 μV) or complete suppression activity intervals of 2–5 seconds in duration [8]. In the EME, the bursts are shorter, and the suppression periods are much longer [11]; the S-B pattern in OS occurs in both wakefulness and sleep, while the S-B pattern in EME, which usually is present only during sleep [9].

The S-B pattern may vary in configuration and the interhemispheric synchronization of the bursts; they may predominate in one hemisphere, especially when associated with lateralized structural anomalies, such as focal cortical dysplasia or hemimegalencephaly [11]. During the suppression periods, focal epileptiform discharges can be observed [12].

The S-B pattern may persist beyond the first year of life, or it may progress to hypsarrhythmia between 3 and 6 months of age; it's coinciding with the development of epileptic spasms in the WS context [11]. The early transition to hypsarrhythmia is more common in the OS, while in the EME the S-B can continue in the infancy until a transient evolution to hypsarrhythmia in the middle and late infancy [10]. There are reports of evolution to the slow spike-wave pattern characteristic of LGS.

2.3.3 Ictal EEG

During tonic spasms, EEG shows desynchronization with or without rapid activity [8]. By means of video-electroencephalography (video-EEG) with electromyographic recordings from deltoid muscles, we observe that each burst is to be associated with tonic contraction of variable duration [13]. The erratic myoclonus of EME habitually has no EEG correlate, whereas limb/axial myoclonus are usually associated with bursts of spikes and polyspikes.

Complex stereotyped movements that are difficult to classify as either spasms or myoclonias are also associated with bursts of activity. There is no correlation between the duration of the burst and the type of seizure [11]. Focal seizures and subclinical phenomena are associated with focal discharges of spikes or sharp wave [8].

2.3.4 EEG differential diagnosis

A discontinuous EEG pattern with resemblances to S-B can be seen in neonatal hypoxic ischemic encephalopathy, but in this condition, the pattern is generally transient and can be reactive. Treatment for neonatal status epilepticus, such as midazolam, sufentanil, and fentanyl infusion, may exhibit a pattern evocative of S-B.

2.4 Etiology

The etiologies of OS are diverse, including specific genetic mutations, cortical brain malformations, mitochondrial disorders, nonketotic hyperglycinemia, and severe perinatal hypoxic-ischemic injury. On the other hand, EE vitamin-responsive disorders need to be ruled out as a potential underlying etiology; in certain cases the cause is unknown.

The most frequent genetic abnormalities linked with OS are aristaless-related homeobox (ARX) gene mutations at Xp22.13, cyclin-dependent kinase-like 5 (CLDK5) (STK9) gene at Xp22, solute carrier family 25 [mt carrier, glutamate carrier-1/GC-1] member 22 (SLC25A22) gene at 11p15.5, STXBP1 (MUNC18-1) gene microdeletion at 9 q33.3-q34.11, KCNQ2 gene mutations, SCN2A gene mutations, and GABRA1 gene mutations [14].

EME is usually associated with inherited metabolic disorders, such as nonketotic hyperglycinemia, organic acidemias, Zellweger syndrome, and molybdenum cofactor deficiency [15]. Until the report of Cohen in 2014, in two siblings with early myoclonic encephalopathy, born to consanguineous parents of Arab Muslim origin, a potential mutation of SLC25A22 should be considered in infants presenting as EME, severe microcephaly, and autosomal recessive inheritance with negative metabolic workup [16].

Several of the genes may manifest as phenotypes that overlap not only with OS and EME but also with other EEs such as West syndrome [14].

Box 1 shows differences between early epileptic encephalopaties [17].

EME	OS
Clinical Early myoclonus progressively becoming erratic, fragmented, and massive, followed by focal seizures and rarely tonic spasms	*Clinical* Characterized by tonic spasms, focal seizures, and rarely massive myoclonus; this is never erratic
EEG The S-B pattern is continuous in both awake and sleep states	*EEG* The S-B pattern is limited or more distinct during sleep
Etiology Structural brain abnormalities, a few metabolic, non-familial. Genes found: ARX, STXBP1, KCNQ2, and PNKP	*Etiology* Cryptogenic, familial, and metabolic. Genes found: ErbB4 and SEC25A22

OS, Ohtahara syndrome; EME, early myoclonic encephalopathy; S-B, suppression-burst; ARX, aristaless-related homeobox

Box 1.
Differences between early infantile epileptic encephalopathy (EME) and Ohtahara syndrome (OS).

2.5 Treatment and prognosis.

There is no specific treatment efficacious for these epileptic syndromes. For OS, adrenocorticotropic hormone (ACTH)/corticosteroids, vigabatrin, levetiracetam, zonisamide, phenobarbitone, rufinamide, and ketogenic diet should be tried. Resective surgery may be useful in cases of focal cortical dysplasia or hemimegalencephaly. Patients diagnosed as EME should receive a trial of pyridoxine. In cases with nonketotic hyperglycinemia, oral administration of ketamine, tryptophan, and dextromethorphan, in combination with benzoate, may improve the neurological symptoms [18]. Vigabatrin and sodium channel blocker AEDs should be avoided in the myoclonic phase of EME.

Prognosis in both syndromes is very poor, and the response to treatment is very disappointing. About half of patients die within weeks or months from onset, and the others progress with severe neurological impairments. Two-thirds of the survived OS patients develop infantile spasms, around 3–7 months, and numerous advances to LGS after 1 year of age [18]. In EME, the erratic myoclonus will improve spontaneously with time, and then they will carry on having focal seizures, despite its treatment.

3. Infantile spasms (IS) and West syndrome (WS)

3.1 Overview

West syndrome (WS) was first described by Dr. WJ West of Tunbridge, United Kingdom, in 1841, in a letter addressed to the editor of *The Lancet*. West reports the characteristic clinical features in his own son. In 1952, Gibbs and Gibbs describe hypsarrhythmia, the characteristic electroencephalographic feature of WS [1]. WS is an age-dependent epilepsy that usually starts in the first year of life, most frequently between the first 3 and 9 months of life; however spasms can also affect older children but rarely beyond the age of 2 years. Even though the triad of epileptic spasms in cluster, developmental regression, and hypsarrhythmia on the EEG defines WS, it is not always associated with the classical hypsarrhythmic EEG pattern, and patients do not always have developmental regression at the beginning of the disease [19]. The recent ILAE classification included the term "epileptic spasms" (ES), rather than "infantile spasms," when this seizure type is observed at other ages. Hypsarrhythmia can also be incidentally recorded in the absence of spasms.

3.2 Seizures: symptoms and semiology

ES are a seizure type, characterized by short-term muscle contractions that affect predominate proximal and truncal muscles which lead to abrupt flexion, extension, or mixed movements. According to EEG-EMG polygraphy records, an epileptic spasm reaches the full contraction more slowly than myoclonia but faster than a tonic seizure [20]. Usually, ES occurs in clusters but may be isolated. Clusters of ES increase progressively in frequency and intensity, reach a peak, and then gradually decline before they stop.

Some ES are limited to making only grimaces, deviation of the eye, and nodding; they can also be subclinical; it's called "subtle" ES. On the other hand, ES may be asymmetric, or asynchronous, concomitant with various focal manifestations that may implicate the limbs, head, or eyes; sometimes ES may express with compartmental and vegetative features. If ES is preceded or followed by, or interspersed with, focal seizures, it suggests a focal lesion [21].

3.3 Electroencephalography

3.3.1 Background

Continuously abnormal during the wakefulness and sleep.

3.3.2 Interictal abnormalities

A typical interictal presentation in WS, hypsarrhythmia, refers to a high-voltage (hypsos = height), disorganized, and chaotic (without any discernible normal background rhythm = arrhythmia) EEG pattern. At onset, hypsarrhythmia may be present only during the drowsiness and light sleep, but it soon grows into profuse during the wakefulness.

Sometimes epileptic discharges appear to be focal or multifocal, however, without a rhythmic or organized pattern. This electrical manifestation is almost continuous, although in initial stages, background activity can be observed intermittently. Hypsarrhythmia predominates in the posterior regions; rarely, posterior predominance is observed, especially after the first year of life [11]. This pattern of hypsarrhythmia reaches its peak in stage 1 of sleep, is less persistent in stages II and III of sleep (as multifocal spikes and sharp discharges), and disappears completely in REM sleep.

Different variants of hypsarrhythmia have been reported further than its typical presentation; these include (1) hypsarrhythmia with increased interhemispheric synchronization, (2) asymmetric hypsarrhythmia, (3) hypsarrhythmia with episodes of voltage attenuation, (4) hypsarrhythmia with a consistent focus of epileptic discharges or focal slowing, and others [22].

When the EEG shows atypical hypsarrhythmia, an underlying structural origin can be suspected; for example, predominating focal discharges or slow complexes could indicate a focal lesion, diffuse high-voltage theta-alpha activity may indicate lissencephaly or pachygyria, and persistent asymmetry or asynchrony may suggest a focal lesion or agenesis of the corpus callosum.

3.3.3 Ictal EEG

Ictal activity associated with ES includes a diffuse high-amplitude triphasic slow wave, a low-amplitude brief fast discharge, or a short-lasting diffuse flattening of ongoing activity [13, 20]. A transient disappearing or reduction of the hypsarrhythmic pattern could be seen during a cluster of ES. Patients with brain lesions may show an asymmetry of the ictal high-amplitude slow wave because of the more involved hemisphere. Focal or unilateral fast discharges directly preceding the high-voltage slow wave are greatly suggestive of focal cortical lesion [11].

3.4 Etiology

WS etiology can be genetic, structural or metabolic, or unknown. Prenatal and perinatal etiologies explain more than 40% of the cases; they include central nervous system malformations, neurocutaneous syndromes (especially tuberous sclerosis), metabolic disorders, hypoxic-ischemic encephalopathy, central nervous system infections, and other acquired conditions [23].

Underlying etiology may be genetic, either chromosomal abnormalities or single-gene defects. The mutations in specific genes are ARX, GAMT, ALG13, CDKL5, SCN2A, STXBP1, SCN1A, ALG13, GABRB3, DNM1, SCN8A, MAGI2, ACADS, WDR45, and GABRA1 [23, 24].

3.5 Treatment and prognosis

The key short-term aims of therapy are the rapid abolition of ES and the elimination of hypsarrhythmia. Effective treatment is associated with better outcome, at least in patients where the underlying pathology is not responsible for significant neurological deterioration. Therefore, children with WS, who are developmentally normal prior to spasms, continue to be normal after successful early treatment; on the other hand, children with WS, who have some cognitive problems prior to spasms, remain to have cognitive deficits, even after successful treatment related to the underlying pathology [25].

Other factors that contribute to unfavorable outcome are onset at age < 3 months, psychomotor retardation, existence of other seizure types, persistence of abnormal EEG features, mild to gross neurologic deficits, significant computed tomography/MRI findings, and long duration of therapy. All unfavorable prognostic factors seem to relate to the underlying pathology; some symptomatic cases may develop autism or LGS [26].

With the exception of IS in the setting of tuberous sclerosis complex (TSC), there is relatively broad consensus that hormonal therapy is the most effective class of initial treatment for IS [27]; but the best agent, dose, and length of treatment are not clear. The most studied medications are natural adrenocorticotropic hormone (ACTH, a 39 amino acid peptide), synthetic ACTH (sACTH, a truncated peptide spanning the first 24 N-terminal residues), prednisolone, and prednisone (the prodrug of prednisolone).

The highest short-term response rates (freedom from ES and hypsarrhythmia on treatment day 14) have been observed with ACTH administered at high dose (150 U/m^2 body surface areas per day, divided into two daily doses) [28]. Although some authors reported that short-term response was far superior with this regimen of ACTH in comparison to prednisolone at dose of 2 mg/kg/day [29], a sequence of studies has suggested that higher dose regimens of prednisolone are as effective as ACTH. In the UKISS study, no difference in response rate between prednisolone (40–60 mg/day) and a "moderate" dose of sACTH (0.50–0.75 mg on alternate days) was observed, although treatment allocation was not randomized [30]. Likewise, in a debatably underpowered retrospective analysis, Kossoff and colleagues reported that efficacy of high-dose prednisolone (40–60 mg/day) was similar to historical experience with high-dose natural ACTH [31]. In other relatively small study evaluating short-term efficacy of very high-dose prednisolone (8 mg/kg/day; max 60 mg/day) followed by high-dose natural ACTH in prednisolone nonresponders, the EEG-confirmed response to prednisolone (63%) was analogous to the reported ACTH response in most current studies [25].

More recently, in a large-scale prospective observational study led by the National Infantile Spasms Consortium (United States) without randomized treatment distribution, Knupp and colleagues reported that response rates to natural ACTH (most with high-dose protocol; 150 U/m^2/day) and oral corticosteroids (most with high-dose prednisolone; 40–60 mg/day) were statistically indistinct [32]. In the only modern randomized controlled trial comparing high-dose prednisolone (40–60 mg/day) with moderate-dose sACTH (0.5–0.75 mg on alternate days), Wanigasinghe and colleagues found that response to prednisolone was superior, though the response rate to sACTH was inexplicably low [33].

Given the cost of a typical course of ACTH exceeds 100,000 USD, a typical course of prednisolone costs less than 100 USD; many of treatment protocols for WS begin with prednisolone/prednisone and leave ACTH as an alternative for patients without response to this drug.

All hormonal therapies exhibit similar—and important—adverse event profiles. The main risk is immunosuppression, which can be severe and potentially lethal, as well as hypertension, with the potential to yield congestive heart failure [34]. As such, avoidance of infectious contacts and screening for asymptomatic hypertension are key safety measures to be endorsed during any course of hormonal therapy. In addition, most clinicians prescribe antibiotic prophylaxis for pneumocystis pneumonia, screen for asymptomatic hyperglycemia, monitor serum potassium given modest risk of hypokalemia, and also screen for adrenal or pituitary insufficiency after a course of hormonal therapy.

Vigabatrin (VGB) is an irreversible inhibitor of γ-aminobutyric acid (GABA) transaminase, with proven efficacy in the treatment of IS in several randomized, controlled trials [35, 36]. Nevertheless, short-term response rates to VGB are considerably lower in comparison to the hormonal therapies. With respect to long-term outcomes, the superiority of hormonal therapy is not as clear [37, 38]. Although a large-scale trial of VGB versus high-dose hormonal therapy has not been undertaken in a TSC cohort, several studies indeed suggest that response to VGB is substantially higher among patients with WS associated with TSC in comparison to patients with other etiologies [39–41]. There is broad consensus that patients with IS in the setting of TSC should receive first-line treatment with VGB [27].

Overall, VGB is moderately effective (and highly effective in the setting of TSC) and confers moderate risk. The threat of visual field loss is relatively low and perhaps diminished by short courses of therapy; the risk of reversible and habitually asymptomatic MRI toxicity is moderately high and dose-dependent [41].

The hypothesis that combination therapy is superior to either therapy alone was proven in the International Collaborative Infantile Spasms Study (ICISS) [42], in which the investigators randomized new-onset patients with IS to receive either hormonal therapy (prednisolone or sACTH) alone or in combination with VGB. The combination therapy group exhibited superior response rates with respect to clinical outcome (parent-reported freedom from ES on days 14–42), electroclinical outcome, and time to cessation of ES.

A minority of children with IS are good candidates for surgical resection [43]. The etiologies best suitable to surgical resection include cortical dysplasia, cortical tubers in TSC, and various acquired structural lesions, for example, unifocal stroke or hemorrhage. The role of nonresective surgical approaches (e.g., corpus callosotomy) is not well established in these patients [43].

There are rare occasions in which a specific metabolic etiology of IS prompts a specific therapeutic intervention, either as an alternative or adjunct to first-line therapy [44]; the most notable examples include pyridoxine (vitamin B6) dependency (treated with pyridoxine or leucovorin), pyridoxal-5-phosphate deficiency (treated with pyridoxal-5-phosphate), glucose transporter type 1 (Glut1) deficiency (treated with the ketogenic diet), and nonketotic hyperglycinemia (ameliorated to some extent by sodium benzoate and other interventions to promote central glycine clearance) [45].

Other treatments are supported by very limited reports of efficacy. It includes traditional antiseizure drugs such as topiramate, zonisamide, valproic acid, felbamate, and benzodiazepines clonazepam and nitrazepam. Among nonpharmacologic therapies, numerous studies suggest substantial efficacy for treatment of IS with the ketogenic diet; most of these are retrospective, and none has utilized placebo controls or unbiased outcome assessment. Prognosis depends on etiology and is better in children without apparent structural cause. In nearly half of the patients, WS evolves into LGS or multifocal epilepsies.

4. Severe myoclonic epilepsy in infancy (Dravet syndrome)

4.1 Overview

Severe myoclonic epilepsy of childhood was described in 1978 by Charlotte Dravet and included among epileptic encephalopathies in the 2001 proposal [3]. However, the acceptance that DS is a channelopathy of the SCN1A gene, as well as the presence of neurological deterioration in the early stages of the disease, has questioned whether the deterioration is really due to epileptic seizures or due to channelopathy [46].

Estimated prevalence of Dravet syndrome (DS) is about 1% of epilepsy syndromes in infancy and childhood, being more frequently in male. According to different descriptions of the natural course during of DS childhood, two phases have been identified: early phase (first year of life) and a steady phase (from 2 to 5 years of life); the electroclinical features are different between these phases. Early phase is characterized by long hemi- or generalized convulsive seizures, typically related with fever, while in the steady phase, seizures that predominate are myoclonic seizures (MS), atypical absences, and complex partial seizures (CPS); also, events of nonconvulsive status may occur. Cognitive development slows down progressively causing moderate/severe intellectual disability generally after the age of 4–5 years. Most patients develop ataxia, pyramidal signs, and hypotony, which persist to adulthood.

Seizure behavior should vary in time; association between seizures and fever may be absent; also CPS and MS may begin in the early phase. Diagnosis of DS may be delayed because of the variability in evolution, the seizure polymorphism, and the non-specific EEG features. Long-term prognosis is always bad, pharmacoresistance is the rule, and most patients go on severely cognitively impaired.

4.2 Seizures: symptoms and semiology

The typical picture is previously healthy children who begin with seizures in the first year of life; its seizures should be unilateral or generalized convulsive (clonic or tonic-clonic), are commonly prolonged (more than 10 min), and could be progressed into status epilepticus (SE). Seizures are usually triggered by fever, or occur after immunization, but may also be afebrile. In the second or third year of life, other types of seizure, generally afebrile, can occur [47] in the absence of MS, which starts later [48].

The seizure pattern changes over time; SE is the most problematic through the first 2 years of life and decreases in frequency after 5 years of age. In early childhood, frequent nonconvulsive seizures may negatively impact neurodevelopment. In the adolescent and adult years, brief but frequent nocturnal generalized convulsive seizures are the most common and place the patient at risk of sudden unexpected death in epilepsy (SUDEP). The details of seizures observed in DS are described then:

A. Convulsive seizures

1. Unilateral with clear hemiclonic or tonic convulsions that may alternate sides in the same patient can offer a significant sign to early diagnosis.

2. Generalized tonic-clonic seizure (GTCS).

3. Falsely generalized (FG) and unstable seizures. FG are bilateral convulsive with asymmetric clonic or tonic movements and postures, at times predominating on one side or changing sides during the seizure.

B. Focal seizures, commonly CPC, are accompanied with autonomic features like pallor, cyanosis, respiratory changes, and drooling and oral automatisms, with eyelid or distal jerks. These seizures are short (few minutes) but can progress into a unilateral or generalized motor seizure.

C. Myoclonic seizures (MS) should manifest like massive axial movements with falls or as a few jerks; erratic myoclonias are not rare.

D. Atypical absences (AA) could appear frequently linked with a myoclonic component.

E. Nonconvulsive status epilepticus (NCSE) or obtundation status is prolonged episodes (hours or days) of diminishing of consciousness with loss of contact or variably reduced responsiveness and somnolence, with erratic or segmental myoclonus. This NCSE may be initiated, punctuated, or terminated by GTCS or be combined with axial myoclonic, myoclonic-atonic, or clonic seizures.

F. Tonic seizures are rare and may be triggered by intermittent photic stimulation (IPS), visual patterns, hot water immersion, and physical effort.

Sensitivity to photic or pattern stimulation is noted in approximately 40% of patients, particularly in younger children.

Worsening of seizures or SS may be provoked by blocking sodium channels AEDs, such as carbamazepine, phenytoin, lamotrigine, and vigabatrin.

In adults, seizures are more frequent during sleeping, especially long-lasting clonic seizures or short tonic-clonic seizures, while MS, AA, and focal seizures have a tendency to remit.

4.3 Electroencephalography

EEG abnormalities are non-specific, but interictal EEG is useful for differential diagnosis; however sequential EEG recordings may show the evolution of DS, whereas ictal recordings with EMG polygraphy document seizure polymorphism [11].

4.3.1 Background

In wakefulness state background activity is normal at onset, despite the frequent seizures; diffuse or asymmetric slowing may be seen if EEG is performed immediately after a seizure or may remain on for a few days. During sleeping normal patterns, initially after the first year, there is usually a gradual slowing of the background activity, more obvious if seizures are frequent. Physiological sleep phenomena and organization mostly remain conserved, except numerous nocturnal seizures occur.

4.3.2 Interictal abnormalities (IA)

It may be present at the beginning (22% of patients) and grow during the evolution (77%) [48]. Generalized focal and multifocal abnormalities, spikes, and spike-wave or polyspike-wave discharges, symmetric or not, predominate over the frontal and central areas, but occur over the temporal and occipital areas, too. IA is typically greater during sleeping [48, 49]. The evolution of the EEG aspects with age is not always similar and being dependent on the number and duration of seizures.

4.3.3 Ictal EEG

- Unilateral seizures. The ictal discharge is characterized by rhythmic (2–3/second) bilateral slow waves of higher amplitude over the hemisphere contralateral to the clinical manifestations and intermixed with 10/second recruiting rhythms. In others, the EEG pattern can onset over the frontal or frontal-central regions of one hemisphere, or with bilateral asymmetric onset, but always predominant over the frontal areas.

- Falsely generalized and unstable seizures. In this type of seizures, the EEG discharge is of bilateral symmetric or asymmetric onset with a slow spike, occasionally followed by a brief attenuation, and fast activities intermixed with slow waves. Whereas, the ictal discharge change topographically in a same seizures, in unstable seizures [47].

- In CPS ictal EEG consists of a rhythmic sequence of fast polyspikes intermixed with theta activity during the last part of the seizure, involving the temporal-parietal-occipital region of one hemisphere for the duration of the seizure [47].

- MS are accompanied by generalized spike or polyspike-wave discharges at 3 Hz or more, lasting 1–3 seconds and of higher voltage over the central-parietal areas.

- AA are linked with generalized regular or irregular spike-wave discharges at 2–3.5 Hz, lasting 3–10 seconds.

- In obtundation status EEG background activity is substituted by diffuse delta slow waves, superimposed with multifocal spikes and spike-waves, sharp waves, and generalized spike-and-wave discharges preponderating over frontal-central areas.

- Tonic seizures are associated with diffuse discharges of polyspikes at 8–9 Hz [15].

4.4 Etiology

DS is a channelopathy due to mutation in the SCN1A gene which encodes the alpha 1 subunit of the voltage-gated sodium (Nav1.1) channel reported in 80% of patients [50]. Almost half of SCN1A mutations are truncations, and most DS SCN1A mutations are de novo [51]. SCN1A mutations are not pathognomonic of DS; it could be observed in a spectrum of febrile epilepsy syndromes, which ranges from genetic epilepsy with febrile seizures plus (GEFS+) to DS. The mutations in the SCN1A gene also constitute a risk factor for SUDEP by causing cardiac and respiratory dysfunctions [52]. Another gene implicated in DS is GABRA1 [53].

4.5 Treatment and prognosis

The aim of treatment in patients with DS is reducing seizure frequency, minimizing comorbidities, limiting antiepileptic drug toxicity, and avoiding seizure-related injury and SUDEP [54]. A greater degree of cognitive and behavioral impairment has been associated to higher frequencies of seizures [55, 56].

It is prominent that seizures are triggered by hyperthermia and less frequently by photosensitivity or pattern sensitivity; thus antipyretics for fever, minimizing warm baths or exercising on warm days, and avoiding photosensitivity triggers are recommended [54].

Sodium channel-blocking drugs such as carbamazepine, oxcarbazepine, lamotrigine, and phenytoin should also be avoided because they can aggravate seizures.

Valproic acid, clobazam, topiramate, levetiracetam, and stiripentol are the drugs of choice. Stiripentol combined with valproic acid and clobazam, as well as topiramate, give promising results [54, 57, 58]. The ketogenic diet is an alternative with good results for several patients, achieving a reduction of the seizures by 50% or more [59, 60].

The prognosis for children with DS is poor; the complete cessation of epileptic seizures is not achievable in these patients. Since the onset of disease, the neurological status worsens, and about 10–20% of afflicted children will die prematurely [61, 62]. Early mortality, sometimes due SUDEP, occurs in about 10% of patients. However, the outcome, in at least some children, improves with early diagnosis and appropriate therapeutic intervention.

5. Epilepsy of infancy with migrating focal seizures (EIMFS)

5.1 Overview

EIMFS, previously called malignant migrating partial seizures of infancy, is a rare and severe condition describe in 1995 [63]. EIMFS is characterized by focal "migrating" or "random" seizures beginning within the first 6 months of life, severe global developmental delay, and acquired microcephaly. Epilepsy is highly pharmacoresistant. At onset brain MRI is typically normal, but later it may show delayed myelination, thin corpus callosum, and cerebral atrophy [64]. Patients with intractable seizures have a progressive deterioration with major axial and limb hypotonia, loss of visual contact, and loss of other motor and social skills. Pyramidal and/or extrapyramidal features with athetotic movements may appear; about 18% of the patients died [65].

De novo KCNT1 mutations have been reported in about 50% of patients with sporadic EIMFS [64–66].

5.2 Seizures: symptoms and semiology

It is accepted that the natural history of the EIMFS goes through three distinct phases [63]. The first phase starts in the first 6 months of life and lasts a few weeks or months; patients have sporadic seizures with frequency every few weeks or months. Seizures used to be focal motor with quick generalization or associated with autonomic features like apnea, flushing, or cyanosis [63, 67]. The second phase, called "stormy phase," arises between 1 and 12 months; seizures become more frequent, occurring in clusters several times a day or being practically continuous for several days. Seizure consists of lateral deviation of the head and eyes, twitches of the eyelids, unilateral clonic or tonic jerks of one or both limbs, apnea, flushing and/or cyanosis of the face, chewing movements, and secondary tonic-clonic seizures [68]. Additionally, clinical manifestations may be "subtle" or absent even with the long duration of seizures.

The age at onset of the third phase is variable, from the end of the first year to the fifth year of age. This phase is typically seizure-free, even if interposing illnesses can trigger recurrent seizures or SS. Some patients can evolve to a WS [63, 65].

Migrating focal seizures (MFS) are seizures which occur usually in clusters that last for a few days and are then followed by a few weeks or months of recovery. Within a cluster, seizures are very frequent and may even extend to SS. Clusters increase in frequency within the first 2 years of life.

5.3 Electroencephalography

5.3.1 Background

EEG is usually normal during the first months apart from slowing for many hours after long-lasting seizures. As the disease progresses, background activities become gradually diffusely slower with decline of physiological features. Activity may show alternating asymmetries, with slow activity that change from one hemisphere to another [63]. In seizure-free periods, sleep and wakefulness are obviously differentiated; nevertheless sleep spindles are rare, asynchronous, and asymmetric.

5.3.2 Interictal abnormalities

Interictal abnormalities are usually absent at onset; spikes rapidly grow in frequency and develop multifocal within a few months; multifocal spike-and-wave activities do not show any specific pattern and are not activated in sleep.

5.3.3 Ictal EEG

Epileptic discharges (ED) sequentially involve different areas of the brain, such as describing a random migration, without a specific pattern. The ictal pattern is characterized by rhythmic monomorphic activity in the alpha-theta frequency range, although delta waves, spikes, and spike-waves can also be observed. It is common for epileptic activity to remain limited to one region for a period of time and then decrease in frequency until stop, with a tendency to progressively involve an adjacent area. ED is continued with slow postictal activity without prolonged voltage decrement [63, 68]. When epileptic seizures are frequent, ED changes from one region to another and from one hemisphere to another so that consecutive focal epileptic discharges overlap resulting in a continuous and changing multifocal ictal activity and a very complex epileptic status pattern [11].

5.4 Treatment

Migrating partial seizures are usually refractory to pharmacologic treatment though some cases have responded to bromide (60–80 mg/kg/day), with a termination of the seizures for several months after almost 3 weeks of therapy [69]. Even so, one should be aware of a potential bromoderma tuberosum, which could be appearing with high doses of potassium bromide therapy [70]. Intravenous levetiracetam (60 mg/kg) rapidly interrupted migrating partial status in two children with a good tolerability and safety [71]. Other successful treatments include a combination of sodium bromide, stiripentol, and levetiracetam [72], rufinamide and acetazolamide [73, 74], and stiripentol associated with clonazepam.

6. Epilepsy with myoclonic-atonic seizures (EMAS) or Doose syndrome

6.1 Overview

In 1970, Herman Doose reported seizures in 51 previously normal children between 1 and 5 years of age described as myoclonic and astatic, frequently combined with absences and GTCS and tonic seizures [75]. Doose suggested a genetic etiology [76] and later refined his criteria and emphasized that tonic seizures are rare [77].

In 1989, the ILAE recognized the syndrome of myoclonic-astatic epilepsy with a genetic predisposition, and in 2010 the term changed to "epilepsy with myoclonic-atonic seizures" (EMAS). Features that define EMAS are (1) normal development previous to the start of seizures; (2) onset between 7 months and 6 years of age, of myoclonic, myoclonic-atonic, or atonic seizures; and (3) EEG with generalized spike or polyspike-and-wave discharges.

EMAS represents 1–2% of cases with childhood epilepsy and shows a variable clinical course and age-dependent spectrum. Onset peaks at about 3 years and is more prevalent in boys, ratio about 2:1. A long-term follow-up study showed a common evolution which was classified, according to the definitive seizure outcome, into favorable, intermediate, and unfavorable forms [78]. Cumulative percentage remission reached 40% within 6 months, 63% within 1 year, and 89% within 3 years after seizure onset [78]. Even in children with a favorable clinical course, seizures can be initially pharmacoresistant, sometimes demanding additional ACTH or ketogenic diet; in unfavorable patients, epilepsy remains refractory to treatment with the occurrence of long-lasting episodes of NCSE. Cognition is habitually normal during the first months of the disease, although patients are often severely hyperkinetic; intellectual outcomes range from favorable to unfavorable [79, 80].

6.2 Seizures: symptoms and semiology

The main seizure types range from myoclonic to atonic. MS, atonic seizures (before called astatic), and myoclonic-atonic seizures typically occur a few days or weeks after the onset of GTCS or clonic seizures.

It is common for the first seizures to be clonic seizures or GTCS, which occur in normal children; sometimes they can be preceded by febrile seizures (FS). In a few months, the frequency of crises increases gradually and AA may appear. Nonconvulsive SS may be of myoclonic-atonic, myoclonic, or AA type and may be resistant to treatment. Some patients with a poor outcome may have brief tonic seizures.

The types of seizures observed in EMAS are:

1. Epileptic drop attacks or seizures that cause falls, which can be of three different types taking account the postural change, the temporal sequence of falling, and EMG polygraphy.
    - Myoclonic flexor seizures with sudden flexion or extension of the head and trunk.
    - Myoclonic-atonic seizures with initial change as the myoclonic flexor type, but following falling is produced by loss of muscle tone.
    - Atonic seizures with sudden slumping or collapsing to the floor as a result of transient loss of muscle tone.
2. Generalized clonic seizures occur during both wakefulness and sleep. The clonic component commonly appears as the repetition of massive MS. Clonic movements habitually increase in frequency and may become very rapid resulting in a "clonic vibratory" seizure that usually ends with gradually decreasing frequency of the clonic jerks.
3. GTCS, in which clonic component is preceded by a tonic phase lasting a few seconds.

4. Some patients may have prolonged recurrent AA with associated blurring of consciousness and often random segmental myoclonus or head nodding.

5. NCSE which consists of a cluster of myoclonic-astatic, MS, or AA. Clinically, we observe loss of contact or somnolence. Patients may have salivating and speech trouble ranging from dysarthria to mutism. Sometimes, erratic myoclonus in the face, the upper limbs, the eyelids, mouth, tongue, and fingers should be observed, associated with ataxic, hypotonia, tremor, and difficulty in walking.

6. Generalized tonic seizures with or without few clonic components occur during sleeping. When predominant, these seizures are associated with unfavorable outcome; they are resistant to treatment. When the tonic phase is preceded by a myoclonic jerk, seizures are termed "myotonic."

6.3 Electroencephalography

6.3.1 Interictal background

Background activity is normal at the onset of the disease. A characteristic 4–7-Hz diffuse theta rhythm, usually predominating over the central-parietal areas (central theta waves), is often present, intermixed with normal waking activities and increasing during the drowsiness. In some children, background may be diffusely slow. During sleeping, physiological features are usually seen at the onset, while diffuse slowing with loss of sleep architecture can occur during the evolution, mainly in the severe forms of the spectrum [11].

6.3.2 Interictal abnormalities

In wakefulness there may be no epileptiform discharges. If this is present, generalized spike-waves discharges are at 2–3 Hz, predominant over the frontal-central areas. They may show not consistent asymmetries between the hemispheres. Focal or multifocal spikes may also be present; these are rarely abundant and may predominate on one side, but not consistently so, and are not associated with focal slowing [11]. During sleeping, focal and generalized spike-wave discharges may increase and acquire a typical polyspike component.

6.3.3 Ictal EEG

Generalized bilaterally synchronous single or multiple spike-and-wave discharges with 2–4 Hz frequency are commonly associated with all three seizures types that produce drop attacks, although spike-wave discharges are briefer for myoclonus.

The EMG correlate of the jerk is a burst of muscle activity lasting 100 ms; this is followed by a post-myoclonic silent period of EMG inhibition that lasts for 60–500 ms, which is synchronous for the recorded muscles and time-locked to the onset of the slow wave [78]. Both the brisk jerk and the post-myoclonic silent period concur to produce the typical drop.

AA corresponds of generalized irregular spike-wave discharges at 1.5–3 Hz. During NCSE, EEG shows no normal background activity, is characterized by diffuse and irregular spikes and slow waves persisting continuously throughout the episode, and is in combination with erratic myoclonus recorded on the EMG. Generalized tonic seizures correspond to burst of generalized spikes during sleep and eventually wakefulness.

6.4 Etiology

Patients with Doose syndrome have probably a multifactorial inheritance, some of the first to be diagnosed with SCN1A mutations, but others have also been found to have sodium channel subunit beta-1 (SCN1B) and gamma-aminobutyric acid receptor subunit gamma-2 (GABRG2) mutations. However, these genes have not been found consistently in sporadic cases [79].

6.5 Treatment

Ethosuximide is reported to be one of the more effective antiepileptic drugs (AED), especially when absence seizures are the primary seizure type. Valproic acid and lamotrigine are also beneficial; however, lamotrigine probably cause paradoxical worsening in individuals for whom myoclonic seizures are prominent [79]. Levetiracetam and zonisamide have been anecdotally used and may be helpful [23]. The ketogenic diet is a widely reported therapy for Doose syndrome and may be the most efficacious treatment; expert consensus guideline for optimal use of the ketogenic diet listed Doose syndrome as one of the principal indications for this treatment [79]. Seizure remission has been reported even without changes to medication, which suggest that spontaneous remission of seizures does occur.

7. Lennox-Gastaut syndrome (LGS)

7.1 Overview

LGS is an electroclinical syndrome defined by the Marseille School between 1966 and 1972 but was first reported by Lennox and Davis as an epilepsy starts in childhood and characterized by diffuse slow spike-waves (SSW) at <2.5 Hz and several types of seizures including tonic seizures, atypical absences, and "drop attacks" [81]. The electroclinical description proposed by Beaumanoir and adopted by the ILAE Classification Commission in 1989 concerns 2–4% of childhood epilepsies and affects boys more frequently than girls [81]. In about 70–75% of patients, LGS is associated with a variety of inherited or acquired structural anomalies or chromosomal disorders, whereas in the other 25–30%, there is no identifiable etiology [82]. Electroclinical phenotype is similar in spite of the different etiologies because of a common underlying mechanism [83]; functional neuroimaging has indicated that epileptic activity in LGS recruits widespread areas of association cortex and that tonic seizures are expressed through the reticular formation of the pons [84]. Other epileptic syndromes like frontal epilepsies with secondary bilateral synchrony, EMAS, DS, late-onset ES, atypical benign partial epilepsy of childhood, and ring chromosome 20 epilepsy syndrome are the differential diagnoses; thus, an exhaustive evaluation of the medical history along with an EEG during the wakefulness and sleep is very important for the accurate diagnosis of the syndrome.

7.2 Seizures: symptoms and semiology

Seizures start from 1 to 10 years but more frequently between 1 and 8 years; however, onset may occur in younger or older ages, even into adulthood. LGS may follow other types of epileptic syndromes, such as focal epilepsies, OS, and WS.

Diagnosis of LGS requires the following features: (1) many types of seizure, but inevitably include tonic seizures (TS) and atypical absences (AA), (2) cognitive impairment, and (3) typical interictal and ictal EEG patterns.

TS are mandatory for the diagnosis of LGS; they are diurnal and nocturnal, facilitated in NREM sleep, and typically occur in clusters. TS consist of sudden flexion of the neck and body, raising of the arms in flexion or extension, extension of the legs, and contraction of the face muscles. It continuing of the eyes and autonomic manifestations (apnea and facial flushing tachycardia), and can culminate as diffuse tremor (rapid, small-amplitude jerks affecting the whole body). They are axial and involve typically the proximal parts of the limbs, symmetrically or with unilateral predominance. TS can produce sudden falling, associated or not with brief loss of consciousness; the distal limb muscles are relatively spared.

AA is the second most common seizure, present in about 75% of patients. The main clinical manifestation is a brief lapse in consciousness, although some awareness may be preserved [82]; they are subtle and difficult to recognize without concurrent formal assessment of cognition and responsiveness. They are of long duration with the EEG discharge lasting >20 seconds, but their onset and termination are not always clinically discernible. Associated clinical features may include eyelid and mouth myoclonias and a decrease in muscle tone that may lead to a fall.

"Drop attacks" (sudden falls) are also frequent, affect 30–60% of patients, and are habitually related with a brief tonic seizure or an epileptic spasm [81]; the definition of seizure type that cause sudden falls most be requiring Video-EEG and polygraphic recording.

Drop attacks, and other types of seizures observed in LGS, are not specific to this syndrome; these are tonic-clonic, focal, myoclonic, and myoclonic-atonic. Episodes of SE may occur in about 60% of patients, consisting of alteration of consciousness with continuous SSW, and may be linked with serial tonic seizures [83].

7.3 Electroencephalography

7.3.1 Background

EEG is variable depending on etiology (structural, chromosomal, or idiopathic) and age, ranging from almost normal to, most often, poorly structured without physiological features and generally altered by continuous interictal abnormalities.

7.3.2 Interictal abnormalities

Generalized interictal features during the wakefulness and sleep are mandatory for diagnosis of LGS [11].

In wakefulness, high-amplitude, diffuse, and synchronous SSW at 1.5–2.5 Hz is typical. Slow SSW has maximal amplitude over frontal areas and ranges in duration from a few seconds to a few minutes or sub-continuous. The complexes typically consist of a spike (duration < 70 ms) or a sharp wave (70–200 ms), followed first by a positive deep and then by a negative wave (300–500 ms) [81]. Such stimuli, as eye opening, noise, calling the patient's name, and pain, tend to decline the occurrence or terminate SSW [81]; on the other hand, relaxation and drowsiness favor their occurrence. Hyperventilation (HV) and intermittent photic stimulation (IPS) usually have little influence on the SSW activity.

Characteristic features during sleeping are:

- SSW discharges that are activated during slow sleep, with more marked tendency toward bilateral synchrony than in wakefulness.
- Bursts of high-amplitude generalized polyspikes and polyspike-waves.

- "Paroxysmal fast activity" (PFA), which consists of sequences of rhythmic activity at 10–25 Hz and lasts for a few seconds (2–10 seconds) during NREM sleep. PFA is an essential diagnostic criterion.

These may be subclinical or accompanied by subtle change of axial muscle tone, which is detectable only by EMG electrodes as the ictal expression of a tonic seizure [81]. Interictal abnormalities and seizures decrease in REM sleep.

Focal abnormalities are usually present in patients with structural lesions; they are non-specific and depend on the underlying pathology: focal or multifocal spikes, spike-waves, polyspikes, slow waves, and focal bursts of rapid rhythms.

7.3.3 Ictal EEG

EEG pattern associated with typical seizures of LGS are:

- TS correspond to fast bilateral rhythmic spikes at 15–25 Hz. Amplitude is low at onset but increases as the discharge progresses, preponderating over the anterior areas and the vertex; occasionally diffuse slow waves follow after the end of the seizure [81].

- AA is concomitant with an irregular, diffuse, high-amplitude, more or less symmetric SSW that predominates over the frontal areas. AA may be difficult to differentiate from the interictal SSW pattern.

7.4 Etiology

LGS is classified as genetic, structural or metabolic, or unknown. Approximately 70% of children with LGS have symptomatic. The underlying etiologies include a history of encephalitis, meningitis, tuberous sclerosis, brain malformations (e.g., cortical dysplasias), birth asphyxia, and trauma. LGS may also follow the diagnosis of West syndrome [23]. If unknown, then it can be either idiopathic or cryptogenic. Idiopathic refers to unknown etiology with the underlying cause being suspected as genetic; in contrast to cryptogenic, the underlying cause is also not known but is presumed to be structural or metabolic. The causative role of mutations in other genes (such as GABRB3, ALG13, SCN8A, STXBP1, DNM1, FOXG1, or CHD2) has been elucidated in recent exome studies or in case reports in patients with LGS without a history of infantile spasms [85].

7.5 Treatment and prognosis

The long-term prognosis varies and has not improved using new AED as compared with earlier prescribed drugs [86].

Valproate is a first-choice drug, which has an effect in multiple seizure types including drop attacks; useful combinations are with clobazam, ethosuximide, lamotrigine, levetiracetam, topiramate, zonisamide, and rufinamide. We should avoid too many drugs as well as carbamazepine, oxcarbazepine, and vigabatrin, which may deteriorate some types of seizures. Felbamate carries the risk of aplastic anemia and hepatic failure and is used in exceptional cases [17].

Alternative treatment options for LGS include ketogenic diet, vagal nerve stimulation (VNS) or thalamic electrical stimulation, and corpus callosotomy (CC) [87]. VNS and CC showed more than 50% reduction in seizure frequency in patients with LGS. A study showed that CC may be more beneficial than VNS only in "drop attack" seizures [87], while another study did not show any significant difference between the two procedures [88].

Prognosis is typically poor with children having seizures into adulthood and 75–95% with intellectual disability and behavioral and psychiatric disorders [82]. The risk of death is increased, compared with their peers of the same age, usually due to seizures and falls.

8. Encephalopathy with electrical status epilepticus during slow sleep (ESES)

8.1 Overview

The term "electrical status epilepticus during sleeping" which was first described by Tassinari [1] refers to the EEG pattern (continuous spike-wave complexes exclusively during non-rapid eye movement (NREM) sleep), with a spike-wave index accounting for at least 80–85% of slow sleep. Other concept, "continuous spikes and waves during sleeping" (CSWS) are considered synonymous of ESES, but indicates both, EEG features and clinical neuropsychological characteristics, of this EE [89, 90].

Encephalopathy with ESES is an EE characterized by seizures of various types and neurological deterioration in cognitive, motor, and behavioral areas. The encephalopathy is caused by a prominent activation of epileptic abnormalities during NREM sleep [11]. Anti-seizure drugs, immune modulatory agents, and surgery [91] have been used to treat conditions associated with ESES. In spite of the long-term favorable outcome of epilepsy and ESES, the prognosis is protected because of the persistence of severe cognitive and behavioral disturbances in about a half of the patients.

8.2 Seizures: symptoms and semiology

ESES syndrome is manifest with epilepsy and encephalopathy:

1. Epilepsy onset can fluctuate from 2 to 12 years, with a peak at about 4–5 years, and can appear before the identification of ESES pattern. Mostly, seizures are present during ESES, but in others there is no history of clinical seizures at any time. Semiology and frequency of seizures can vary; the presence of TS during sleeping excludes this diagnosis. Three groups of seizures type have been proposed: [11].
    - Motor seizures, rare and nocturnal during the evolution of the syndrome
    - Unilateral partial motor seizures or secondary TCGS, principally occurring during sleeping
    - Rare nocturnal seizures in which AA develops during the course of ESES, often associated with negative myoclonus or atonic components leading to sudden falls
2. Encephalopathy manifests at the beginning or the worsening of neuropsychological troubles, which include global cognitive regression and various degrees of language impairment (acquired aphasia), behavioral disorders (hyperactivity, attention deficits, and disturbances of personality), and deterioration of motor skills (dystonia, dyspraxia, ataxia, and negative myoclonus) [11].

8.3 Electroencephalography

8.3.1 Background

During the wakefulness, it depends on the underlying etiology.

8.3.2 Interictal abnormalities

During the wakefulness, the EEG is characterized by focal or multifocal slow spikes, frequently intermixed with diffuse slow spikes and waves. In some children, the interictal EEG pattern may be similar to those observed in idiopathic focal epilepsies; in other cases, a background asymmetry, the presence of polyspikes or repetitive fast spikes, or other features may indicate underlying structural pathologies (e.g., disorders of neuronal migration). These interictal EEG abnormalities may increase when ESES starts; in addition, diffuse bursts of 2–3-Hz spike-and-wave discharges may appear [11].

The typical EEG pattern consisted of continuous or sub-continuous slow spike-and-waves, at 1.5–2.5 Hz, persisting through all NREM sleep; it appears immediately after patients fall asleep. This EEG pattern is commonly observed between 4 and 14 years and develops 1 or 2 years after the onset of seizures.

The epileptic discharges can vary from mainly focal (frontal, centrotemporal, etc.) or multifocal to unilateral, or diffuse (occasionally with shifting from a unilateral to a diffuse pattern in the same patient). In the original description, a spike-wave index (SWIs), ranging from 85 to 100% and measured during overnight sleep EEG recording, was considered an essential feature for the diagnosis [92]; however, SWIs under 85% have been used for the diagnosis of ESES syndrome as well [11].

8.4 Etiology

The good outcome is the rule, independent of the etiology and is observed besides cortical malformations such as multilobar polymicrogyria. ESES syndrome has been associated with a few genes including neuroserpin/SRPX2 and ataxin 1/ATX1 [23]; most recently, pathogenic de novo involves genes previously associated with autism (MDGA2 and SHANK3), seizures (GRIN2A), or language impairment (CDH13) [93]. Furthermore, SLC9A6 mutations have been found in patients with Christianson syndrome and CSWS [94]. The reason for manifestation of ESES in most patients is not known [23].

9. Landau-Kleffner syndrome (LKS)

9.1 Overview

The first description of the Landau and Kleffner syndrome (LKS) is due to William Landau and Frank Kleffner, who in 1957 reported six children with different types of seizures and acquired aphasia [2]. No other descriptions were made until the 1980s, when different authors described several new cases [95].

LKS is a type of ESES syndrome which manifests with an acquired epileptic aphasia (auditory agnosia) that occurs in the child with already developed age-appropriate speech. Like ESES, LKS is characterized by epileptic EEG pattern particularly prominent during sleeping, with or without manifest clinical seizures. Although in the first descriptions LKS is not related to brain organic lesions, patients with LKS may have congenital or acquired brain lesions [11].

9.2 Epileptic aphasia and seizure symptoms and semiology

LKS appear usually from 2 to 8 years of age; almost 60% of cases have epilepsy as the first symptom, while aphasia in the rest. Aphasia is a verbal auditory agnosia with a subacute onset, followed by rapid reduction of spontaneous speech, with perseverations, paraphasias, phonological errors, and verbal stereotypies; it can progress to mutism. Aphasia frequently has a course with remissions and exacerbations, usually related to quantitative variations of paroxysmal activity during sleeping [2, 96, 97]. The duration of the language disorder is very variable, though if it persists unchanged for more than a year, spontaneous recovery is rare. After a flexible time, aphasia stabilizes and regularly recovers before adulthood [98].

Although between 70 and 80% of patients present with epileptic seizures, these tend to be rare, sometimes a single seizure, which often occurs during sleeping. The seizures present clinical heterogeneity that includes subtle motor events such as ocular flicker, ocular deviation, simple motor focal seizures, AA, unilateral motor seizures, and, eventually, GTCS. CPSs are uncommon, while tonic seizures have never been reported. The course of the epilepsy is typically benign and seizures respond excellent to AED. Seizures eventually disappear over time, generally by about the age of 15 years [98].

9.3 Electroencephalography

9.3.1 Background

Normal.

9.3.2 Interictal paroxysmal abnormalities

9.3.2.1 Wakefulness

High-amplitude repetitive spikes and spike-waves with variable topography over time. Unilateral discharges are more common early in the course of LKS, habitually located in the temporal regions (>50% of the children) or in the parietal-occipital regions (around 30% of the children). Generalized spike-wave discharges have also been reported.

9.3.2.2 Sleep

At the beginning of sleep, epileptic discharges (ED) are also initiated. The ED can be partial, often on posterior temporal topography. Unilateral subclinical discharges can be detected alternating between both hemispheres. During the development of the disease, the EEG of the sleep will show a pattern of bilateral spike-wave activity, continuous or sub-continuous, during more than 85% of the NREM sleep time (ESES syndrome) [97]. LKS is a clinical subtype included in the wide spectrum of the clinical manifestations of ESES syndrome.

9.4 Etiology

In most patients the cause of LKS remains unknown. Autoimmune etiology has been suspected because of minor immunological irregularities reported in a number of patients and because of the response of LKS patients to immunotherapy [23]. Mutations in GRIN2A (16p13.2) have been reported as a major genetic cause of LKS and of the syndrome known as epileptic encephalopathy with continuous spikes and waves during slow-wave sleep (CSWS) [99]. Children with LKS have, most of the time, a normal development until the start of language regression. Seizures of LKS often respond well to treatment with AED, but the speech and language impairments often persist, despite seizure control [100]. Occasional cases can be secondary to structural lesions such as benign temporal lobe tumors with improvement after focal resection [101].

9.5 Treatment of encephalopathies with CSWS, including LKS

The aim of treatment is to stop seizures and eliminate epileptic discharges in the EEG; this will prevent and reverse cognitive decline in the idiopathic group and will prevent any further deterioration predetermined by the underlying pathology [18]. For it, early diagnosis and rapid appropriate and effective treatment are required.

Seizures in LKS are easier to control than seizures in CSWS. Many old and new AEDs are effective, depending on the seizure types. Valproate, sulthiame, benzodiazepines, ethosuximide, levetiracetam, lamotrigine, intravenous immunoglobulin (IVIG), corticosteroids, and ketogenic diet could be effective. The sodium channel-blocking AEDs are contraindicated [17]. In some cases, with severe linguistic impairment, subpial intracortical transections have been successful.

10. Conclusion

Epileptic encephalopathy is defined as a condition where the epileptic activity itself may contribute to the severe neurological and cognitive impairment seen, over and above that would be expected from the underlying pathology alone. The epilepsy syndromes at high risk of this are a disparate group of conditions characterized by epileptic seizures that are difficult to treat and developmental delay. Knowledge of the various severe epilepsy syndromes is vital to understanding the rationale for treatment.

Conflict of interest

The authors declare no conflicts of interest.

DOI: http://dx.doi.org/10.5772/intechopen.85378

Author details

Otman Fernandez-Concepcion* and Melvin Lopez-Jimenez
Baca Ortiz Hospital, Quito, Ecuador

*Address all correspondence to: otmanfc@gmail.com

References

[1] Capovilla G, Wolf P, Beccaria F, Avanzini G. The history of the concept of epileptic encephalopathy. Epilepsia. 2013;**54**(Suppl 8):2-5

[2] Landau WM, Kleffner FR. Syndrome of acquired aphasia with convulsive disorder in children. Neurology. 1957;**7**(8):523-530

[3] Engel J, International League Against Epilepsy (ILAE). A proposed diagnostic scheme for people with epileptic seizures and with epilepsy: Report of the ILAE task force on classification and terminology. Epilepsia. 2001;**42**(6):796-803

[4] Engel J. Report of the ILAE classification core group. Epilepsia. 2006;**47**(9):1558-1568

[5] Berg AT, Berkovic SF, Brodie MJ, Buchhalter J, Cross JH, van Emde BW, et al. Revised terminology and concepts for organization of seizures and epilepsies: Report of the ILAE commission on classification and terminology, 2005-2009. Epilepsia. 2010;**51**(4):676-685

[6] Beal JC, Cherian K, Moshe SL. Early-onset epileptic encephalopathies: Ohtahara syndrome and early myoclonic encephalopathy. Pediatric Neurology. 2012;**47**(5):317-323

[7] Ohtahara S, Ohtsuka Y, Yamatogi Y, Oka E. The early-infantile epileptic encephalopathy with suppression-burst: Developmental aspects. Brain & Development. 1987;**9**(4):371-376

[8] Yamatogi Y, Ohtahara S. Early-infantile epileptic encephalopathy with suppression-bursts, Ohtahara syndrome; its overview referring to our 16 cases. Brain & Development. 2002;**24**(1):13-23

[9] Ohtahara S, Yamatogi Y. Ohtahara syndrome: With special reference to its developmental aspects for differentiating from early myoclonic encephalopathy. Epilepsy Research. 2006;**70**(Suppl 1):S58-S67

[10] Guerrini R, Aicardi J. Epileptic encephalopathies with myoclonic seizures in infants and children (severe myoclonic epilepsy and myoclonic-astatic epilepsy). Journal of Clinical Neurophysiology. 2003;**20**(6):449-461

[11] Koutroumanidis M, Arzimanoglou A, Caraballo R, Goyal S, Kaminska A, Laoprasert P, et al. The role of EEG in the diagnosis and classification of the epilepsy syndromes: A tool for clinical practice by the ILAE neurophysiology task force (part 2). Epileptic Disorders. 2017;**19**(4):385-437

[12] Al-Futaisi A, Banwell B, Ochi A, Hew J, Chu B, Oishi M, et al. Hidden focal EEG seizures during prolonged suppressions and high-amplitude bursts in early infantile epileptic encephalopathy. Clinical Neurophysiology. 2005;**116**(5):1113-1117

[13] Fusco L, Vigevano F. Ictal clinical electroencephalographic findings of spasms in West syndrome. Epilepsia. 1993;**34**(4):671-678

[14] Hwang S-K, Kwon S. Early-onset epileptic encephalopathies and the diagnostic approach to underlying causes. Korean Journal of Pediatrics. 2015;**58**(11):407-414

[15] Nabbout R, Desguerre I, Sabbagh S, Depienne C, Plouin P, Dulac O, et al. An unexpected EEG course in Dravet syndrome. Epilepsy Research. 2008;**81**(1):90-95

[16] Cohen R, Basel-Vanagaite L, Goldberg-Stern H, Halevy A, Shuper A, Feingold-Zadok M, et al. Two siblings with early infantile myoclonic encephalopathy due to mutation in

the gene encoding mitochondrial glutamate/H+ symporter SLC25A22. European Journal of Paediatric Neurology. 2014;**18**(6):801-805

[17] Covanis A. Epileptic encephalopathies (including severe epilepsy syndromes). Epilepsia. 2012;**53**(Suppl 4):114-126

[18] Covanis A. Clinical management of epileptic encephalopathies of childhood and infancy. Expert Review of Neurotherapeutics. 2014;**14**(6):687-701

[19] Scheffer IE, Berkovic S, Capovilla G, Connolly MB, French J, Guilhoto L, et al. ILAE classification of the epilepsies: Position paper of the ILAE Commission for Classification and Terminology. Epilepsia. 2017;**58**(4):512-521

[20] Vigevano F, Fusco L, Pachatz C. Neurophysiology of spasms. Brain & Development. 2001;**23**(7):467-472

[21] Watanabe K, Negoro T, Okumura A. Symptomatology of infantile spasms. Brain & Development. 2001;**23**(7):453-466

[22] Hrachovy RA, Frost JD. Infantile spasms. Handbook of Clinical Neurology. 2013;**111**:611-618

[23] Shbarou R, Mikati MA. The expanding clinical spectrum of genetic pediatric epileptic encephalopathies. Seminars in Pediatric Neurology. 2016;**23**(2):134-142

[24] Epi4K Consortium, Epilepsy Phenome/Genome Project, Allen AS, Berkovic SF, Cossette P, Delanty N, et al. De novo mutations in epileptic encephalopathies. Nature. 2013;**501**(7466):217-221

[25] Hussain SA, Shinnar S, Kwong G, Lerner JT, Matsumoto JH, Wu JY, et al. Treatment of infantile spasms with very high dose prednisolone before high dose adrenocorticotropic hormone. Epilepsia. 2014;**55**(1):103-107

[26] Fisher RS, Cross JH, French JA, Higurashi N, Hirsch E, Jansen FE, et al. Operational classification of seizure types by the international league against epilepsy: Position paper of the ILAE commission for classification and terminology. Epilepsia. 2017;**58**(4):522-530

[27] Pellock JM, Hrachovy R, Shinnar S, Baram TZ, Bettis D, Dlugos DJ, et al. Infantile spasms: A U.S. consensus report. Epilepsia. 2010;**51**(10):2175-2189

[28] Oguni H, Yanagaki S, Hayashi K, Imai K, Funatsuka M, Kishi T, et al. Extremely low-dose ACTH step-up protocol for West syndrome: Maximum therapeutic effect with minimal side effects. Brain & Development. 2006;**28**(1):8-13

[29] Baram TZ, Mitchell WG, Tournay A, Snead OC, Hanson RA, Horton EJ. High-dose corticotropin (ACTH) versus prednisone for infantile spasms: A prospective, randomized, blinded study. Pediatrics. 1996;**97**(3):375-379

[30] Lux AL, Edwards SW, Hancock E, Johnson AL, Kennedy CR, Newton RW, et al. The United Kingdom infantile spasms study comparing vigabatrin with prednisolone or tetracosactide at 14 days: A multicentre, randomised controlled trial. Lancet. 2004;**364**(9447):1773-1778

[31] Kossoff EH, Hartman AL, Rubenstein JE, Vining EPG. High-dose oral prednisolone for infantile spasms: An effective and less expensive alternative to ACTH. Epilepsy & Behavior. 2009;**14**(4):674-676

[32] Knupp KG, Coryell J, Nickels KC, Ryan N, Leister E, Loddenkemper T, et al. Response to treatment in a prospective national infantile spasms cohort. Annals of Neurology. 2016;**79**(3):475-484

[33] Wanigasinghe J, Arambepola C, Sri Ranganathan S, Sumanasena S, Attanapola G. Randomized, single-blind, parallel clinical trial on efficacy of oral prednisolone versus intramuscular corticotropin on immediate and continued spasm control in west syndrome. Pediatric Neurology. 2015;**53**(3):193-199

[34] Riikonen R, Donner M. ACTH therapy in infantile spasms: Side effects. Archives of Disease in Childhood. 1980;**55**(9):664-672

[35] Appleton RE, Peters AC, Mumford JP, Shaw DE. Randomised, placebo-controlled study of vigabatrin as first-line treatment of infantile spasms. Epilepsia. 1999;**40**(11):1627-1633

[36] Elterman RD, Shields WD, Mansfield KA, Nakagawa J, US Infantile Spasms Vigabatrin Study Group. Randomized trial of vigabatrin in patients with infantile spasms. Neurology. 2001;**57**(8):1416-1421

[37] Lux AL, Edwards SW, Hancock E, Johnson AL, Kennedy CR, Newton RW, et al. The United Kingdom infantile spasms study (UKISS) comparing hormone treatment with vigabatrin on developmental and epilepsy outcomes to age 14 months: A multicentre randomised trial. Lancet Neurology. 2005;**4**(11):712-717

[38] Darke K, Edwards SW, Hancock E, Johnson AL, Kennedy CR, Lux AL, et al. Developmental and epilepsy outcomes at age 4 years in the UKISS trial comparing hormonal treatments to vigabatrin for infantile spasms: A multi-Centre randomised trial. Archives of Disease in Childhood. 2010;**95**(5):382-386

[39] Vigevano F, Cilio MR. Vigabatrin versus ACTH as first-line treatment for infantile spasms: A randomized, prospective study. Epilepsia. 1997;**38**(12):1270-1274

[40] Chiron C, Dumas C, Jambaqué I, Mumford J, Dulac O. Randomized trial comparing vigabatrin and hydrocortisone in infantile spasms due to tuberous sclerosis. Epilepsy Research. 1997;**26**(2):389-395

[41] Schwarz MD, Li M, Tsao J, Zhou R, Wu YW, Sankar R, et al. A lack of clinically apparent vision loss among patients treated with vigabatrin with infantile spasms: The UCLA experience. Epilepsy & Behavior. 2016;**57**(Pt A):29-33

[42] O'Callaghan FJK, Edwards SW, Alber FD, Hancock E, Johnson AL, Kennedy CR, et al. Safety and effectiveness of hormonal treatment versus hormonal treatment with vigabatrin for infantile spasms (ICISS): A randomised, multicentre, open-label trial. Lancet Neurology. 2017;**16**(1):33-42

[43] Suzuki Y, Baba H, Toda K, Ono T, Kawabe M, Fukuda M. Early total corpus callosotomy in a patient with cryptogenic West syndrome. Seizure. 2013;**22**(4):320-323

[44] Salar S, Moshé SL, Galanopoulou AS. Metabolic etiologies in West syndrome. Epilepsia Open. 2018;**3**(2):134-166

[45] Debus OM, Kurlemann G, Study Group. Sulthiame in the primary therapy of West syndrome: A randomized double-blind placebo-controlled add-on trial on baseline pyridoxine medication. Epilepsia. 2004;**45**(2):103-108

[46] Dravet C. The core Dravet syndrome phenotype. Epilepsia. 2011;**52**(Suppl 2):3-9

[47] Bureau M, Dalla BB. Electroencephalographic characteristics of Dravet syndrome. Epilepsia. 2011;**52**(Suppl 2):13-23

[48] Specchio N, Balestri M, Trivisano M, Japaridze N, Striano P, Carotenuto A,

et al. Electroencephalographic features in dravet syndrome: Five-year follow-up study in 22 patients. Journal of Child Neurology. 2012;**27**(4):439-444

[49] Caraballo RH, Fejerman N. Dravet syndrome: A study of 53 patients. Epilepsy Research. 2006;**70**(Suppl 1):S231-S238

[50] Nieh SE, Sherr EH. Epileptic encephalopathies: New genes and new pathways. Neurotherapeutics. 2014;**11**(4):796-806

[51] Nabbout R, Gennaro E, Dalla Bernardina B, Dulac O, Madia F, Bertini E, et al. Spectrum of SCN1A mutations in severe myoclonic epilepsy of infancy. Neurology. 2003;**60**(12):1961-1967

[52] Kalume F. Sudden unexpected death in Dravet syndrome: Respiratory and other physiological dysfunctions. Respiratory Physiology & Neurobiology. 2013;**189**(2):324-328

[53] Helbig I, Tayoun AAN. Understanding genotypes and phenotypes in epileptic encephalopathies. Molecular Syndromology. 2016;**7**(4):172-181

[54] Wirrell EC. Treatment of Dravet syndrome. The Canadian Journal of Neurological Sciences. 2016;**43**(Suppl 3): S13-S18

[55] Wolff M, Cassé-Perrot C, Dravet C. Severe myoclonic epilepsy of infants (Dravet syndrome): Natural history and neuropsychological findings. Epilepsia. 2006;**47**(Suppl 2):45-48

[56] Ragona F, Brazzo D, De Giorgi I, Morbi M, Freri E, Teutonico F, et al. Dravet syndrome: Early clinical manifestations and cognitive outcome in 37 Italian patients. Brain & Development. 2010;**32**(1):71-77

[57] Chiron C, Marchand MC, Tran A, Rey E, d'Athis P, Vincent J, et al. Stiripentol in severe myoclonic epilepsy in infancy: A randomised placebo-controlled syndrome-dedicated trial. STICLO study group. Lancet. 2000;**356**(9242):1638-1642

[58] Chhun S, Troude P, Villeneuve N, Soufflet C, Napuri S, Motte J, et al. A prospective open-labeled trial with levetiracetam in pediatric epilepsy syndromes: Continuous spikes and waves during sleep is definitely a target. Seizure. 2011;**20**(4):320-325

[59] Caraballo RH. Nonpharmacologic treatments of Dravet syndrome: Focus on the ketogenic diet. Epilepsia. 2011;**52**(Suppl 2):79-82

[60] Laux L, Blackford R. The ketogenic diet in Dravet syndrome. Journal of Child Neurology. 2013;**28**(8):1041-1044

[61] Sakauchi M, Oguni H, Kato I, Osawa M, Hirose S, Kaneko S, et al. Retrospective multiinstitutional study of the prevalence of early death in Dravet syndrome. Epilepsia. 2011;**52**(6):1144-1149

[62] Genton P, Velizarova R, Dravet C. Dravet syndrome: The long-term outcome. Epilepsia. 2011;**52**(Suppl 2): 44-49

[63] Coppola G, Plouin P, Chiron C, Robain O, Dulac O. Migrating partial seizures in infancy: A malignant disorder with developmental arrest. Epilepsia. 1995;**36**(10):1017-1024

[64] Barcia G, Fleming MR, Deligniere A, Gazula V-R, Brown MR, Langouet M, et al. De novo gain-of-function KCNT1 channel mutations cause malignant migrating partial seizures of infancy. Nature Genetics. 2012;**44**(11): 1255-1259

[65] McTague A, Appleton R, Avula S, Cross JH, King MD, Jacques TS, et al. Migrating partial seizures of infancy: Expansion of the electroclinical, radiological and pathological disease

spectrum. Brain. 2013;**136**(Pt 5): 1578-1591

[66] Ohba C, Kato M, Takahashi N, Osaka H, Shiihara T, Tohyama J, et al. De novo KCNT1 mutations in early-onset epileptic encephalopathy. Epilepsia. 2015;**56**(9):e121-e128

[67] Caraballo RH, Fontana E, Darra F, Cassar L, Negrini F, Fiorini E, et al. Migrating focal seizures in infancy: Analysis of the electroclinical patterns in 17 patients. Journal of Child Neurology. 2008;**23**(5):497-506

[68] Coppola G. Malignant migrating partial seizures in infancy: An epilepsy syndrome of unknown etiology. Epilepsia. 2009;**50**(Suppl 5):49-51

[69] Okuda K, Yasuhara A, Kamei A, Araki A, Kitamura N, Kobayashi Y. Successful control with bromide of two patients with malignant migrating partial seizures in infancy. Brain & Development. 2000;**22**(1):56-59

[70] Nabatame S, Saito Y, Sakuma H, Komaki H, Nakagawa E, Sugai K, et al. Bromoderma in a patient with migrating partial seizures in infancy. Epilepsy Research. 2010;**91**(2-3):283-288

[71] Cilio MR, Bianchi R, Balestri M, Onofri A, Giovannini S, Di Capua M, et al. Intravenous levetiracetam terminates refractory status epilepticus in two patients with migrating partial seizures in infancy. Epilepsy Research. 2009;**86**(1):66-71

[72] Djuric M, Kravljanac R, Tadic B, Mrlješ-Popovic N, Appleton RE. Long-term outcome in children with infantile spasms treated with vigabatrin: A cohort of 180 patients. Epilepsia. 2014;**55**(12):1918-1925

[73] Vendrame M, Poduri A, Loddenkemper T, Kluger G, Coppola G, Kothare SV. Treatment of malignant migrating partial epilepsy of infancy with rufinamide: Report of five cases. Epileptic Disorders. 2011;**13**(1):18-21

[74] Irahara K, Saito Y, Sugai K, Nakagawa E, Saito T, Komaki H, et al. Effects of acetazolamide on epileptic apnea in migrating partial seizures in infancy. Epilepsy Research. 2011;**96**(1-2):185-189

[75] Doose H, Gerken H, Leonhardt R, Völzke E, Völz C. Centrencephalic myoclonic-astatic petit mal. Clinical and genetic investigation. Neuropädiatrie. 1970;**2**(1):59-78

[76] Kaminska A, Oguni H. Lennox-Gastaut syndrome and epilepsy with myoclonic-astatic seizures. Handbook of Clinical Neurology. 2013;**111**:641-652

[77] Doose H. Myoclonic-astatic epilepsy. Epilepsy Research Supplement. 1992;**6**:163-168

[78] Oguni H, Hayashi K, Imai K, Funatsuka M, Sakauchi M, Shirakawa S, et al. Idiopathic myoclonic-astatic epilepsy of early childhood-nosology based on electrophysiologic and long-term follow-up study of patients. Advances in Neurology. 2005;**95**: 157-174

[79] Kelley SA, Kossoff EH. Doose syndrome (myoclonic-astatic epilepsy): 40 years of progress. Developmental Medicine and Child Neurology. 2010;**52**(11):988-993

[80] Trivisano M, Specchio N, Cappelletti S, Di Ciommo V, Claps D, Specchio LM, et al. Myoclonic astatic epilepsy: An age-dependent epileptic syndrome with favorable seizure outcome but variable cognitive evolution. Epilepsy Research. 2011;**97**(1-2):133-141

[81] Markand ON. Lennox-Gastaut syndrome (childhood epileptic encephalopathy). Journal of Clinical Neurophysiology. 2003;**20**(6):426-441

[82] Camfield PR. Definition and natural history of Lennox-Gastaut syndrome. Epilepsia. 2011;**52**(Suppl 5):3-9

[83] Arzimanoglou A, French J, Blume WT, Cross JH, Ernst J-P, Feucht M, et al. Lennox-Gastaut syndrome: A consensus approach on diagnosis, assessment, management, and trial methodology. Lancet Neurology. 2009;**8**(1):82-93

[84] Archer JS, Warren AEL, Jackson GD, Abbott DF. Conceptualizing Lennox-Gastaut syndrome as a secondary network epilepsy. Frontiers in Neurology. 2014;**5**:225

[85] Mastrangelo M. Lennox-Gastaut syndrome: A state of the art review. Neuropediatrics. 2017;**48**(3):143-151

[86] Crumrine PK. Management of seizures in Lennox-Gastaut syndrome. Paediatric Drugs. 2011;**13**(2):107-118

[87] Lancman G, Virk M, Shao H, Mazumdar M, Greenfield JP, Weinstein S, et al. Vagus nerve stimulation vs. corpus callosotomy in the treatment of Lennox-Gastaut syndrome: A meta-analysis. Seizure. 2013;**22**(1):3-8

[88] You SJ, Kang H-C, Ko T-S, Kim HD, Yum M-S, Hwang YS, et al. Comparison of corpus callosotomy and vagus nerve stimulation in children with Lennox-Gastaut syndrome. Brain & Development. 2008;**30**(3):195-199

[89] Holmes GL, Lenck-Santini P-P. Role of interictal epileptiform abnormalities in cognitive impairment. Epilepsy & Behavior. 2006;**8**(3):504-515

[90] Parisi P, Spalice A, Nicita F, Papetti L, Ursitti F, Verrotti A, et al. "Epileptic encephalopathy" of infancy and childhood: Electro-clinical pictures and recent understandings. Current Neuropharmacology. 2010;**8**(4):409-421

[91] Loddenkemper T, Cosmo G, Kotagal P, Haut J, Klaas P, Gupta A, et al. Epilepsy surgery in children with electrical status epilepticus in sleep. Neurosurgery. 2009;**64**(2):328-337. Discussion 337

[92] Patry G, Lyagoubi S, Tassinari CA. Subclinical "electrical status epilepticus" induced by sleep in children. A clinical and electroencephalographic study of six cases. Archives of Neurology. 1971;**24**(3):242-252

[93] Lesca G, Rudolf G, Bruneau N, Lozovaya N, Labalme A, Boutry-Kryza N, et al. GRIN2A mutations in acquired epileptic aphasia and related childhood focal epilepsies and encephalopathies with speech and language dysfunction. Nature Genetics. 2013;**45**(9):1061-1066

[94] Zanni G, Barresi S, Cohen R, Specchio N, Basel-Vanagaite L, Valente EM, et al. A novel mutation in the endosomal Na+/H+ exchanger NHE6 (SLC9A6) causes Christianson syndrome with electrical status epilepticus during slow-wave sleep (ESES). Epilepsy Research. 2014;**108**(4):811-815

[95] Dulac O. Epileptic encephalopathy. Epilepsia. 2001;**42**(Suppl 3):23-26

[96] Mantovani JF, Landau WM. Acquired aphasia with convulsive disorder: Course and prognosis. Neurology. 1980;**30**(5):524-529

[97] Hirsch E, Marescaux C, Maquet P, Metz-Lutz MN, Kiesmann M, Salmon E, et al. Landau-Kleffner syndrome: A clinical and EEG study of five cases. Epilepsia. 1990;**31**(6):756-767

[98] Deonna T, Peter C, Ziegler AL. Adult follow-up of the acquired aphasia-epilepsy syndrome in childhood. Report of 7 cases. Neuropediatrics. 1989;**20**(3):132-138

[99] Lesca G, Rudolf G, Labalme A, Hirsch E, Arzimanoglou A, Genton P,

et al. Epileptic encephalopathies of the Landau-Kleffner and continuous spike and waves during slow-wave sleep types: Genomic dissection makes the link with autism. Epilepsia. 2012;**53**(9):1526-1538

[100] Caraballo RH, Cejas N, Chamorro N, Kaltenmeier MC, Fortini S, Soprano AM. Landau-Kleffner syndrome: A study of 29 patients. Seizure. 2014;**23**(2):98-104

[101] Mikati MA, El-Bitar MK, Najjar MW, Rbeiz JJ, Barada WH, Najjar VF, et al. A child with refractory complex partial seizures, right temporal ganglioglioma, contralateral continuous electrical status epilepticus, and a secondary Landau-Kleffner autistic syndrome. Epilepsy & Behavior. 2009;**14**(2):411-417

Chapter 7

Malignant Migrating Partial Seizures of Infancy (Coppola-Dulac Syndrome)

Alexey Kholin

Abstract

Malignant migrating partial seizures of infancy (MMPSI) is a rare and usually an unrecognized epileptic syndrome of infancy. The first publication was presented by Coppola and colleagues in 1995, and Dulac in 2005 summarized 24 patients' follow-up in the Saint Vincent de Paul Hospital in Paris. Clinical cases have demonstrated a new epileptic syndrome, different from previously described forms of epileptic encephalopathies of infancy for the whole world of epileptology. Seizure onset before the age of 6 months but commonly start within a few weeks of birth. In the age of 1 to 10 months seizures become very frequent, polymorphic and usually get clustered nature; mental and motor retardation is clear observed. Clinical manifestation of seizures may include head and eyes version, lateralized clonic eyelid twitchings, fixed gaze, tonic tension or clonias of one limb or hemispasms, axial tonic spasms, chewing or sucking movements, episodes of apnea, flushing, hypersalivation, and secondary generalized seizures. MMPSI could be also considered as a special type of infantile status epilepticus. Video-EEG monitoring plays the most important role in the MMPSI diagnosis. Ictal EEG patterns involve different areas of the cerebral cortex of both hemispheres; initial zone of ictal patterns shifts from one region to another. MMPSI is a drug-resistant epilepsy with serious prognosis.

Keywords: malignant migrating partial seizures of infancy, Coppola-Dulac syndrome, status epilepticus in infancy, epileptic encephalopathy

1. Introduction

Malignant migrating partial seizures of infancy (MMPSI) is a rare and usually an unrecognized epileptic syndrome of infancy. The International League Against Epilepsy defines this form of epilepsy as follows: seizure onset in the first 6 months of life, occurrence of almost continuous migrating polymorphous focal seizures, combined with multifocal ictal EEG discharges, and progressive deterioration of psychomotor development [1–3]. Exact criteria of MMPSI are not defined and are being developed. According to the draft of the Classification of the Epilepsies 2001, this syndrome refers to presumably symptomatic neocortical focal epilepsy. In the new Classification of the Epilepsies 2017 (ILAE 2017), MMPSI has not found a separate place, but it is implied that it includes in a group of developmental and epileptic encephalopathy.

This severe form of epilepsy was recently described. The first publication about migrating partial seizures of infancy was presented by Coppola and colleagues in 1995 [1], and then personal observations were done by Gerard et al. [4] and by Okuda et al. [5]. Veneselli et al. summarized previous observations and added three own cases [6]. Coppola et al. in their remarkable report (1995) based on neuropediatric department at the René Descartes University (Paris) presented 14 clinical cases of infants of both sexes with previously undescribed epileptic syndrome characterized by virtually continuous multifocal seizures. According to the classical authors description, the first seizures occurred average at the age of 3 months without any significant previous events. During the period from 1 to 10 months, seizures became very frequent. Seizures were focal and had different clinical characteristics; EEG revealed multiple epileptiform discharges arising independently and with migration during subsequent seizures from one cortical region to another. Patients had regression of psychomotor development, tetraparesis and severe muscular hypotonia of axial muscles. Three of 14 patients died: one at the age of 7 months, and other at the age of 7 and 8 years. Seizures were completely ceased only in two patients. In most cases the cause of the disease was not identified; and there were no family cases [1].

In 2005, Dulac summarized 24 patients' follow-up (the largest number of verified cases in the world) in the Saint Vincent de Paul Hospital in Paris. Marsh et al. [25] reported another six cases of MMPSI observed in the Philadelphia Children's Hospital University of Pennsylvania who met the criteria described by Coppola. Presented clinical cases have demonstrated a new epileptic syndrome, different from previously described forms of epileptic encephalopathies of infancy for the whole world epileptology [3].

Synonyms of this epileptic syndrome in the world scientific literature are malignant migrating partial seizures of infancy, migrating partial seizures of infancy, malignant epilepsy of infancy with migrating multifocal seizures, Coppola-Dulac syndrome, and most genetic verified cases, which can be referred to early infantile epileptic encephalopathy type 14 (EIEE14).

2. Etiology

In most MMPSI cases, etiology remains unknown; familial cases are rare. In observation by Dulac, relatives in 3 of 24 patients had febrile convulsions, and 4 patients had family history of epilepsy [3]. Multiple tests for inherited metabolism defects had negative results [7].

2.1 Monogenic mutations with Mendelian type of inheritance

The first genetic sequencing for identification mutations specific for MMPSI was carried out by Coppola et al. [8]. Was performed automatic sequencing of genes of potassium (KCNQ2, KCNQ3) and sodium (SCN1A, SCN2A) ion channels in three children with MMPSI but no mutation have been found. Mutational screening of chloride (CLCN2) ion channel gene revealed a homozygous mutation G2003C (exon 17), leading to a Ser/Thr substitution at the codon 668, in two of the three patients. But the same variation has been found in 38 out of 100 control alleles [8].

At present time a number of monogenic mutations were identified in patients with malignant migrating partial seizures of infancy. In catalog of human genes and genetic disorders – Online Mendelian Inheritance in Man (OMIM), we could find the following positions for MMPSI phenotype (**Table 1**):

Phenotype OMIM classification	Phenotype OMIM number	Gene/ locus	Gene OMIM number	Location	Mutation variants	Inheritance	References
Early infantile epileptic encephalopathy type 3 (EIEE3)	609304	SLC25A22	609302	11p15.5	gly110arg; (.0003)	AR	Poduri et al. [9]
Early infantile epileptic encephalopathy type 6 (EIEE6)	607208	SCN1A	182389	2q24.3	ala1669gly (.0023) arg862gly (.0024)	AD	Freilich et al. [10] Carranza Rojo et al. [11]
Early infantile epileptic encephalopathy type 13 (EIEE13)	614558	SCN8A	600702	12q13.13	phe846ser	AD	Ohba et al. [12]
Early infantile epileptic encephalopathy type 14 (EIEE14)	614959	KCNT1	608167	9q34.3	arg428glm (.0001) ala934thr (.0002) arg474his (.0003) ile760met (.0004) phe932ile (.0009) gly288ser (.0010)	AD	Barcia et al., [13] Vanderver et al. [14] Ishii et al. [15]
Early infantile epileptic encephalopathy type 16 (EIEE16)	615338	TBC1D24	613577	16p13.3	phe229ser (.0005) + cys156ter (.0006)	AR	Milh et al. [18]
Progressive microcephaly with seizures and cerebral and cerebellar atrophy (MSCCA)	615760	QARS	603727	3p21.31	tyr57his (.0003) + arg515trp (.0004)	AR	Zhang et al. [19]

Table 1.
Monogenic mutations as etiological factors of malignant migrating partial seizures of infancy

2.1.1 Early infantile epileptic encephalopathy type 3 (EIEE6; 609304)

Poduri et al. [9] reported about two sibs (brother and sister), born of consanguineous Saudi Arabian parents, with EIEE3 presenting MMPSI phenotype. EEG showed abnormal spikes in various brain regions. Neurological signs included hypotonia and brisk tendon reflexes; psychomotor development was delayed and subsequently arrested. Brain MRI was normal in the boy but showed delayed myelination and diffuse thinning of the corpus callosum in his sister. Two sibs had polymorphic seizures including bilateral and hemiclonic convulsions, flushing of the face, "staring," and eventually bilateral eyelid blinking. The seizures in both children were refractory to treatment. The boy developed seizure onset at 1 week of age and died at 14 months; the girl presented first seizures at 2 weeks of age and died at 47 months of age. They also had two healthy brothers. The research team analyzed consanguineous pedigree (parents are cousins) and obtained DNA from affected and unaffected family members, analyzed single nucleotide polymorphism (SNP) 500 K data to identify regions with evidence for linkage, performed whole-exome sequencing, analyzed homozygous variants in regions of linkage to identify a candidate gene, and performed functional studies of the candidate gene SLC25A22. In affected siblings, a homozygous c.328G-C transversion in the SLC25A22 gene was identified, resulting in a gly110-to-arg (G110R; 609302.0003) substitution at a highly conserved residue in the third transmembrane helix [9].

2.1.2 Early infantile epileptic encephalopathy type 6 (EIEE6; 607208)

It is a well-known fact that mutation in SCN1A is a leading etiological factor for severe myoclonic epilepsy of infancy (Dravet syndrome). OMIM genetic classification is early infantile epileptic encephalopathy type 6 (607208) with autosomal dominant inheritance. Nevertheless, Freilich et al. [10] have found a novel mutation in the SCN1A gene in the girl with MMPSI who died at the age of 9 months from recurrent status epilepticus (SE). This girl had a severe phenotype, with onset of seizures at age 10 weeks, progression to refractory recurrent seizures by age 5 months, SE of migrating multifocal seizures confirmed by EEG monitoring, progressive microcephaly, and profound psychomotor delay. By sequencing genomic DNA from blood, the heterozygous missense mutation c.C5006C > A transversion in the SCN1A gene, resulting in an ala1669-to-glu (A1669E; 182389.0023), which further was confirmed in brain DNA, was identified. The resulting amino acid substitution p.A1669E alters an evolutionarily conserved residue in an intracellular linker of domain 4 of the SCN1A sodium channel protein [10].

In a scientific group of Epilepsy Research Centre, Department of Medicine, University of Melbourne, Australia, Carranza Rojo et al. [11] have investigated 15 unrelated children with MMPSI for mutations in genes associated with infantile epileptic encephalopathies (SCN1A, CDKL5, STXBP1, PCDH19, and POLG). One girl with seizure onset at 2 weeks had heterozygous missense mutation de novo 2584C-G transversion in exon 14 of the SCN1A gene, resulting in an arg862-to-gly (R862G; 182389.0024) that affects the sodium channel by substitution in the voltage sensor segment S4 of the second protein domain. She had epilepsy onset of alternative hemiclonic seizures (Dravet-like onset) at the age of 2 weeks with developing status epilepticus of multifocal migrating seizure. Also, the girl had acquired microcephaly, developmental regression, and severe intellectual disability with much more severe phenotype than children with Dravet syndrome. And, another girl who developed MMPSI at the age of 2 months had de novo 11.06 Mb deletion of chromosome 2q24.2q31.1 encompassing more than 40 genes that included SCN1A. Screenings of CDKL5, STXBP1, and PCDH19 and the three common European mutations of POLG were negative [11].

Along with Dravet and MMPSI syndromes, mutation in SCN1A gene has been also associated with generalized epilepsy with febrile seizures plus type 2 (604403), familial febrile seizures type 3A (604403), and familial hemiplegic migraine type 3 (609634). All the diseases have autosomal dominant inheritance.

2.1.3 Early infantile epileptic encephalopathy type 13 (EIEE13; 614558)

Ohba et al. [12] identified in seven unrelated patients with early-onset epileptic encephalopathies seven different de novo heterozygous missense mutations in the SCN8A gene, and one of them had MMPSI. In a 5-year-old bedridden severe delayed and profound intellectual disabled Japanese boy by whole-exome sequencing, de novo previously not described mutation in SCN8A gene c.2537 T > C (p.Phe846Ser) was detected. He developed apnea seizures from the age of 2 months and further at 4 months demonstrated migrating hemiclonic convulsions increasing up to status epilepticus of multifocal migrating seizures. MRI has shown mild atrophy of the cerebellum and thin corpus callosum. High-dose combined antiepileptic therapy with phenobarbital, phenytoin, and lamotrigine, ketogenic diet, and vagus nerve stimulator (VNS) implantation are temporarily and partially effective [12].

Voltage-dependent sodium channels, such as SCN8A, are responsible for the initial membrane depolarization that occurs during generation of action potentials in most electrically excitable cells. Mutations in KCNT1 aside from EIEE13 also determine benign familial infantile seizures type 5 (OMIM 617080) and cognitive impairment with or without cerebellar ataxia (OMIM 614306) with autosomal dominant inheritance.

2.1.4 Early infantile epileptic encephalopathy type 14 (EIEE14; 614959)

Barcia et al. in 2012 had identified four different de novo heterozygous mutations in the KCNT1 gene (608167.0001–608167.0004) in 6 of 12 unrelated pediatric patients (50%) with clinically manifestation as MMPSI. The gene KCNT1 encodes a sodium-activated potassium channel that is widely expressed at the nervous system. Its activity contributes to the slow hyperpolarization as the neuronal membrane potential that follows repetitive firing. The C-terminal cytoplasmic domain interacts with a protein network, including FMRP (fragile X mental retardation protein), suggesting additional functions [13].

OMIM genetic classification for this type of MMPSI is early infantile epileptic encephalopathy type 14 (614959). At present time, the following allelic variants of KCNT1 gene mutation in patients with MMPSI were identified:

ARG428GLN (608167.0001 KCNT1). It was founded by Barcia et al. [13] in three unrelated patients of French origin and was identified as de novo heterozygous 1283G-A transition in exon 13 of the KCNT1 gene, resulting in an arg428-to-gln substitution at a highly conserved residue in the cytoplasmic C-terminal domain.

ALA934THR (608167.0002 KCNT1). In a child of French origin with MMPSI, Barcia et al. [13] identified a de novo heterozygous 2800G-A transition in exon 24 of the KCNT1 gene, resulting in an ala934-to-thr substitution at a highly conserved residue in the cytoplasmic C-terminal domain. The mutation was shown to cause constitutive activation of the sodium-activated potassium channel, mimicking the effects of phosphorylation of the C-terminal domain by protein kinase C activation.

ARG474HIS (608167.0003 KCNT1). It was identified in a patient of French origin with MMPSI by Barcia et al. [13] as de novo heterozygous 1421G-A transition in exon 15 of the KCNT1 gene, resulting in an arg474-to-his substitution at a highly conserved residue.

ILE760MET (608167.0004 KCNT1). It was also founded by Barcia et al. [13] in a child of Ukrainian origin with early clinical manifestation of MMPSI and was identified as de novo heterozygous 2280C-G transversion in exon 20 of the KCNT1 gene, resulting in an ile760-to-met substitution at a highly conserved residue.

All these mutations were identified by exome sequencing and also were confirmed by Sanger sequencing. Mutations were not found in 200 controls or in several large control databases [13].

PHE932ILE (608167.0009 KCNT1). Vanderver et al. [14] identified in an Australian boy the de novo heterozygous c.2794 T-A transversion in the KCNT1 gene, resulting in a phe932-to-ile substitution at a highly conserved residue in the cytoplasmic C-terminal domain. This mutation was found by whole-exome sequencing, confirmed by Sanger sequencing, and was not present in the 1000

Genomes Project or Exome Sequencing Project databases. Seizure onset was at age of 1 month with refractory myoclonic seizures that progressed to different polymorphic seizure types and status epilepticus. He also had microcephaly and severe developmental stagnation. Brain imaging showed serious delayed myelination, and EEG demonstrated background slowing with multifocal interictal discharges and occasional periods of burst suppression. The patient doesn't have classical MMPSI characteristics and survived (last observation at the age of 10) with a decrease of pharmacoresistant seizures at the age of 7 [14].

GLY288SER (608167.0010 KCNT1). Ishii et al. in two unrelated Japanese girls with MMPSI identified a de novo heterozygous c.862G-A transition in the KCNT1 gene, resulting in a gly288-to-ser substitution at a highly conserved residue in the pore region of the channel [15].

Kawasaki et al. described three infants with malignant migrating partial seizures with KCNT1 mutations accompanied by massive systemic to pulmonary collateral arteries with life-threatening hemoptysis and heart failure [16].

Madaan with colleagues from Child Neurology Division, Department of Pediatrics, All India Institutes of Medical Sciences (New Delhi, India), in 2018 identified a child with MMPSI who had a novel heterozygous missense mutation in exon 10 of the KCNT1 gene (chr9:138650308; c.808C > C/G (p.Q270E)). Neither quinidine nor ketogenic diet could control his seizures, and the child succumbed to his illness at 9 months of age [17].

My personal observation consists of two Russian girls with MMPSI having KCNT1 mutations: one with gly288ser (608167.0010 KCNT1) and the other with previously not described mutations c.1066C > T (arg356trp) in exome 12 (chr9:138656907C > T, rs752514808). So, it seems that KCNT1 is a major disease-associated gene for the MMPSI phenotype.

It is interesting that mutations in KCNT1 also determine another form of epilepsy – nocturnal frontal lobe epilepsy type 5. But the mutation is different from the cases of MMPSI and is marked .0005–.0008 (ARG928CYS, TYR796HIS, ARG398GLN, and MET896ILE).

2.1.5 Early infantile epileptic encephalopathy type 16 (EIEE14; 615338)

Milh et al. [18] identified compound heterozygosity for two mutations in exon 2 of the TBC1D24 gene (686 T-C transition, resulting in a phe229-to-ser, 613577.0005, and 468C-A transversion, resulting in a cys156-to-ter, 613577.0006) in two sisters with malignant migrating partial seizures of infancy. These girls early developed clonic seizures in the second month of life and subsequently demonstrated prolonged, almost continuous migrating seizures of different types with severe neurologic deterioration and lack of psychomotor development [18].

OMIM genetic classification for this type of MMPSI – early infantile epileptic encephalopathy type 16 (615338). The screening of TBC1D24 in an additional set of eight MMPSI patients observed by Milh and colleagues was negative. The TBC1D24 gene encodes a member of the Tre2-Bub2-Cdc16 (TBC) domain-containing RAB-specific GTPase-activating proteins, which coordinates peripheral membrane Rab proteins and other GTPases for the proper transport of intracellular vesicles. Coimmunoprecipitation studies showed that the phe229ser mutation impaired the interaction of TBC1D24 with adenosine diphosphate (ADP)-ribosylation factor 6 (ARF6, 600,464), and overexpression of the mutant protein in primary cortical neurons abolished the ability of TBC1D24 to increase neurite length and arborization, consistent with a loss of function [18].

Mutation in TBC1D24 gene has been also associated to infantile familial myoclonic epilepsy (OMIM 605021, autosomal recessive inheritance), DOORS syndrome (deafness, onychodystrophy, osteodystrophy, mental retardation, and seizures syndrome – OMIM 220500) with autosomal recessive inheritance, and also autosomal recessive deafness type 86 (614617), and autosomal dominant deafness type 65 (616044).

2.1.6 Progressive microcephaly with seizures and cerebral and cerebellar atrophy (MSCCA; 615760)

Zhang et al. [19] in four patients from two unrelated families with progressive microcephaly, intractable seizures, and cerebral and cerebellar atrophy (MSCCA; 615,760) identified compound heterozygous mutations in the QARS gene (603727.0001–603727.0004). The mutations were found by whole-exome sequencing and confirmed by Sanger sequencing. QARS (or GLnRS; 603,727) is a class I aminoacyl-tRNA synthetase. Aminoacyl-tRNA synthetases are enzymes that charge tRNAs with their cognate amino acids. The specificity of this reaction determines the fidelity of mRNA translation. At least one synthetase exists in the cytoplasm for each amino acid. QARS is essential for normal brain development. Studies in patient cells and expression of recombinant variants in *E. coli* showed that all four mutations caused a severe loss of QARS catalytic activity, consistent with a loss-of-function effect. Homozygous loss of QARS in zebrafish caused decreased brain and eye size and extensive cell death in the brain. Two sibs observed by Zhang et al. [19], born of unrelated French parents, had clinical and EEG signs of malignant migrating partial seizures of infancy and compound heterozygous mutations in the QARS gene, a c.169 T-C transition, resulting in a tyr57-to-his (603727.0003) substitution at a highly conserved residue in the N-terminal domain, and a c.1543C-T transition, resulting in an arg515-to-trp (603727.0004) substitution at a highly conserved residue in the catalytic domain. Patient cells showed decreased aminoacylation activity of QARS compared to control. Expression of recombinant arg515trp (.0004) in *E. coli* resulted in no QARS catalytic activity, whereas tyr57his (.0003) decreased QARS activity to less than 10% that of controls. In addition, the arg515trp mutation appeared to cause protein misfolding and aggregation, resulting in decreased expression of the soluble mutant protein [19].

2.1.7 Rhizomelic chondrodysplasia punctata type 2 (RCDP2; 222765)

On personal observation of MMPSI patients, one Russian boy with clinical and electroencephalographic pattern of mixed form (MMPSI and early myoclonic encephalopathy) had rhizomelic chondrodysplasia punctata type 2 (RCDP2; 222,765) from the group of peroxisomal metabolic diseases [20]. Rhizomelic chondrodysplasia punctata type 2 (RCDP2) is caused by homozygous or compound heterozygous mutation in the DHAPAT gene (GNPAT; 602,744), which encodes acyl-CoA:dihydroxyacetonephosphate acyltransferase, on chromosome 1q42. This peroxisomal disorder is characterized by disproportionately short stature primarily affecting the proximal parts of the extremities, a typical facial appearance including a broad nasal bridge, epicanthus, high-arched palate, micrognathia, dysplastic external ears, eye abnormalities-cataract and coloboma, congenital contractures, dwarfism, hypotonia, and severe mental retardation. Biochemically, plasmalogen synthesis and phytanic acid alpha-oxidation are defective.

2.2 Chromosome aberrations

At 2010 group of genetics from the Department of Pediatrics, University of Michigan (Ann Arbor, Michigan, USA), has found de novo 598 kb 16p11.2 microduplication in a boy with refractory MMPSI, who has developed seizures in 4 months and also has spastic quadriparesis, severe global developmental delay, hypotonia, and microcephaly [21].

In 2012 Poduri and colleagues from the Department of Neurology of Children's Hospital Boston (Massachusetts, USA) in a patient, born of consanguineous Palestinian parents, with clinical manifestation as MMPSI, identified a homozygous 486-kb deletion on chromosome 20p12.3 encompassing the promoter region and exons 1, 2, and 3 of the PLCB1 gene. The deletion breakpoints were mapped from 8,094,049–8,094,072 to 8,580,261–8,580,284 (GRCh37). The breakpoints lie within two LINE nuclear elements and likely arose from nonallelic homologous recombination. PLCB1 gene (607,120; locus 20p12.3) is responsible for early infantile epileptic encephalopathy type 12 (EIEE12; 613,722). Phospholipase C-beta (PLCB) catalyzes the generation of inositol 1,4,5-trisphosphate (IP3) and diacylglycerol (DAG) from phosphatidylinositol 4,5-bisphosphate (IP2), a key step in the intracellular transduction of many extracellular signals. The PLCB1 gene encodes a mammalian PLCB isoform that is expressed in cerebral cortex, hippocampus, amygdala, lateral septum, and olfactory bulb [22].

2.3 Other etiological factors

Most cases of MMPSI are considered as unknown etiology (cryptogenic). But also MMPSI had its symptomatic analogs including cases considered as dual pathology [1–3, 20, 23].

In two of three cases for the first time presented by Coppola et al., neuropathologic brain examination showed marked loss of hippocampal neurons in combination with gliosis in the CA1 sector of hippocampal pyramidal layer [1, 23].

Personal observation of 35 cases with MMPSI contains 12 children with symptomatic clinical-electroencephalographic copies of MMPSI (5 boys and 7 girls). Only two infants had cerebral dysgenesis: lissencephaly-pachygyria in one girl and polymicrogyria in another girl. Other ten children had severe perinatal hypoxic-ischemic CNS disturbances (four of them mixed with perinatal infections-cytomegalovirus, ureaplasma, chlamydia, herpes type 1) that caused serious brain damage, tetraparetic spastic form of cerebral palsy, and severe retardation in combination with epileptic encephalopathy. Their clinical and video-EEG signs demonstrated MMPSI picture.

3. Clinical signs

At the present time, at least about 100 cases of MMPSI appear to be described in the world literature. However, the number of publications has been steadily growing in recent years. Obviously, this serious disease is more common than diagnosed due to the low clinicians' awareness. In the structure of patients with onset of status epilepticus before 3 years of age (n = 267), a group of children with MMPSI consisted 4.9% (n = 13), and in the structure of infant with SE (n = 147) – 8.8% [24].

Both sexes are equally susceptible. According to Dulac, 20 children with MMPSI included 9 girls and 11 boys [3]. Disease onset varies in age from 1 week to 7 months of life (average – 3 months) [1, 4]. According to Marsh et al., seizures onset varied from the first days to 3 months (average – 25 days) [25].

In most cases, pattern of the first seizure includes motor component of one limb or half of the body; and 50% of the patients develop secondary generalization. In some cases after seizure onset, their frequency uncontrolled rapidly rises to status epilepticus. However, seizures could have longer duration, but at onset seizures often go unrecognized. Cases with autonomic manifestation (episodes of apnea, short blackouts with cyanosis or redness) are difficult to diagnose [3]. Thus, in observation by Gerard et al. [4], epileptic seizures with diffuse erythema and sweating with subsequent hiccups were reported as gastroesophageal reflux, and only a few weeks later, addition of focal seizures was noted, which made diagnosis obvious [4]. According to observations by Dulac, the initial period of the disease usually lasts from 1 week to 3 months (average – 45 days). During this period, seizures may be quite rare, for example, once a week [3].

In the age of 24 days to 10 months (mean 4.5 months), seizures become very frequent and polymorphic but usually are still focal. Seizures usually get clustered (serial) nature, mental and motor retardation is clear. Clinical manifestation of seizures may include head and eye version, lateralized eyeball twitching, fixed gaze, clonic eyelid twitching, tonic tension or clonic spasms of one limb or hemispasms, axial tonic spasms, chewing or sucking movements, episodes of apnea, flushing, hypersalivation, and secondary generalized seizures. One patient may have multiple different combinations of seizures. Typically, seizure duration is 1–4 minutes, but in some cases, it may persist up to several 1 of minutes, until the status epilepticus development. As far as the disease progresses, secondary generalized seizures became more frequent. Seizures are almost continuous or occur as a series 5–30 times per day, mainly on awakening and when falling asleep. Seizure periods may alternate with clear periods when seizures occur within 2–5 days continuously, and then there are several "light" days (the cyclic course of disease) [1–3, 26].

It should be considered that many seizures are hardly noticeable visually and often remain unrecognized for parents and medical staff. In particular, these are "volatile" paroxysms, as short episodes of apnea, episodes of eyes closing or eyes deviation, episodes of facial flushing, etc. Only video-EEG monitoring can prove the epileptic genesis of paroxysmal phenomena.

The course of the disease and the severity of clinical symptoms often have undulating pattern: a period of severe illness and permanent seizures may continue for several weeks, and then it is replaced by a relatively favorable period of the temporary seizure regression and some improvement in cognitive and motor functions. This phenomenon generates additional difficulties in controlling the quality of care as it is quite difficult to differentiate in which case the decrease in frequency and severity of seizures is a true response to therapy and in which case it is subject to the course of the disease.

Under personal observation of patients with MMPSI, age of seizure onset ranged from the 1st day of postnatal life up to 6 months of life. MMPSI were characterized by marked polymorphism (**Table 2**) and high frequency of epileptic seizures and were in fact a special form of infantile status epilepticus (SE) in the form of migrating multifocal SE. All patients had five or more types of epileptic seizures.

Neurological findings in MMPSI children marked with neurological impairment from birth-severe central tetraparesis, often with muscular hypotonia in the axial and limb muscles [1], microcephaly, strabismus, and athetoid hyperkinesis [25]-are common. Many patients in dynamics are unable to walk and sit without support and in severe cases are also unable to control the vertical head position, drink, and swallow. In all cases, there is mental retardation, usually severe, and visual agnosia [3].

Personal patients with MMPSI (n = 35) in neurological status had a high representation of various disorders: high level of stigmatization was observed in 15

Seizure types	Patients (n)	%
Tonic versive seizures	35	100
Tonic spasms	33	94.3
Ophthalmo-tonic seizures	35	100
Ophthalmo-clonic seizures	11	31.4
Atonic seizures	23	65.7
Dialeptic (pseudoabsences)	19	54.3
Pharyngo-oral seizures	18	51.4
Tongue clonus	7	20
Hemiclonic	19	54.3
Jacksonian march	11	31.4
Automotor	8	22.9
Apnea with cyanosis	14	40
Autonomic with vomiting	5	14.3
Focal myoclonic	18	51.4
Bilateral myoclonic	13	37.1
Fragmentary "erratic" myoclonus	5	14.3
GTCS	14	40
SE of migratory minor motor seizures	**35**	**100**
SE of inhibitory seizures	**12**	**34.3**
Hemiconvulsive SE	**11**	**31.4**
SE of tonic spasms	**10**	**28.6**
Myoclonic SE	**9**	**25.7**
SE of GTCS	**8**	**22.9**

Table 2.
Epileptic seizure types in patients with malignant migrating partial seizures of infancy (n=35)

patients (42.8%), 13 patients (37.1%) had microcephaly, and optic nerve atrophy was observed in 27 patients (77.1%). Disorders of bulbar innervation were observed in all patients, while in nine children (25.7%), these impairments were bulbar syndrome, and in 26 children (74.3%) – pseudobulbar syndrome. All patients with MMPSI had changes in the muscle tone: 10 children (28.6%) had spastic hypertonus, 16 children (45.7%) had diffuse muscle hypotonia, and 9 children had dystonic changes (25.7%). Severe movement disability with tetraparesis was formed in all of the children with MMPSI. Neurological disorders were expressed at birth (n = 16, 45.7%) or developed with the onset of seizures (n = 19, 54.3%) and tended to a steady progression in all the patients. All children with MMPSI had delay of motor and mental development (n = 35, 100%), up to a complete development stop in 26 infants (74.3%).

4. Electroencephalographic findings and neuroimaging

4.1 EEG and video-EEG monitoring

Diffuse slowing of the main background activity is typical that is revealed in the first EEG recordings. At first epileptic cause of these EEG phenomena may remain undetected, especially if symptoms include only short autonomic paroxysms. Epileptiform disorders in disease onset are rare. However, in 3 of 14 patients in the observation by Gerard et al. [4], originally normal background EEG was observed; later, slowing with variable asymmetry was recorded in all cases. Often, slow-wave accentuation in one of the EEG recordings is more pronounced in one hemisphere, while the later study may reveal dominating slow-wave lateralization from the opposite side. Multiregional spikes without clear activation during sleep are registered in all cases during development of the disease. However, pathognomonic interictal EEG pattern in MMPSI is absent. During the period relatively free of seizures, stage differentiation in the structure of sleep EEG may persist, but sleep spindles are rare and usually asymmetric [3]. When seizures become very frequent, interictal activity is almost absent.

Ictal EEG patterns involve different areas of the cerebral cortex in the course of successive seizures. Ictal pattern is a rhythmic activity of alpha and theta range, occurring in one region with adjacent regions involvement during seizure, followed by a gradual decrease of the frequency characteristics. Caraballo with colleagues, analyzing 17 infants with MMPSI, had distinguished three different EEG patterns: 8 cases with alternating simple focal motor seizures at onset, and the ictal EEG pattern was characterized by recurrence of rhythmic focal spikes or rhythmic sharp theta or alpha activity in the Rolandic region; 5 cases with complex focal seizures and progressive appearance of polymorphic theta-delta in temporo-occipital regions recurring independently; and 4 cases with focal complex seizures with motor manifestations and ictal EEG with flattening or fast activity in frontotemporal region followed by unilateral fast polyspikes in alternating clusters in both hemispheres. Correlations between these three patterns with severity or prognosis were not found [27]. Electro-clinical seizure patterns last from 1 to 4 minutes. Multiple subclinical ictal EEG patterns lasting from 30 seconds to 1 minute are also typical [1]. Observations show an alternative cortical section of both hemispheres' involvement in epileptogenesis, which implies the presence of a diffuse pathological process in the cerebral cortex [3].

When seizures become very frequent, initial zone of ictal pattern shift from one region to another and from one hemisphere to another occurs. As a result, extended, migratory ictal activity, which forms a complex EEG pattern of status epilepticus, develops [1–3].

Video-EEG monitoring plays the most important role in the MMPSI diagnosis, as it is able to detect a correlation between ictal pattern localization of and clinical characteristics of seizure. Thus, ictal pattern in the frontal region produces clinical signs in the form of tonic tension or clonic spasms in the contralateral limb; ipsilateral automatisms or a versive seizure with alternating tonic phenomena and fencing posture are possible. EEG pattern is localized in perirolandic area and manifests with contralateral clonus of the lips, tongue, facial muscles, and hypersalivation. Temporal EEG patterns clinically manifest with broad "frozen" gaze ("staring" phenomenon) and oro-alimentary automatisms. Ictal EEG patterns originating from occipital cortex correlate with lateralized clonic eyes and head twitching. In the case of parietal pattern, nonspecific motor activity is possible; sometimes, a child seems "listening" to his/her inner feelings. The above phenomena are contrary to a prevailing opinion that there is no clear clinical-electroencephalographic correlation of focal ictal patterns in infants and rather suggest the opposite.

As child grows, the amplitude of ictal activity tends to increase with growing involvement of the frontal lobes; many seizures become secondarily generalized. The phenomenon of secondary bilateral synchronization typically occurs after only a few weeks from the onset [1]. However, Gerard et al. [4] in the last observations found a delay of bilateral synchronization and additional foci of epileptiform activity generation, at least up to 2 months from the onset (possibly as antiepileptic drug effect) [4]. At this stage detection of early drug resistance may result to a wrong decision about surgical treatment. Extended video-EEG monitoring also has a considerable importance in this category of patients, because visualization of seizures originating from the same cortex area does not mean that all seizures originate only from this area [28].

Despite the various topographies, ictal EEG patterns of all episodes are very similar and correspond to rhythmic activity of the alpha or theta range, prone to the spread and involving all large cortex areas [7].

EEG in personal patients (n = 35) was characterized by diffuse slowing of background activity, while in the developed stage, background EEG was almost completely replaced by continuous ictal patterns. In the initial stages of the disease, interictal record revealed regional or multiregional epileptiform discharges with formation of multifocal independent spike foci (MISF) pattern. Most cases of MMPSI (20 patients, 57.1%) initially had MISF with transformation in MMPSI as frequency of epileptic seizures increased and migratory status developed. In seven cases (20%), monofocal epilepsy was initially observed, followed by addition of extra foci, new types of seizures, and increase of multifocal ictal events up to SE. At eight infants (22.9%), the first properly done EEG investigation fixed the multiregional SE pattern with its preservation in dynamic video-EEG studies and negative prognosis for live.

Ictal EEG patterns in the developed stage of MMPSI involved different areas of the cerebral cortex during a series of seizures, which could overlap each other in cases when ictal pattern in one area is not yet over, but the same pattern appeared in other cortical areas. There may be a complex picture, combining postictal changes in one region of the cerebral cortex, initial ictal pattern in another area, and developed ictal pattern in the third. Typical EEG pattern of MMPSI is presented in a series of electroencephalograms (**Figures 1–7**). In general, ictal pattern

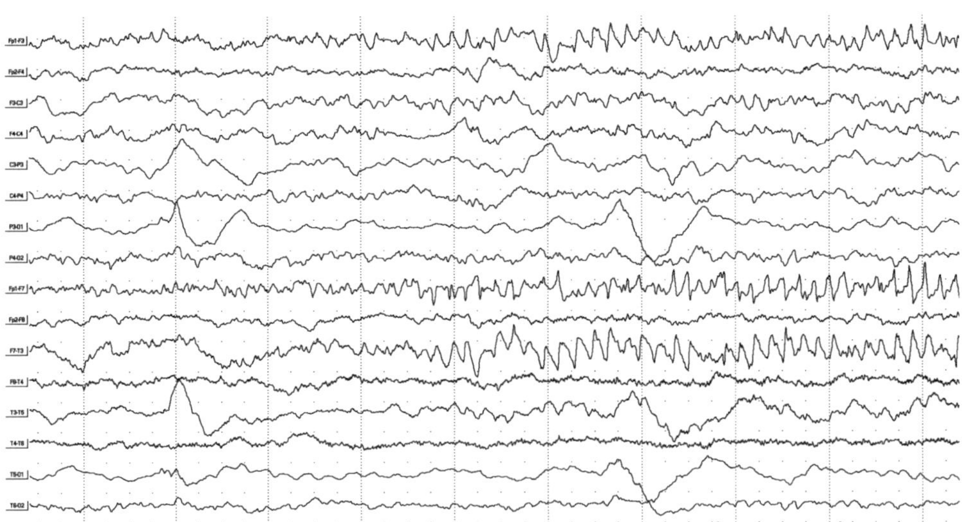

Figure 1.
Patient G.E., 1 year old. Diagnosis: Malignant migrating partial seizures of infancy. EEG during status seizures. Emergence of regional ictal EEG pattern in the left frontal region in the form of fast epileptiform activity and transformation to regular activity of theta range with amplitude increase and sharp wave inclusion. In the left parietal, posterior temporal region is seen delta-accentuation after the previous seizure. Manifestation: Right-sided tonic seizure with oro-facial and versive components.

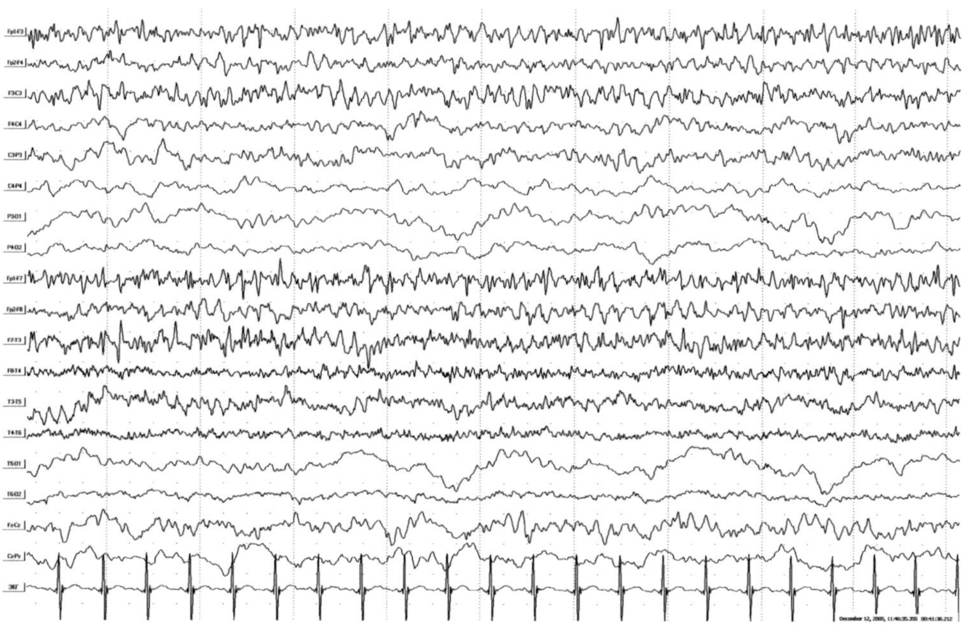

Figure 2.
The same patient. Continuation of ictal EEG. Ictal epileptiform activity involves neighboring regions and same areas of the right hemisphere, but with maintenance of left-sided lateralization. Manifestation: Bilateral tonic seizure.

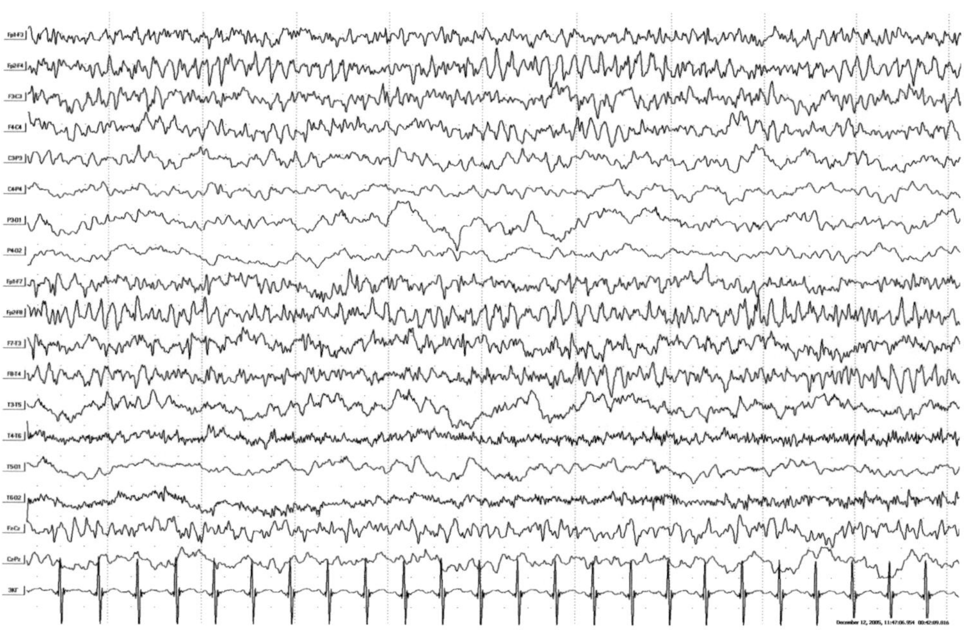

Figure 3.
The same patient. Continuation of ictal EEG. Ictal epileptiform activity in the frontal areas changes to the right-sided lateralization. Manifestation: Transformation to asymmetric tonic seizure with left-sided accentuation.

demonstrates migration of paroxysmal ictal characteristics from one region to another, without formation of stable interregional relations. Probably, only due to ictal pattern migration, patients are able to stay in SE of focal seizures for a long time without development of life-threatening cerebral edema.

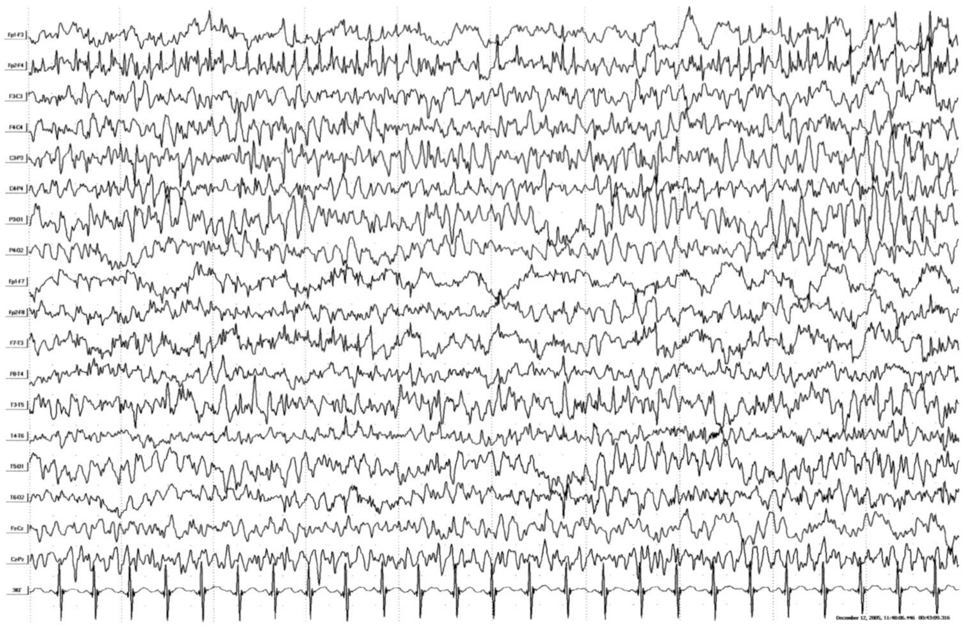

Figure 4.
The same patient. Continuation of ictal EEG. Diffuse spread of ictal epileptiform activity with multiple spikes. On this background, emergence of regional accentuation of ictal pattern in the left parietal-posterior temporal region. Manifestation: Transformation to generalized tonic seizure with clonic component.

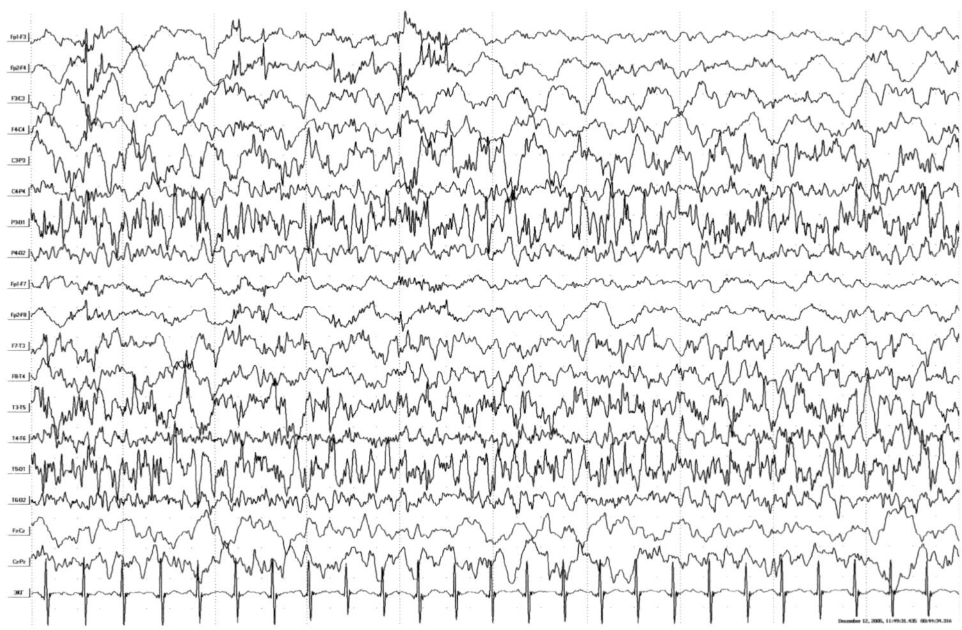

Figure 5.
The same patient. Continuation of ictal EEG. Slowing down of frequency characteristics of the diffuse ictal pattern with transformation to the delta slowing. In the opposite left parietal-posterior temporal region, activation of the regional ictal pattern with regionally accentuated polyspikes and spike-wave complexes is seen. Manifestation: Transformation to asymmetric tonic seizure with right-sided clonic component.

The following variants of ictal patterns have been identified in patients with MMPSI: regional "saw tooth" activity of alpha and theta range; "lafa" runs were obligate ictal patterns and were detected at all patients with MMPSI; frequently

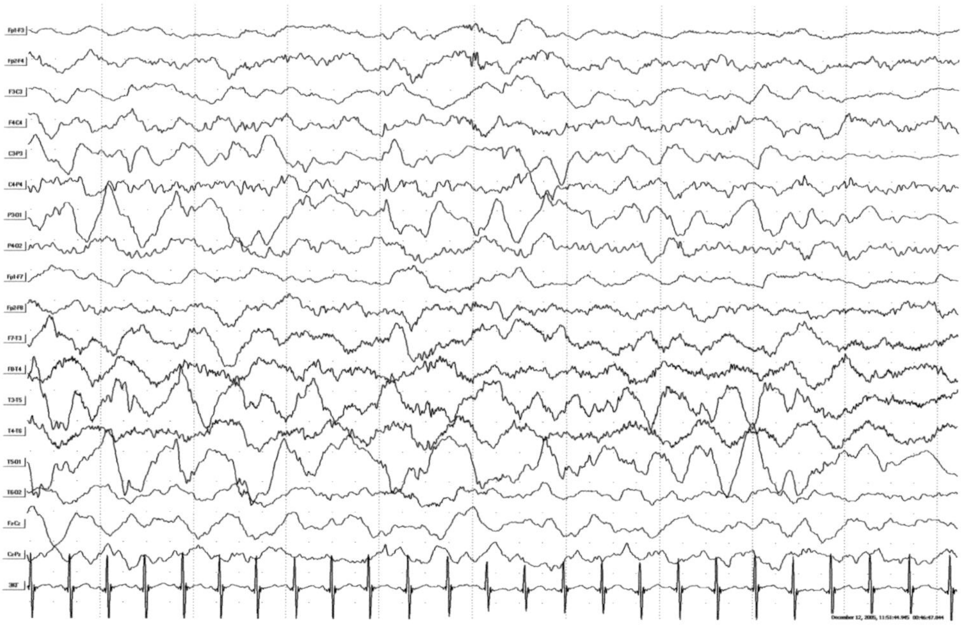

Figure 6.
The same patient. Continuation of ictal EEG. Shift of ictal pattern in the left parietal-posterior temporal region to the delta slowing with slow epileptiform complexes. At the same time in the right hemisphere, emergence of a new ictal pattern in the form of low-amplitude fast activity (lafa). Manifestation: Short-term decrease of clinical ictal severity.

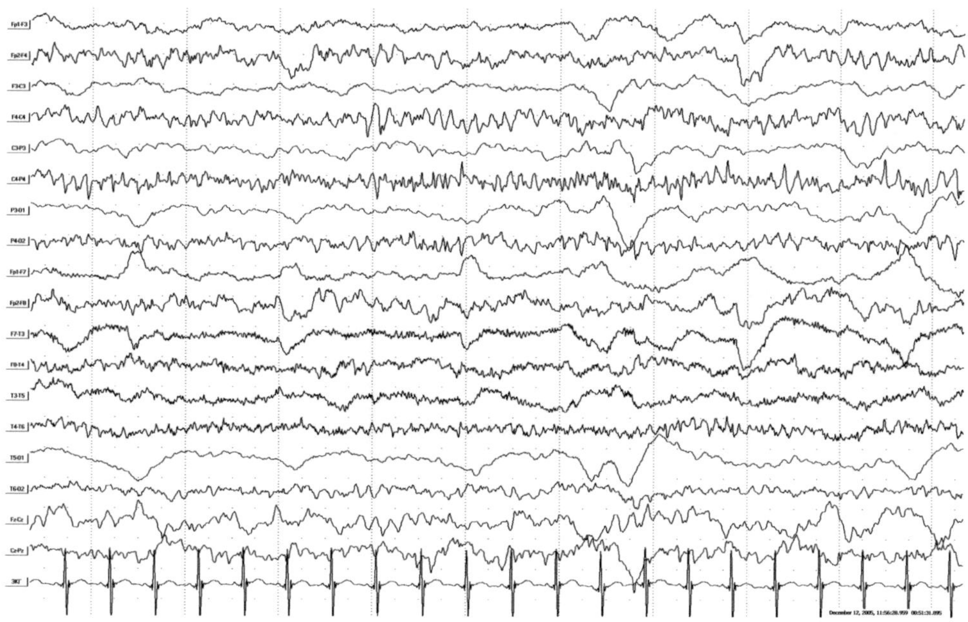

Figure 7.
The same patient. Continuation of ictal EEG. Ictal pattern in the right hemisphere in the form of regular alpha-theta activity with frontal-central accentuation. Postictal changes in the left hemisphere in the form of depression of the bioelectric activity with delta rhythm dominance. Manifestation: Asymmetrical tonic seizure with left-sided accentuation.

runs of fast regular spike-wave complexes were also identified; and runs of slow regular spike-wave complexes (rarely), and diffuse spike- and polyspike-wave discharges.

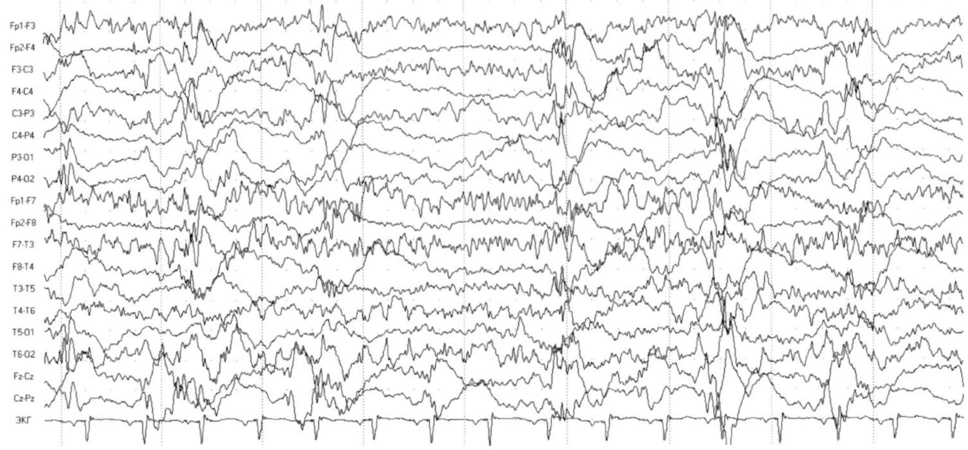

Figure 8.
Patient P.S., age 1 year and 1 month old. Ictal EEG. Diagnosis: Mixed form of MMPSI + EME.EEG reveals combination of suppression-burst pattern with polyspike waves and focal ictal patterns in the left frontal and right temporal areas independently.

Along with "classical" EEG pattern of MMPSI, atypical mixed variants were observed in the manner of superposition of continuous migratory multiregional SE pattern to suppression-burst pattern with diffuse polyspike-wave discharges (**Figures 8–10**). Five of these infants (three boys and two girls) had a special mixed form of epilepsy in the form of MMPSI combination with early myoclonic encephalopathy (EME) with the presence of multiple fragmented "erratic" myoclonus along with migrating focal status seizures.

Such mixed form with transformation of EME into MMPSI was also described by specialists from the Department of Pediatrics of the Taipei City Hospital Zhongxing Branch (Taipei, Taiwan) in a female neonate [29].

4.2 Neuroimaging

According to the world literature, CT and MRI changes are absent, and the majority of MMPSI cases are regarded as cryptogenic. Atrophic changes are nonspecific and further are exacerbated by the constant epileptic seizures [1, 25].

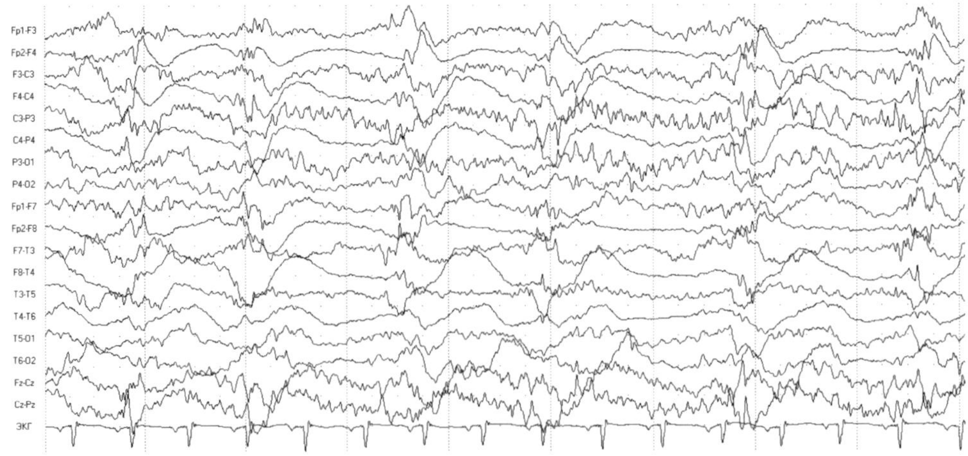

Figure 9.
The same patient. Continuation of ictal EEG. EEG reveals combination of suppression-burst pattern and focal ictal patterns in the left centro-parietal area with central sagittal (vertex accent).

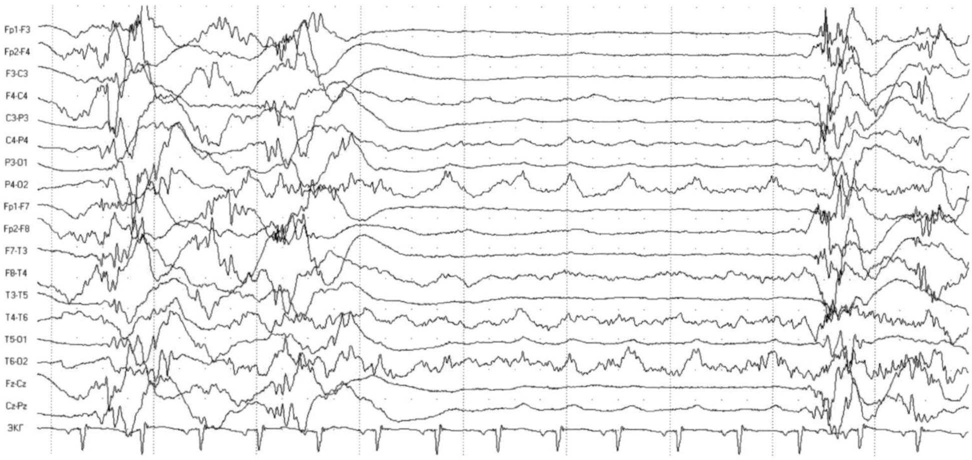

Figure 10.
The same patient. Continuation of ictal EEG. EEG reveals combination of suppression-burst pattern and focal ictal pattern in right occipital-posterior temporal area.

Coppola et al. found left temporal lobe dual pathology in a child with MMRSI, including hippocampal sclerosis and cortical-subcortical blurring [23]. Caraballo et al. reported about mesial temporal lobe sclerosis in 3 of 17 patients [27]. Gross-Tsur et al. presented patients with MMPSI decreased N-acetyl aspartate in the frontal cortex and basal ganglia revealed by MR brain spectroscopy [30].

In cases of cryptogenic MMPSI, minimal or moderate subatrophic changes initially were fixed, sometimes in combination with a moderate delay of myelination, but with progressive cerebral atrophy at 11 children with persistent pharmacoresistant seizures. Dysgenetic brain malformations were found at neuroimaging only in two children with symptomatic analogs of MMPSI in the form of lissencephaly-pachygyria in one girl and polymicrogyria in another girl. Remaining ten patients with symptomatic analogs of MMPSI had a wide range of hypoxic-ischemic CNS lesions in the form of periventricular leukomalacia, parasagittal Chugani necrosis, and diffuse cortical-subcortical atrophy ("walnut" brain).

5. Treatment

MMPSI is a drug-resistant epilepsy form with serious prognosis. Treatment approaches are still developing. Baseline, old, and new antiepileptic drugs in various combinations, as well as corticosteroids, are ineffective [1–3]. However, Dulac observed seizure aggravation during treatment with carbamazepine and vigabatrin in these patients [3]. Perez et al. observed temporary seizure remission in two cases of MMPSI with combination of stiripentol (metabolic drug, inhibitor of several cytochrome P-450 enzymes) and high doses of clonazepam [31]. Hmaimess et al. published about effectiveness of levetiracetam in MMPSI [32]. Okuda et al. [5] reported efficacy of potassium bromide in migrating partial seizures of infancy. A 3-month-old boy and a 4-month-old girl with failure of common antiepileptic drugs reached complete remission of seizures in one case and significant decrease of seizure frequency (95%) in another case due to treatment with potassium bromide 80 mg/kg/day [5]. In all cases of seizure control, gradual improvement in psychomotor development of children was observed that also proves the leading role of epileptiform activity and persistent seizures in the development of epileptic encephalopathy [3].

Chien et al. have stopped erratic myoclonus and suppressive-burst pattern on EEG in a mixed form of EME + MMPSI using dextromethorphan 20 mg/kg [29].

There are different opinions about usefulness of ketogenic diet in MMPSI. So, François et al. proclaimed that seizures in MMPSI are also resistant to ketogenic diet [33]. But specialists from Children's Neuroscience Centre of Royal Children's Hospital (Parkville, Victoria, Australia) published data about efficacy of the ketogenic diet in children with this pharmacoresistant form of epilepsy [34].

Surgical treatment of MMPSI is unreasonable because of diffuse nature of brain damage and lack of clear local structural defect [3]. Theoretically, anterior callosotomy may be offered as a palliative intervention; however, there is no such experience in this form of epilepsy.

A group of scientists from the Pediatric Neurology Department of Azienda Ospedaliera Universitaria (Ancona, Italy) have published about positive experience of vagus nerve stimulation (VNS therapy) in three infants with pharmacoresistant MMPSI [35].

Our cases confirmed that MMPSI are resistant to antiepileptic therapy. Monotherapy had no significant effect in all patients. All patients with MMPSI failed to relieve from epileptic seizures. In 14 MMPSI cases, antiepileptic therapy was completely ineffective (56%), reduction of seizures >50% was observed in seven patients (28%), and only in six patients decrease of seizures was >75% (17.16%). Relatively effective combinations of antiepileptic drugs included valproates with barbiturates (phenobarbital and hexamidine) and benzodiazepines. Clobazam 1 mg/kg was most effective among benzodiazepine groups. In two patients positive effect was observed with combination of levetiracetam, and in one case – with combination of benzodiazepine and topiramate. Phenytoin in two cases caused moderate positive effect with "escape effect." In one patient, frequency of seizures decreased during treatment with potassium bromide (50 mg/kg) but with side effects in the form of hypersomnia. High doses of vitamin B6 in two cases were moderately positive.

Ethosuximide, rufinamide, carbamazepine, and oxcarbazepine have no substantial positive effect. In one case, carbamazepine in cryptogenic focal frontal epilepsy with temporary positive effect caused subsequent aggravation of seizures with appearance of additional foci with clinical and electroencephalographic transformation into MMPSI.

Hormone therapy caused only a temporary moderate positive effect in eight cases and was completely ineffective at other cases.

For emergent relief of SE of hemiconvulsive and secondary generalized tonic-clonic seizures in 15 cases of MMPSI, benzodiazepines (relanium and midazolam) had only a temporary effect in eight or were completely ineffective in seven cases.

Positive effect in SE in MMPSI was observed with sodium oxybate administration at a dose of 100–150 mg/kg, 400 mg/min. This was done in seven cases of hemiconvulsive (n = 3) and secondary generalized tonic-clonic SE (n = 4) resistant to benzodiazepines with a temporary regression (six cases) or a decrease of clinical-EEG paroxysmal events (one case).

In three patients with MMPSI, intravenous valproates caused significant positive effect in relieving SE, especially in cases of tonic-autonomic seizures with episodes of apnea, with aggravation during treatment with benzodiazepines [36]. The recommended dose was 25 mg/kg intravenous over 5 min with the following maintenance infusion – 2 mg/kg/h.

Sodium thiopental (4 mg/kg for 2 min and then infusion of 0.2 mg/kg per minute) is the last chance to stop drug-resistant SE but caused death in one girl due to central inhibition of cardiac activity.

6. Prognosis

MMPSI is a form of epilepsy with poor prognosis. Within a few months after disease onset, frequency and duration of seizures increase up to the serial seizures and status epilepticus. A number of patients die in the first year of life due to multiple prolonged epileptic seizures, development of respiratory distress syndrome, and decorticate rigidity [30]. Based on the generalized clinical observations, mortality in this syndrome is 28% [3]. The results obtained by Marsh et al. are prognostically more favorable: during the 7-year follow-up, all six patients survived; however, psychomotor retardation with severe muscular hypotonia persisted in three of them, and only one patient reached seizure control for a long time [25].

Mortality at personal observed cases was 25.7% (n = 9); however, the expected mortality is higher due to short follow-up (1 year) in more than half of these patients. The oldest of the survived patients with MMPSI is 9 years old; there is gross delay of psychomotor development with unformed verticalization skills, absence of voice activity, spastic tetraparesis, and multiple focal asymmetric tonic, versive, pharyngo-oral, and dialeptic seizures.

Follow-up of patients with MMPSI allowed distinguishing the following subpopulations:

- "Classical" form in the form of marked SE of migrating multifocal seizures is pharmacoresistant with a poor prognosis for psychomotor development, seizures, and life (19 cases, 54.3%).

- Mixed form (MMPSI + EME) with a combination of electro-clinical MMPSI characteristics but also with the presence of fragmented "erratic" myoclonus and suppression-burst pattern with polyspike-wave discharges on EEG (five cases, 14.3%) with also poor prognosis for mental and motor functions, seizures, and life.

- "Moderate" or "mild" form with a consistent evolution from unifocal form to multifocal form with EEG pattern MISF, and then developed expressed MMPSI electro-clinical characteristics, but with a possible regression and decrease in frequency of seizures during combined antiepileptic therapy (six cases, 17.1%).

- "Subtle" form, in the form of only "subtle" minimal motor seizures, inhibitory seizures, multiple ictal patterns during sleep, and leading to awakening (five cases, 14.3%). This form causes a rough developmental delay in infants, but without video-EEG monitoring, it remains unrecognized [20].

7. Conclusions

MMPSI is an independent epileptic syndrome with special clinical-neurophysiological characteristics, distinct from other forms of epilepsy. Diagnosis can be established if there are different types of focal seizures, involving multiple extended EEG and electro-clinical ictal EEG patterns with involvement of several independent areas in both hemispheres. All the patients need complex investigations including dynamic video-EEG monitoring, neuroimaging, and genetic tests (whole-exome sequencing is more preferable).

MMPSI should also be differentiated from the syndrome described by Ohtahara – "severe epilepsy with multiple independent spike foci" (SE-MISF). In the literature, this form is also known as Markand-Blume-Ohtahara syndrome [37]. Unlike MMPSI, this form manifests with predominantly pseudogeneralized seizures: bilateral axial tonic spasms, atypical absences, and myoclonic but focal seizures could also observed. But SE-MISF and MMPSI could have evolutional changes into each other.

Therefore, malignant migrating partial seizures of infancy is the third type of infantile epileptic encephalopathy, along with early encephalopathies with suppression-burst pattern (Aicardi and Ohtahara syndromes) and West syndrome, when the cerebral cortex is more prone to generate epileptic excitation migrating from one area of the cortex to another, without clear interregional organization. This condition is caused by age-dependent features of infant brain with cortex hyperexcitability at a certain stage of evolution [3, 38].

The definition of this syndrome has not been defined in the international classification of epilepsies and epileptic syndromes. The term "malignant migrating partial seizures of infancy" characterizes this form of epilepsy rather as syndrome, so it is proposed to discuss the following title "malignant epilepsy of infancy with migrating multifocal seizures" that may more fully capture the essence of the disease. Taking into account contributions of scientists that first described this form of epilepsy (Coppola) and gave the most detailed description of the clinical and neurophysiological criteria (Dulac), the following definition is proposed: Coppola-Dulac syndrome [39].

Acknowledgements

I would like to express my special thanks to a veteran of World War II, the world's famous coryphaeus of neurology and epileptology, Academician and Professor Vladimir Alexeevich Karlov; to an expert in epilepsy, President of the scientific council of the French Epilepsy Research Foundation, leading specialist of Children's Hospital Necker, Professor Olivier Dulac; to my German teacher and mentor, Professor Hans Holthausen; to my scientific supervisors and epilepsy experts, Professor Konstantin Yurievich Mukhin and Professor Andrey Sergeevich Petrukhin; to the Head of the Department of Neurology, Neurosurgery and Medical Genetics of Pirogov Russian National Research Medical University, Professor Nikolay Nikolaevich Zavadenko; to the Head of the Department of Psychoneurology N2 of the Russian Children Clinical Hospital, Dr. Elena Stepanovna Il'ina; and to all my colleagues. Also, I would like to extend my special thanks to my big family and especially my wife Elena!

Conflict of interest

No conflict of interest.

Author details

Alexey Kholin
Department of Neurology, Neurosurgery and Medical Genetics of Pediatric Faculty, Pirogov Russian National Research Medical University, Moscow, Russia

*Address all correspondence to: drkholin@mail.ru

References

[1] Coppola G, Plouin P, Chiron C, Robain O, Dulac O. Migrating partial seizures in infancy: A malignant disorder with developmental arrest. Epilepsia. 1995;**36**(10):1017-1024

[2] Coppola G. Malignant migrating partial seizures in infancy: An epilepsy syndrome of unknown etiology. Epilepsia. 2009;**50**(Supp. 5):49-51. DOI: 10.1111/j.1528-1167.2009.02121.x

[3] Dulac O. Malignant migrating partial seizures in infancy. In: Roger J, Bureau M, Dravet C, Genton P, Tassinari CA, Wolf P, editors. Epileptic Syndromes in Infancy, Childhood and Adolescence. 4th ed. John Libbey; 2005. pp. 73-76. ISBN: 2-7420-0575-7

[4] Gerard F, Kaminska A, Plouin P, Echenne B, Dulac O. Focal seizures versus focal epilepsy in infancy: A challenging distinction. Epileptic Disorders. 1999;**1**(2):135-139

[5] Okuda K, Yasuhara A, Kamei A, Araki A, Kitamura N, Kobayashi Y. Successful control with bromide of two patients with malignant migrating partial seizures in infancy. Brain & Development. 2000;**22**(1):56-59

[6] Veneselli E, Perrone MV, Di Rocco M, Gaggero R, Biancheri R. Malignant migrating partial seizures in infancy. Epilepsy Research. 2001;**46**(1):27-32

[7] Panayiotopoulos CP. A Clinical Guide to Epileptic Syndromes and their Treatment. Bladon Medical Publishing. Oxford, 2002. pp. 36-49. ISBN: 1904218237

[8] Coppola G, Veggiotti P, Del Giudice EM, Bellini G, Longaretti F, Taglialatela M, et al. Mutational scanning of potassium, sodium and chloride ion channels in malignant migrating partial seizures in infancy. Brain & Development. 2006;**28**(2):76-79. DOI: 10.1016/j.braindev.2005.05.002

[9] Poduri A, Heinzen EL, Chitsazzadeh V, Lasorsa FM, Elhosary PC, LaCoursiere CM, et al. SLC25A22 is a novel gene for migrating partial seizures in infancy. Annals of Neurology. 2013; **74**(6):873-882. DOI: 10.1002/ana.23998

[10] Freilich ER, Jones JM, Gaillard WD, Conry JA, Tsuchida TN, Reyes C, et al. Novel SCN1A mutation in a proband with malignant migrating partial seizures of infancy. Archives of Neurology. 2011;**68**(5):665-671. DOI: 10.1001/archneurol.2011.98

[11] Carranza Rojo D, Hamiwka L, McMahon JM, Dibbens LM, Arsov T, Suls A, et al. De novo SCN1A mutations in migrating partial seizures of infancy. Neurology. 2011;**77**(4):380-383. DOI: 10.1212/WNL.0b013e318227046d

[12] Ohba C, Kato M, Takahashi S, Lerman-Sagie T, Lev D, Terashima H, et al. Early onset epileptic encephalopathy caused by de novo SCN8A mutations. Epilepsia. 2014; **55**(7):994-1000. DOI: 10.1111/epi.12668

[13] Barcia G, Fleming MR, Deligniere A, Gazula V-R, Brown MR, Langouet M, et al. De novo gain-of-function KCNT1 channel mutations cause malignant migrating partial seizures of infancy. Nature Genetics. 2012;**44**:1255-1259. DOI: 10.1038/ng.2441

[14] Vanderver A, Simons C, Schmidt JL, Pearl PL, Bloom M, Lavenstein B, et al. Identification of a novel de novo p. Phe932Ile KCNT1 mutation in a patient with leukoencephalopathy and severe epilepsy. Pediatric Neurology. 2014; **50**(1):112-114. DOI: 10.1016/j. pediatrneurol.2013.06.024

[15] Ishii A, Shioda M, Okumura A, Kidokoro H, Sakauchi M, Shimada S,

et al. A recurrent KCNT1 mutation in two sporadic cases with malignant migrating partial seizures in infancy. Gene. 2013;**531**:467-471. DOI: 10.1016/j.gene.2013.08.096

[16] Kawasaki Y, Kuki I, Ehara E, Murakami Y, Okazaki S, Kawawaki H, et al. Three cases of KCNT1 mutations: Malignant migrating partial seizures in infancy with massive systemic to pulmonary collateral arteries. The Journal of Pediatrics. 2017;**191**:270-274. DOI: 10.1016/j.jpeds.2017.08.057

[17] Madaan P, Jauhari P, Gupta A, Chakrabarty B, Gulati S. A quinidine non responsive novel KCNT1 mutation in an Indian infant with epilepsy of infancy with migrating focal seizures. Brain & Development. 2018;**40**(3): 229-232. DOI: 10.1016/j.braindev.2017.09.008

[18] Milh M, Falace A, Villeneuve N, Vanni N, Cacciagli P, Assereto S, et al. Novel compound heterozygous mutations in TBC1D24 cause familial malignant migrating partial seizures of infancy. Human Mutation. 2013;**34**: 869-872. DOI: 10.1002/humu.22318

[19] Zhang X, Ling J, Barcia G, Jing L, Wu J, Barry BJ, et al. Mutations in QARS, encoding glutaminyl-tRNA synthetase, cause progressive microcephaly, cerebral-cerebellar atrophy, and intractable seizures. American Journal of Human Genetics. 2014;**94**(4):547-558. DOI: 10.1016/j.ajhg.2014.03.003

[20] Kholin AA. The syndrome of malignant migrating partial seizures in infancy or Coppola-Dulac syndrome (19 cases). Zhurnal Nevrologii i Psikhiatrii Imeni S.S. Korsakova. 2013;**113**(3):21-27

[21] Bedoyan JK, Kumar RA, Sudi J, Silverstein F, Ackley T, Iyer RK, et al. Duplication 16p11.2 in a child with infantile seizure disorder. American Journal of Medical Genetics Part A. 2010;**152A**(6):1567-1574. DOI: 10.1002/ajmg.a.33415

[22] Poduri A, Chopra SS, Neilan EG, Elhosary PC, Kurian MA, Meyer E, et al. Homozygous PLCB1 deletion associated with malignant migrating partial seizures in infancy. Epilepsia. 2012; **53**(8):e146-e150. DOI: 10.1111/j.1528-1167.2012.03538.x

[23] Coppola G, Operto FF, Auricchio G, D'Amico A, Fortunato D, Pascotto A. Temporal lobe dual pathology in malignant migrating partial seizures in infancy. Epileptic Disorders. 2007;**9**(2): 145-148. DOI: 10.1684/epd.2007.0106

[24] Kholin AA. Status epilepticus in infancy and early childhood. D.M.thesis. Moscow. 2010. 54 p

[25] Marsh E, Melamed SE, Barron T, Clancy RR. Migrating partial seizures in infancy: Expanding the phenotype of a rare seizure syndrome. Epilepsia. 2005; **46**(4):568, 72. DOI: 10.1111/j.0013-9580.2005.34104.x

[26] Dulac O, Chiron C. Malignant epileptic encephalopathies in children. Baillière's Clinical Neurology. 1996;**5**(4): 765-781

[27] Caraballo RH, Fontana E, Darra F, Cassar L, Negrini F, Fiorini E, et al. Migrating focal seizures in infancy: Analysis of the electroclinical patterns in 17 patients. Journal of Child Neurology. 2008;**23**(5):497-506. DOI: 10.1177/0883073807309771

[28] Kholin AA, Ilina ES, Kolpakchi LM, Fedonuk ID, Mikhailova SV, Semykina LI, et al. Malignant migrating partial seizures in infancy. Clinical observation of 6 cases. Rus. zh. detsk. nevrol. 2007; **2**(2):25-38

[29] Chien YH, Lin MI, Weng WC, Du JC, Lee WT. Dextromethorphan in the treatment of early myoclonic encephalopathy evolving into migrating

partial seizures in infancy. Journal of the Formosan Medical Association. 2012; **111**(5):290-294. DOI: 10.1016/j.jfma.2012.03.007

[30] Gross-Tsur V, Ben-Zeev B, Shalev RS. Malignant migrating partial seizures in infancy. Pediatric Neurology. 2004; **31**(4):287-290. DOI: 10.1016/j.pediatrneurol.2004.05.001

[31] Perez J, Chiron C, Musial C, Rey E, Blehaut H, d'Athis P, et al. Stiripentol: Efficacy and tolerability in epileptic children. Epilepsia. 1999;**40**(11): 1618-1612

[32] Hmaimess G, Kadhim H, Nassogne MC, Bonnier C, van Rijckevorsel K. Levetiracetam in a neonate with malignant migrating partial seizures. Pediatric Neurology. 2006;**34**(1):55-59. DOI: 10.1016/j.pediatrneurol.2005.06.011

[33] François LL, Manel V, Rousselle C, David M. Ketogenic regime as anti-epileptic treatment: Its use in 29 epileptic children. Archives de Pédiatrie. 2003;**10**(4):300-306

[34] Thammongkol S, Vears DF, Bicknell-Royle J, Nation J, Draffin K, Stewart KG, et al. Efficacy of the ketogenic diet: Which epilepsies respond? Epilepsia. 2012;**53**(3):e55-e59. DOI: 10.1111/j.1528-1167.2011.03394.x

[35] Zamponi N, Rychlicki F, Corpaci L, Cesaroni E, Trignani R. Vagus nerve stimulation (VNS) is effective in treating catastrophic 1 epilepsy in very young children. Neurosurgical Review. 2008;**31**(3):291, 7. DOI: 10.1007/s10143-008-0134-8

[36] Kholin AA, Ilina ES, Lemeshko ID, Mukhin KY, Petrukhin AS. Malignant migrating partial seizures of infancy: The experience of treatment of status epilepticus in infancy using intravenous valproate – Convulex (a clinical cases). Zhurnal Nevrologii i Psikhiatrii Imeni S. S. Korsakova. 2010;**110**(3 Supp. 2):17-24

[37] Yamatogi Y, Ohtahara S. Severe epilepsy with multiple independent spike foci. Journal of Clinical Neurophysiology. 2003;**20**(6):442-448

[38] Ohtahara S, Yamatogi Y. Epileptic encephalopathies in early infancy with suppression – Burst. Journal of Clinical Neurophysiology. 2003;**20**(6):398-407

[39] Kholin AA. Malignant migrating partial seizures in infancy or Coppola-Dulac syndrome. Materials of 29th International Epilepsy Congress, Rome. 2011. p. 716

Section 5

Epilepsy - Therapeutic Aspect

Chapter 8

The Role of Nondrug Treatment Methods in the Management of Epilepsy

Natalia Shnayder, Ekaterina Narodova, Valeriya Narodova, Andrey Narodov and Evgeniy Erakhtin

Abstract

The review is devoted to the issue of nondrug epilepsy treatment in the adult population in Russia and abroad. The conducted literature review allowed us to reveal the basic nondrug epilepsy treatment options. However, not all of these options have a sufficient evidence base, and some of them are not always safe. Particularly, methods with low level of evidence include acupuncture and aromatherapy. Further studies are needed to explore the methods aimed to eliminate the epileptic system dominant through the development of a new, more powerful dominant. One of the methods, which can influence the pathogenesis of epilepsy, is physical activity for patients with epilepsy, since epileptiform activity on the EEG is reported to disappear during exercises. The positive results of the application of art therapy (music therapy) are also described in the modern literature. Tempo-rhythm correction methods hold a specific place in neurorehabilitation. There are considerable amount of studies concerning the application of tempo-rhythmic methods in neurology and psychiatry. It can be concluded that these methods are relevant worldwide and can be used in diagnostics and correction of neurological and psychiatric diseases (such as schizophrenia, Parkinson's disease, epilepsy).

Keywords: epilepsy, adults, nonpharmacological treatment, review, tapping

1. Introduction

According to the world statistics, epilepsy takes the third place among overall morbidity after cardiovascular diseases and diabetes mellitus and the third place in neurological morbidity [1]. Therefore, epilepsy is a relevant public health problem both in Russia and abroad [2]. This fact fosters the development and implementation of medicinal and alternative (nondrug) methods of epilepsy treatment around the world. However, current epilepsy treatment options allow achieving remission or reducing the number of seizures only in 60–70% of patients [3].

An important problem of epileptology is ensuring the safety and acceptability of the treatment as well as prevention of adverse drug reaction (ADR) of antiepileptic drugs (AEDs). The emergence of the ASEs can often decrease patients' life quality, thereby offsetting the positive effect of the treatment. Moreover, such ASEs as depression and anxiety (the fear of the coming seizure) may aggravate epileptic seizures [4]. Some ASEs are associated with the AEDs' effects on the liver enzymes.

These effects cause induction or inhibition of the liver enzymes, making other AEDs displaced from protein linkages. These reactions increase the rate of metabolism and cause the reduction of the plasma concentration of ADRs, which may lead to difficulties in the choice of AEDs' dosage. On average, the frequency of ASEs and complications of antiepileptic therapy remains high and varies, according to different authors, from 7 to 25% [5–7].

Therefore, the presence of ADRs requires the immediate withdrawal of AEDs, even if the drug-induced epilepsy remission is achieved. It should be noted that 40% of epileptic patients need polytherapy. This leads to the increase in the ADRs' frequency, adverse drug-drug interactions, and teratogenicity [8]. Also, there are difficulties in assessing the effectiveness of ADRs of a single drug. Drug-drug interactions often decrease antiepileptic treatment efficiency and contribute to the development of ADRs [2, 9, 10].

Consequently, nondrug methods of epilepsy treatment should also be used, both as an additional therapy and (in some cases) as the basic therapy (e.g., vagus nerve stimulation) (see **Table 1**).

The principle of the dominant was introduced in neurophysiology by the outstanding Russian physiologist Uchtomsky in 1911 [11]. Under "the dominant" he meant the dominant reflex system, which determines the integral nature of the functioning of the nerve centers in any period of time and ensures the appropriate behavior of animal and human. He also described the dominants' properties, the main of which were increased excitability, the ability to summation, high resistance, and inertia of excitation. Also, a theory of pathological dominant was suggested. Within this theory, pathological dominant represents sharply enhanced focus of excitation in the central nervous system, caused by "pathogenic effects of the environment."

Later, in 1980, Kryzhanovskii developed the doctrine of "pathological determinant." The latter was described as a "modified formation of the central nervous system, forming a pathological system and determining the nature of its activities" [12]. According to this doctrine, the determinant can form a pathological system in the central nervous system. The feature of the pathological system is the ability to suppress the physiological system. Such pathophysiological mechanisms underlie most neurological disorders. Kryzhanovskii proposed a mechanism of fighting the pathological dominant by introducing another, more powerful dominant [13]. A significant part of the research dedicated to the hand tapping is based on this mechanism.

According to Rudnev, the cyclical nature of movements in wrist tapping is a natural statistical regularity that is a standard you can compare different parameters

Noninvasive methods	Invasive methods
Physical activity	Vagus nerve stimulation
Transcranial magnetic stimulation	Deep brain stimulation
Psychotherapy	Percutaneous stimulation of the trigeminal Nerve
Music therapy	Surgery
Aromatherapy	
Acupuncture	
Referential bioadaptation	
Tapping	

Table 1.
Nondrug methods of epilepsy treatment.

to. Consequently, the study of these biologically appropriate movements makes it possible to establish a pattern of certain rates and rhythms that occurs in the pathology at different levels of the human nervous system [14].

2. Results and their discussion

2.1 Nonpharmacological noninvasive therapy

2.1.1 Psychotherapy

Currently, it is the practice to distinguish three fundamental categories of psychotherapeutic techniques, used in epileptology: rewards/sanctions, self-control, and neurofeedback. "Rewards/sanctions" and "self-control" categories are used for self-induced seizures and for so-called reflective attacks as well as for epileptic seizures, amplifying under the influence of emotional factors. Neurofeedback is a nonpharmacological method of epilepsy treatment with objective registration, amplification, and "feedback" of physiological information to the patient. This method is based on the principle of self-identification of one's own EEG data.

Based on the information from different authors, using neurofeedback can lead to a great reduction in the number of seizures in 50% cases of patients with epileptic risk factors. From this 50%, in 10% of cases, it is possible to completely discontinue AEDs without reappearance of epileptic seizures for 2–3 years and more, and in the remaining 40–50% of cases after the use of the neurofeedback method, it is possible to have pharmacological treatment [15].

2.1.2 Art therapy

There are also art therapy options for epilepsy treatment. For example, there is an actively developing method, based on the creation of therapeutic music to reduce the number of epileptic seizures. This method is based on the theory that epileptic seizures occur because of abnormal synchronization of the brain's electric activity, and the majority of them stop spontaneously. The effect of structured auditory stimuli provides noninvasive galvanic cortex stimulation, which can reduce epileptiform activity [16].

To prove this hypothesis, authors conducted a randomized research, which explored the effectiveness of music therapy for patients diagnosed with epilepsy [17]. Patients were exposed to Mozart's music every night for 1 year. Based on the results of the research, a 17% reduction in the number of epileptic seizures was noticed. The achieved effect remained stable during the next year [18, 19]. In another randomized research, which studied both children and adult patients with epilepsy, it was revealed that 85% of patients had a positive response to music therapy with an average reduction of epileptiform activity index by 31% during the music listening and by 24% after it [20–28].

2.1.3 Aromatherapy

Aromatherapy can be useful (for achieving a state of relaxation) as a component of epilepsy behavioral treatment. However, its use is more justified for the treatment of conditions, accompanying epilepsy, such as anxiety and depression. In the application of aromatherapy for patients with epilepsy, camphora, sage, and rosemary should be avoided because these substances are known to aggravate patients' condition and increase the number of epileptic seizures [10].

In Asia-Pacific region, they actively use acupuncture as a nonpharmacological method of epilepsy treatment. There is data on the use of acupuncture for patients with stroke in order to avoid poststroke epilepsy. Weng et al. showed that patients with stroke receiving acupuncture had significantly less probability of poststroke epilepsy compared to those who did not receive such treatment ($p < 0.0001$). However, defensive effects, associated with acupuncture, need further exploration [29].

Some authors report neuroprotective, anti-inflammatory, and neurotrophic effects of acupuncture and electroacupuncture. These effects are explained by the amplification of recurrent inhibition of the brain cortex and hippocampus with the liberation of different neurotransmitters, including gamma-aminobutyric acid (GABA) and serotonin. However, due to the lack of controlled clinical trials, those methods cannot be recommended as reliably effective and safe in epileptology [30].

2.1.4 Physical activity

Patients with epilepsy experience a range of social restrictions, leading to their external and internal stigmatization. These limitations include the employment problem, driving prohibition, and restriction of *physical activity*. However, it is a well-known fact that physical exercises lead to better functional adaptation [31]. Patients with epilepsy, involved in sport, can receive the same benefits of physical activity as healthy people, including increase in performance efficiency and tolerance, weight loss, and cardiovascular system functioning normalization. Physical activity is also a critical factor in reducing the risks of diabetes mellitus, arterial hypertension, coronary heart disease, obesity, and osteoarthritis. As for psychological advantages, the research in this field found out that physically active patients have better mental health than those leading a sedentary lifestyle [32–34].

Physical activity in early age can cause neuronal reserve's formation, which then will be used during the life course. Consequently, physically active patients have lower risk of developing cognitive impairments associated with epilepsy [35, 36].

Preventive and curative effect of the physical activity in case of epilepsy can be achieved in accordance with several principles, including the principles of consistency, regularity, duration, monitoring, and personalization of the training load. Despite this, it is believed that enhanced muscular activity is accompanied with tachypnea (hyperventilation), which can initiate the seizures.

However, some authors claim that physical activity can reduce the likelihood of seizures. Usually, seizures do not occur while running, swimming, ice skating, skiing, crossing the crowded street, as well as during sport events, although this issue is disputable. On the other side, it is reported that seizures often start when patients are relaxed or sleeping.

The described fact accounts for the development of new dominant excitation areas in the central nervous system (CNS) during vigorous exercises. Due to the negative induction, these areas slow down or inhibit the epileptic area activity, therefore preventing seizure occurrence. It is reported that during physical exercises seizures occur much more rare than during relaxation [31]. The disappearance of epileptiform activity in many patients' EEG during the physical activity proves this theory [37–40].

2.1.5 Ketogenic diet

Ketogenic diet (KD) is a high-fat and low-carbohydrate diet that induces ketosis. Ketosis is a metabolic state where the body uses ketone bodies, made from the breakdown of fatty acids in the liver, rather than carbohydrates as primary source of energy. The classical KD has a fat to carbohydrate plus protein ratio of 3–4:1. Additionally, classical KD can be supplemented with either long- or medium-chain triglycerides (LCT or MCT) to maintain the appropriate ratio and improve effectiveness. The diets appear to be highly effective as 36–85% of the patients with epilepsy experience more than 50% seizure reduction when on KD [41]. Multiple epileptic syndromes, such as glucose transporter 1 (GLUT1) deficiency, are especially responsive to KD [42].

2.1.6 Tapping

Tapping is a psychomotor test that can be used to assess the psychophysiological brain functions, in particular the time perception. Tapping without any external influence reflects the speed of nervous processes and endogenous rhythmic processes of the central nervous system since tapping with the preferred test speed represents a "biological constant" [43, 44].

However, in case of exogenously defined long-term reproduction of the rhythmic intervals, the frequency of stimulation is of importance. A number of studies revealed association between the frequency of exogenous stimulation in case of tapping and body response. Specifically, if stimulation is more than 1 Hz, the leading value is the reaction to time, and at a stimulation frequency less than 1 Hz, the reaction to the stimulus prevails. Therefore, at the frequency of exogenous stimulation of 1 Hz, both reactions acquire an equivalent value.

Despite the long-standing interest in tapping, new developments in this area constantly appear. This is due to the fundamental principles of this technique. In this case we are talking about the doctrine of dominants.

Therefore, tempo-rhythm correction methods hold a specific place in neurorehabilitation. Prototypical techniques of such therapy include movement therapy, music therapy, and logopedic rhythmics [43].

One of the methods of studying the typological features of the nervous system is the "tapping test." The essence of the classical tapping test technique is the application of pencil points on an A4 sheet of paper, pre-drawn into six squares, with the maximum allowable speed. The movement from square to square is carried out by command every 5 seconds, from left to right clockwise [45].

Tapping test is widely used to study the effect of sleep duration on the level of anxiety of different groups of patients [46, 47].

The technique of meridian tapping [or the emotional freedom technique (EFT)] is used as a clinical procedure to alleviate the psychological and physical suffering of the patient. This method is described as "tapping" and is often combined with other nondrug techniques aimed at relieving patient's emotional stress. Such techniques may include acupuncture and aromatherapy. The EFT includes finger tapping on certain points on the face and hands. More than 60 research articles in various journals report 98% of the effectiveness of this technique in various patients with psychological disorders (such as post-traumatic stress disorder, phobias, anxiety, depression), as well as in patients with various somatic diseases (asthma, fibromyalgia, pain, epilepsy). The advantages of this method are its simplicity and safety. Patients can easily learn this technique and use it as a self-help in various pathological conditions. Also, this technique is used by nurses for patients undergoing inpatient treatment [48].

To study neural mechanisms, lying in foundation of rhythm reproduction, authors conducted an EEG during the tapping test. All subjects were divided into two groups of those who were previously trained and those who were not. EEG analysis showed that beta-rhythm in temporal and hippocampal areas in those who were trained beforehand was higher than in those who were not trained. More than that synchronization between frontal and temporal and hippocampal areas on later training stages was higher than on earlier stage. These results show that frontal, temporal, and hippocampal beta-neuron schemes can be studied with auditory motor rhythm [49].

In other studies, it was concluded that the decrease in beta-rhythm in temporal areas is connected with rhythmic movements (in this case, rhythmic hand movements) [50]. It is also supposed that temporal areas play an important role in rhythm reproduction, correlating with frontal areas and basal ganglia, forming a link between auditory stimulus and motor response [51]. It is proven that the hippocampus is connected with the processing of rhythmic information. Moreover, EEG showed the beta-fluctuation in the cerebellum during the processing of sensorimotor information [52].

2.1.7 Transcranial magnetic stimulation

Low-frequency rhythmic transcranial magnetic stimulation (rTMS) leads to a decrease in the cerebral cortex neuronal excitability, while high-frequency rTMS increases their excitability [2]. The mechanisms of rTMS are related to its ability to cause long-term effects of postsynaptic inhibition in excitatory neurotransmitter systems and neuronal excitability reduction through inactivation of the voltage-dependent ion channels [53].

2.2 Nonpharmacological invasive therapy

2.2.1 Percutaneous stimulation of trigeminal nerve

Percutaneous stimulation of trigeminal nerve is a minimally invasive method which is based on exposure of the first trigeminal nerve's branches to electricity. To implement this method in practice, a special system is used which consists of external electric impulse generator and electroconductive plasters. There are few studies which report the use of this method, but most of them consider this method to have a positive clinical effect. During preliminary clinical trials, 57% of patients noticed a 50% or more reduction in the number of seizures [54].

2.2.2 Vagus nerve neurostimulation

Vagus nerve neurostimulation (VNS) is one of the nondrug epileptic treatment methods. The principle of this method is in the chronic electrical stimulation of the left vagus nerve, using an implantable stimulator [55]. The primary candidates for the application of this method are patients with drug-refractory epilepsy (DRE), who cannot get resection surgery.

The main contraindications for this method are pregnancy and lactation, cardiac arrhythmia, bronchial asthma, chronic obstructive pulmonary disease, acute peptic and duodenal ulcer, vasovagal syncope, and type 1 diabetes [56]. Against the background of VNS therapy during the period from 3 months to 3 years, a complete cessation of seizures was revealed in 4.8–17.6% of patients. The decrease in the number of seizures by 50% or more was detected in 27.3–47% of patients, while the decrease in the number of seizures by less than 50% was detected in 23.5% of patients [57–59].

2.2.3 Deep brain stimulation

Deep brain stimulation is an effective therapeutic method for DRE treatment, especially for temporal lobe epilepsy. Thus, according to a randomized study, assessing the effectiveness of hippocampal stimulation in patients with temporal lobe DRE, positive effect in the form of complete disappearance of seizures was found in 50% of patients [60]. According to other studies, it was shown that after

11 years of deep brain stimulation, the attacks were not registered for at least 12 months in only 13.8% of the patients [61].

The principle of this method is in electrode implantation into certain brain structures (target structures), these electrodes being supplied with low-voltage and high-frequency electric current. Due to the impulses, generated by the neurostimulator, the selected brain structures change their functions. Thus, this high-frequency stimulation of the target structures allows reducing the severity of the symptoms and the amount of AEDs taken by the patients as well as bringing the patient back into the society [56].

3. Conclusion

Based on the conducted literature review results, it can be stated that an adequate number of Russian and foreign studies of the analyzed period are dedicated to nonpharmacological epilepsy treatment. Both methods with proven clinical effectiveness and low-reliable treatment options were found in the studied literature.

Most of the authors emphasize a positive influence of physical activity on epileptic patients, including prevention of epileptic seizures. Besides, physical activity is reported to have a positive influence on patients' psychic function, preventing cognitive disorders. However, up until now, physical exercises as an additional therapy are not included in any treatment program for patients with epilepsy. The analysis of the literature showed that it is due to the current concern of neurologists and epileptologists over the occurrence of epileptic seizures in state of hyperventilation.

Those concerns are not unfounded, because hyperventilation can provoke epileptic seizures in a certain group of patients with epilepsy. As a result, it is reasonable not to ban physical activity for all epileptic patients but to limit its intensity for the group of patients, in whom hyperventilation can provoke epileptic seizures. Meanwhile, the fact is reported that during physical exercising the reduction of epileptiform activity occurs on the epileptic patients' EEG. There are also works that prove a positive effect of music therapy, but the issue is still underinvestigated.

All the options for nonpharmacological epilepsy treatment, represented in the present review, are based on the classical theory of Kryzhanovskii about creation and destruction of pathological systems [62]. The author noted that on early stages of the disease the elimination of pathological determinant leads to liquidation of pathological (and, as a result, epileptic) system.

On late stages the fixation of pathological system leads to chronization of pathological process and corresponding neural disorders. The battle with pathological systems, especially with those with complicated and matured forms, is hard and is not always effective. It requires a complex pathogenetic therapy, focused on elimination of pathological determinant (e.g., the elimination of epileptic focus) and normalization of other links of the pathological system. Activation of antiepileptic system, amplification of overall control, and other genetic mechanisms are important as well. It is also known that there is a constant countdown in living system, on which homeostasis is based [63].

According to the theory of Rudnev [14], the so-called internal time is a genetic core of any motor activity, having both populations' and individual characteristics. Internal time is expressed as an individual rhythm. A lot of studies explore individual rhythm, its "maturation" in late ontogenesis, as well as its breaking in different cases of neural disorders [64]. Individual rhythm is a reflection of harmony of brains' work, and its breaking is a sign of disintegration in brain's work. Since there is an established fact that in case of epilepsy a pathological activation of brains' neurons occurs, which is a stress for central neural system, it is possible that the epileptic system occurrence can change patients' individual rhythm.

In reproduction of tapping, there are different brain structures concerned, such as the cerebellum. Taking into account the fact that the cerebellum is an antiepileptic device, its activation during tapping can have a therapeutic effect on epileptic patients. Tempo-rhythm studies focused on epileptic patients could be used for the development of new rehabilitative methods. As a fundamental support of this theory, exploration of dominants involving the opportunity to work out a new dominant for this group of patients with tapping exercises makes these studies relevant. Consequently, research on individual rhythm changes in patients with symptomatic post-surgery epilepsy and comparison of these changes with healthy persons' individual rhythm indicators can help to create a new dominant in the absence of pathological focus and reset remaining epileptic system links, imposing the mode of operation closest to the physiological one and activate antiepileptic system. There is also a concept which states that "seizures lead to seizures." First proposed by doctor William Gowers (1881) and reflecting the concept of epilepsy as a progressing disease [65], this concept remains relevant.

Conflict of interest

The authors declare that they have no conflicts of interest to disclose.

Author details

Natalia Shnayder[1], Ekaterina Narodova[2*], Valeriya Narodova[2], Andrey Narodov[2] and Evgeniy Erakhtin[3]

1 V.M. Bekhterev National Medical Research Center of Psychiatry and Neurology, St Petersburg, Russian Federation

2 Professor V.F. Voino-Yasenetsky Krasnoyarsk State Medical University, Krasnoyarsk, Russian Federation

3 N.S. Karpovich Krasnoyarsk Interdistrict Clinical Hospital of Emergency Care, Russian Federation

*Address all correspondence to: katya_n2001@mail.ru

References

[1] Avakyan GN. Epidemiology of epilepsy and optimization of drug therapy for focal epilepsy. Epilepsy and Paroxyzmal Conditions. 2014;**6**(5):3-5. (In Russian)

[2] Karlov VA. Epilepsy in Children and Adults, Women and Men: A Guide for Doctors. Moscow: Medicine; 2010. 720 p. (In Russian)

[3] Melikyan EG, Gekht AB. Life quality in epileptic patients. Lechebnoe delo. 2011;(1):4-8. (In Russian)

[4] Kalinin VV. Correction of affective and cognitive disorders in epileptic patients and the value of lamotrigine. Neurology, Neuropsychiatry, Psychosomatics. 2013;**5**(2):78-83. (In Russian)

[5] Voronkova KV, Pylaeva OA, Kosyakova ES, Mazalskaya OV, Golosnaya GS, Provatorova MA, et al. Modern principles of epilepsy therapy. Zhurnal Nevrologii i Psikhiatrii Imeni S.S. Korsakova. 2010;(6):24-36. (In Russian)

[6] Zenkov LR. Clinical Epileptology. Moscow: MIA; 2010. 405 p. (In Russian)

[7] Bochanova E. Pharmacogenetics of antiepileptic drugs (literature review). Good Clinical Practice. 2017;**1**:51-55. (In Russian)

[8] Dmitrenko DV, Shnaider NA, Strotskaya IG, Kichkaylo AS, Zobova SN. Mechanisms of valproate-induced teratogenesis. Neurology, Neuropsychiatry, Psychosomatics. 2017;**9**(1S):89-96. DOI:10.14412/2074-2711-2017-1S-89-96. (In Russian)

[9] Kwan P, Arzimanoglou A, Berg AT, Brodie MJ, Allen Hauser W, Mathern G, et al. Definition of drug resistant epilepsy: Consensus proposal by the ad hoc Task Force of the ILAE Commission on Therapeutic Strategies. Epilepsia. 2010;**51**(6):1069-1077. DOI: 10.1111/j.1528-1167.2009.02397.x

[10] Karpova VI, Krushinskaya NS, Mukhin KY. Epilepsy: History, Diagnosis, Practice, Treatment, Advice to Patients. Moscow: System Solutions; 2011. 224 p. (In Russian)

[11] OYu Z, Efimov GB. The Problems of Artificial Intelligence and the Dominant Theory by O.O. Uchtomsky. Mathematical Machines and Systems. Vol. 12008. pp. 98-105. (In Russian)

[12] Kryzhanovskii GN. Determinant Structures in the Pathology of the Nervous System. Medicine: Moscow; 1980. 360 p. (In Russian)

[13] Kryzhanovskii GN. Pathological integrations in the central nervous system. Bulletin of Experimental Biology and Medicine. 1999;**127**(3):219-222. (In Russian)

[14] Rudnev VA. Functional Diagnosis and Recovery of Voluntary Movements in the Pathology of the Central Nervous System. Krasnoyarsk: Publishing House of Krasnoyarsk University; 1982. 160 p. (In Russian)

[15] Sterman MB, Egner T. Foundation and practice of neurofeedback for the treatment of epilepsy. Applied Psychophysiology and Biofeedback. 2006;**31**(1):21-35. DOI: 10.1007/s10484-006-9002-x

[16] Fisher RS. Therapeutic devices for epilepsy. Annals of Neurology. 2012;**71**(2):157-168. DOI: 10.1002/ana.22621

[17] Bodner M, Turner RP, Schwacke J, Bowers C, Norment C. Reduction of seizure occurrence from exposure to auditory stimulation in individuals with neurological handicaps: A

randomized controlled trial. PLoS One. 2012;**7**(10):e45303. DOI: 10.1371/journal.pone.0045303

[18] Mehndiratta P, Sajatovic M. Treatments for patients with comorbid epilepsy and depression: A systematic literature review. Epilepsy Behavior. 2013;**28**(1):36-40. DOI: 10.1016/j.yebeh.2013.03.029

[19] Schmidt D, Sillanpaa M. Evidence-based review on the natural history of the epilepsies. Current Opinion in Neurology. 2012;**25**(2):159-163. DOI: 10.1097/WCO.0b013e3283507e73

[20] Dastgheib SS, Layegh P, Sadeghi R, Foroughipur M, Shoeibi A, Gorji A. The effects of Mozart's music on interictal activity in epileptic patients: Systematic review and meta-analysis of the literature. Current Neurology and Neuroscience Reports. 2014;**14**(1):420. DOI: 10.1007/s11910-013-0420-x

[21] Cardamone L, Salzberg MR, O'Brien TJ, Jones NC. Antidepressant therapy in epilepsy: Can treating the comorbidities affect the underlying disorder? British Journal of Pharmacology. 2013;**168**(7):1531-1554. DOI: 10.1111/bph.12052

[22] Bozzi Y, Borrelli E. The role of dopamine signaling in epileptogenesis. Frontiers in Cellular Neuroscience. 2013;**7**:157. DOI: 10.3389/fncel.2013.00157

[23] Rocha L, Alonso-Vanegas M, Villeda-Hernandez J, Mujica M, Cisneros-Franco JM, Lopez-Gomez M, et al. Dopamine abnormalities in the neocortex of patients with temporal lobe epilepsy. Neurobiology of Disease. 2012;**45**(1):499-507. DOI: 10.1016/j.nbd.2011.09.006

[24] Raglio A, Farina E, Giovagnoli AR. Can music therapy alleviate psychological, cognitive, and behavioral impairment in epilepsy? Epilepsy Behavior. 2014;**31**:7-8. DOI: 10.1016/j.yebeh.2013.10.008

[25] Modi AC, Rausch JR, Glauser TA. Early pediatric antiepileptic drug nonadherence is related to lower long-term seizure freedom. Neurology. 2014;**82**(8):671-673. DOI: 10.1212/WNL.0000000000000147

[26] Tavakoli F, Hoseini SE, Mokhtari M, Vahdati A, Razmi N, Vessal M. Role of music in morphine rewarding effects in mice using conditioned place preference method. Neuro Endocrinology Letters. 2012;**33**(7):709-712

[27] Lin LC, Juan CT, Chang HW, Chiang CT, Wei RC, Lee MW, et al. Mozart K.448 attenuates spontaneous absence seizure and related high-voltage rhythmic spike discharges in long evans rats. Epilepsy Research. 2013;**104**(3):234-240. DOI: 10.1016/j.eplepsyres.2012.11.005

[28] Tasset I, Quero I, García-Mayórgaz ÁD, del Río MC, Túnez I, Montilla P. Changes caused by haloperidol are blocked by music in Wistar rat. Journal of Physiology and Biochemistry. 2012;**68**(2):175-179. DOI: 10.1007/s13105-011-0129-8

[29] Weng SW, Liao CC, Yeh CC, Chen TL, Lane HL, Lin JG, et al. Risk of epilepsy in stroke patients receiving acupuncture treatment: A nationwide retrospective matched-cohort study. BMJ Open. 2016;**6**(7):e010539. DOI: 10.1136/bmjopen-2015-010539

[30] Yi PL, Jou SB, Wu YJ, Chang FC. Manipulation of epileptiform electrocorticograms (ECoGs) and sleep in rats and mice by acupuncture. Journal of Visualized Experiments. 2016;(118). DOI: 10.3791/54896

[31] Astashenko OI. Encyclopedia of Therapeutic Movements in Various Diseases: Joints, Back and Spine, Gynecological and Urological,

Heart and Blood Vessels, Liver and Gastrointestinal Tract. St. Petersburg: Vector; 2009. 306 p. (In Russian)

[32] Arida RM, Cavalheiro EA, Scorza FA. From depressive symptoms to depression in people with epilepsy: Contribution of physical exercise to improve this picture. Epilepsy Research. 2012;**99**(1-2):1-13. DOI: 10.1016/j.eplepsyres.2011.10.012

[33] Sitnikov IY, Mikhailova NV, Savinov SV, Abedimova RA, Akchurina YE, Bondareva IV, et al. Physical load and epilepsy. Neurosurgery and Neurology of Kazakhstan. 2015;**41**(4):13-17. (In Russian)

[34] Nass RD, Meiling S, Andrié RP, Elger CE, Surges R. Laboratory markers of cardiac and metabolic complications after generalized tonic-clonic seizures. BMC Neurology. 2017;**17**(1):187. DOI: 10.1186/s12883-017-0965-4

[35] Tutkun E, Ayyildiz M, Agar E. Short-duration swimming exercise decreases penicillin-induced epileptiform ECoG activity in rats. Acta Neurobiologiae Experimentalis (Wars). 2010;**70**(4):382-389

[36] Gomes da Silva S, de Almeida AA, Silva Araújo BH, Scorza FA, Cavalheiro EA, Arida RM. Early physical exercise and seizure susceptibility later in life. International Journal of Developmental Neuroscience. 2011;**29**(8):861-865. DOI: 10.1016/j.ijdevneu.2011.07.011

[37] Arida RM, Scorza FA, Cavalheiro EA. Favorable effects of physical activity for recovery in temporal lobe epilepsy. Epilepsia. 2010;**51**(Suppl 3):76-79. DOI: 10.1111/j.1528-1167.2010.02615.x

[38] Arida RM, Scorza FA, Gomes da Silva S, Schachter SC, Cavalheiro EA. The potential role of physical exercise in the treatment of epilepsy. Epilepsy Behavior. 2010;**17**(4):432-435. DOI: 10.1016/j.yebeh.2010.01.013

[39] Vancini RL, de Lira CA, Scorza FA, de Albuquerque M, Sousa BS, de Lima C, et al. Cardiorespiratory and electroencephalographic responses to exhaustive acute physical exercise in people with temporal lobe epilepsy. Epilepsy Behavior. 2010;**19**(3):504-508. DOI: 10.1016/j.yebeh.2010.09.007

[40] de Lima C, Vancini RL, Arida RM, Guilhoto LM, de Mello MT, Barreto AT, et al. Physiological and electroencephalographic responses to acute exhaustive physical exercise in people with juvenile myoclonic epilepsy. Epilepsy Behavior. 2011;**22**(4):718-722. DOI: 10.1016/j.yebeh.2011.08.033

[41] Ye F, Li X, Jiang W, Sun H, Liu J. Efficacy of and patient compliance with a ketogenic diet in adults with intractable epilepsy: A meta-analysis. Journal of Clinical Neurology. 2015;**11**:26-31

[42] Kass HR, Winesett SP, Bessone SK, Turner Z, Kossoff EH. Use of dietary therapies amongst patients with GLUT1 deficiency syndrome. Seizure. 2016;**35**:83-87. DOI: https://doi.org/10.1016/j.seizure.2016.01.011

[43] Bykov YN. Cerebral integrated mechanisms (Message 2). Siberian Medical Journal (Irkutsk). 2001;**2**:4-9. (In Russian)

[44] Pogelt B, Roth N, Poget A. Automated rhythmic movements and their control under different experimental conditions. Biomedica Biochimica Acta. 1984;**43**(4):485-491

[45] Kolomiets OI, Petrushkina NP, Bykov EV, Yakubovskaya IA. Functional state characteristics of central nervous system among sportsmen with different orientation of the training process. The Russian Journal of Physical Education and Sport. 2017;**12**(2):217-225. DOI: 10.14526/01_2017_225. (In Russian)

[46] 9i, De Gennaro L, Violani C, Braibanti P, Bertini M. A finger-tapping

task and a reaction time task as behavioral measures of the transition from wakefulness to sleep: Which task interferes less with the sleep onset process. Sleep. 1997;**20**(4):301-312

[47] Mazzetti M, Bellucci C, Cipolli C, Pizza F, Russo PM, Tuozzi G, et al. Age-related differences in sleep-dependent consolidation of motor skills in patients with narcolepsy type 1. Sleep Medicine. 2016;**24**:80-86. DOI: 10.1016/j.sleep.2016.06.015

[48] Rancour P. The emotional freedom technique: Finally, a unifying theory for the practice of holistic nursing, or too good to be true? Journal of Holistic Nursing. 2017;**35**(4):382-388. DOI: 10.1177/0898010116648456

[49] Edagawa K, Kawasaki M. Beta phase synchronization in the frontal-temporal-cerebellar network during auditory-to-motor rhythm learning. Scientific Reports. 2017;7:42721. DOI: 10.1038/srep42721

[50] Fujioka T, Trainor LJ, Large EW, Ross B. Internalized timing of isochronous sounds is represented in neuromagnetic β oscillations. Journal of Neuroscience. 2012;**32**(5):1791-1802. DOI: 10.1523/jneurosci.4107-11.2012

[51] Patel AD, Iversen JR. The evolutionary neuroscience of musical beat perception: The Action Simulation for Auditory Prediction (ASAP) hypothesis. Frontiers in Systems Neuroscience. 2014;**8**:57. DOI: 10.3389/fnsys.2014.00057

[52] Salmi J, Pallesen KJ, Neuvonen T, Brattico E, Korvenoja A, Salonen O, et al. Cognitive and motor loops of the human cerebro-cerebellar system. Journal of Cognitive Neuroscience. 2010;**22**(11):2663-2676. DOI: 10.1162/jocn.2009.2138

[53] Funke K, Ben-Ali A. Modulation of cortical inhibition by rTMS–Findings obtained from animal models. The Journal of Physiology. 2011;**589**(Pt18):4423-4435. DOI: 10.1113/jphysiol.2011.206573

[54] Hsu WY, Cheng CH, Lin MW, Shih YH, Liao KK, Lin YY. Antiepileptic effects of low frequency repetitive transcranial magnetic stimulation: A meta-analysis. Epilepsy Research. 2011;**96**(3):231-240. DOI: 10.1016/j.eplepsyres.2011.06.002

[55] Khachatryan VA, Mamatkhanov MR, Lebedev KE. Vagostimulation in the system of surgical treatment of epilepsy. Pediatric Neurosurgery and Neurology. 2012;(2-3):152-161. (In Russian)

[56] Balabanova AI, Bavdurnuy AA, Bolba MV, Belova EV, Rakhmanina OA, Muravjov SA. Life style and non-medication treatment methods of epilepsy. Medical Science and Education of Ural. 2015;**16**(2-1):139-145. (In Russian)

[57] Vaiman M. Treatment of Epilepsy with Vagus Nerve Stimulation: The Israeli Experience. [Internet]. 2013. Available from: http://www.medines.net/cms/28-статьи/143-лечение-эпилепсии-стимуляцией-блуждающего-нерва-израильский-опыт.html [Accessed: September 27, 2018]. (In Russian)

[58] Lipatova LV, Skoromets TA, Gromov SA, Tabulina SD, Vtorov AV, Bondareva MM, et al. Experience of using vagus nerve stimulation to treat drug resistant epilepsy. Neurology, Neuropsychiatry, Psychosomatics. 2014;**6**(1Suppl):18-21. DOI: 10.14412/2074-2711-2014-1S-18-21. (In Russian)

[59] Sufianov AA, Orlov AS, Matveev EI, Lebedeva DI. Experience with use of chronic neurostimulation of vagus nerve in treatment of pharmacoresistant epilepsy. Epilepsy and Paroxyzmal Conditions. 2012;**4**(3):48-49. (In Russian)

[60] Cukiert A, Cukiert CM, Burattini JA, Mariani PP, Bezerra DF. Seizure outcome after hippocampal deep brain stimulation in patients with refractory temporal lobe epilepsy: A prospective, controlled, randomized, double-blind study. Epilepsia. 2017;**58**(10):1728-1733. DOI: 10.1111/epi.13860

[61] Kim SH, Lim SC, Kim J, Son BC, Lee KJ, Shon YM. Long-term follow-up of anterior thalamic deep brain stimulation in epilepsy: A 11-year, single center experience. Seizure. 2017;**52**:154-161. DOI: 10.1016/j.seizure.2017.10.009

[62] Kryzhanovskii GN. Fundamentals of General Pathophysiology. Moscow: Medical News Agency; 2011. 253 p. (In Russian)

[63] Moiseeva NI. Some methodological aspects of the study of the concept of time in biology. In: Bekhtereva NP, editor. Methodological Questions of the Time of Theoretical Medicine. Leningrad: Medicine; 1975. pp. 87-117. (In Russian)

[64] Narodova EA, Prokopenko SV, Narodova VV, Narodov AA. Rehabilitation of the patients with complex motor aphasia during the ischemic insult. Journal of New Medical Technologies. 2012;**1**. [Internet]. Available from: http://medtsu.tula.ru/VNMT/Bulletin/E2012-1/3938.pdf [Accessed: September 27, 2018]. (In Russian)

[65] Kwan P, Schachter SC, Brodie MJ. Current concepts: Drug-resistant epilepsy. New England Journal of Medicine. 2011;**365**(10):919-926. DOI: 10.1056/NEJMra1004418

Chapter 9

Ketogenic Diet Therapies in Children and Adults with Epilepsy

Matthew Charles Lee Phillips

Abstract

Despite a wide array of anti-epileptic drugs and the option of surgery, one-third of children and adults with epilepsy continue to suffer from drug-resistant seizures. Many of these patients may benefit from a ketogenic diet, a non-pharmacologic therapy proven to improve seizure control in epilepsy. Ketogenic diets aim to mimic the metabolic profile of fasting, and probably improve seizure control through a variety of mechanisms that collectively stabilize synaptic function. Although many similarities exist with regards to patient selection, patient preparation, and diet implementation in children compared to adults, there are also important differences. The most conspicuous challenge to the more widespread use of ketogenic diets in children and adults with epilepsy is a lack of access to ketogenic services in many regions of the world. Moreover, the culinary and social restrictions associated with conventional ketogenic diets pose a significant barrier to their use in adults.

Keywords: ketogenic, diet, children, adults, epilepsy

1. Introduction

Epilepsy is defined by recurrent, spontaneous seizures arising from hyperexcitable neurons in the brain. Yet despite a wide array of anti-epileptic drugs and the option of surgery, approximately one-third of children and adults with epilepsy continue to experience drug-resistant seizures [1]. Many of these patients may be candidates for a ketogenic diet, a well-established, non-pharmacologic therapeutic option proven to improve seizure control in epilepsy [2, 3].

The origins of ketogenic diets derive from the ancient practice of fasting [4], widely acknowledged as effective in treating epilepsy since the 5th century BC; indeed, until the 19th century, epilepsy was believed to be a disease of "eating too much" [5]. Depending on a person's body fat stores, fasting can be maintained for a considerable length of time (the record for a single continuous fast is 382 days) [6]. However, since everyone must eventually eat, fasting is not a feasible long-term solution for seizure control in epilepsy.

In 1921, Wilder addressed this problem by developing a high-fat, low-carbohydrate diet designed to mimic the metabolic profile of fasting [4]. The high-fat, low-carbohydrate nature of the diet elevated blood ketones and lowered blood glucose levels, producing a metabolic profile similar to that of a multi-day fast. Unlike fasting, Wilder's diet provided adequate long-term nutrient intake, thus preventing malnutrition and promoting healthy long-term growth and development. Since the diet increased hepatic ketogenesis, it became known as a "ketogenic diet."

2. Ketogenic diets

In essence, a ketogenic diet is any high-fat, adequate-protein, low-carbohydrate diet that forces the body to burn fats—not carbohydrates—as the primary energy source [7, 8]. During this process, the liver converts fats into ketone bodies, or "ketones" (organic molecules that readily serve as energy substrates for non-hepatic organs, particularly brain, heart, and skeletal muscle) [9]. The three endogenous ketones are acetone, acetoacetate, and beta-hydroxybutyrate (BHB) [7]; BHB is the primary blood ketone. During a sustained ketogenic diet, the blood BHB level is elevated, and lies within the range of 0.5–8 mmol/L, constituting a state of "physiological ketosis" (in contrast to pathological ketoacidosis, which is associated with a blood BHB level of 15–20 mmol/L or higher, and a concomitant lowering of blood pH) [10].

2.1 Mechanisms of ketogenic diets in epilepsy

Ketogenic diets appear to improve seizure control through a variety of mechanisms that collectively stabilize neuron synaptic function (**Table 1**) [7, 8]. It is not known whether the key mediators of improved seizure control are the ketones themselves, or additional metabolic changes induced by the diets [11].

2.1.1 Ketones as key mediators of seizure control

The most conspicuous metabolic change induced by a ketogenic diet is elevated blood ketone levels [7]. While it is well-documented that ketones enhance neuron energetics, accumulating evidence suggests they may also play direct and indirect roles in reducing neuron excitability, exerting direct antiseizure effects, and decreasing generation of reactive oxygen species and inflammatory mediators [7, 8, 11]. Thus, there are multiple avenues by which ketones may contribute to improved seizure control; they are not just "energy molecules" [11].

Ketones enhance intracellular adenosine triphosphate (ATP) levels and bioenergetic capacity by increasing mitochondrial oxidative phosphorylation [12]. The oxidation of acetoacetate and BHB feeds acetyl-CoA directly into the Krebs cycle

General mechanism	Specific mechanism
Enhanced neuron energetics	Enhanced neuron ATP production
	Stimulated mitochondrial biogenesis
Reduced neuron excitability	Hyperpolarized potassium channels
	Altered glutamate to GABA ratio
	Increased extracellular adenosine
Direct antiseizure effects	Ketone-mediated antiseizure effects
	Raised medium-chain fatty acids
	Reduced glucose metabolism
Other mechanisms	Reduced oxidative stress
	Reduced inflammation

ATP = adenosine triphosphate; GABA = γ-aminobutyric acid.

Table 1.
Mechanisms through which ketogenic diets may stabilize synaptic function.

through anaplerosis (the replenishing of depleted metabolic cycle intermediates) [7], which increases the turnover of the Krebs cycle, generating additional protons and electrons that are channeled to the electron transport chain where they may be used to enhance ATP production [12].

Ketones may also inhibit neuronal excitability. ATP-dependent potassium channels, which hyperpolarize the cell membrane, are activated by ketones, decreasing spontaneous cell firing rates [13]. Moreover, acetoacetate concentrations well within the range produced by a ketogenic diet inhibit vesicle loading of the excitatory neurotransmitter glutamate, resulting in reduced glutamate release into the synapse and enhanced synthesis of the inhibitory neurotransmitter γ-aminobutyric acid (GABA) [14]. It is thought that the ensuing altered glutamate to GABA ratio reduces neuron excitability.

Studies dating back to the 1930s also support the direct antiseizure effects of ketones [15, 16]. In mice, acetone and acetoacetate raise seizure thresholds, resulting in fewer seizures [15, 16]. Although BHB did not appear to contribute to antiseizure effects in these earlier studies, more recent studies indicate that BHB probably does play a direct antiseizure role, and that its effects may have been previously missed for methodological reasons [11].

Lastly, ketones may influence seizure control by lowering cell oxidative stress and inflammation [11]. BHB inhibits histone deacetylases (enzymes that remove acetyl groups from lysine residues on histones, allowing DNA to wrap tightly and preventing gene expression), resulting in upregulated anti-oxidant genes and reduced oxidative stress in kidney cells [17]. Moreover, BHB inhibits the assembly of the immune sensor nucleotide oligomerization domain (NOD)-like receptor protein 3, a multi-protein complex that controls the release of various inflammatory mediators [18].

2.1.2 Additional metabolic changes that may mediate seizure control

Emerging evidence suggests that a number of additional metabolic changes induced by ketogenic diets may also contribute to enhanced neuron energetics, reduced neuron excitability, and direct antiseizure effects, improving seizure control [7, 8].

Ketogenic diets can improve seizure control in patients with mitochondrial disorders [19]. This observation may be partly explained by the action of the medium-chain fatty acid, decanoic acid, on peroxisomal proliferator-activated receptor γ, which stimulates neuronal mitochondrial biogenesis [19]. The increased mitochondrial biomass enhances neuron ATP production capacity and cell energy reserves.

Ketogenic diets may also alter brain levels of the neurotransmitter adenosine. The disruption of adenosine signaling induces seizures; this effect is reversible by a ketogenic diet [20]. This observation suggests that the diet increases extracellular adenosine levels, activating inhibitory adenosine A1 receptors and reducing neuron hyperexcitability [7].

Lastly, ketogenic diets may exert direct antiseizure effects by raising medium-chain fatty acid levels and decreasing glucose metabolism [7, 8]. The medium-chain fatty acid, decanoic acid, blocks seizure-like activity in animals [21]. Moreover, since the antiseizure effects of ketogenic diets can be rapidly reversed by glucose infusions, decreased glucose metabolism is thought to contribute to seizure control. The mechanism for this effect could be partially explained by the observation that ketogenic diets induce a reduction in glycolysis, subsequently repressing the expression of brain-derived neurotrophic factor, a known pro-convulsant [7].

2.2 Conventional ketogenic diets in epilepsy

To date, four major, "conventional" ketogenic diets are supported by published evidence in the treatment of children and adults with epilepsy (**Table 2**) [2, 3]. The primary difference between each diet lies in the ratio of fat to protein plus carbohydrate, described by weight or by calorie intake.

2.2.1 The classic ketogenic diet (CKD)

Created by Wilder in the 1920s [1], the CKD is the oldest of all ketogenic diet therapies and in its purest form consists of 80% fat by weight (roughly equivalent to 90% fat by caloric intake), translating to a 4:1 ratio of fat to protein plus carbohydrate, although a 3:1 ratio or lower can often be used [2]. In the CKD, the fat source consists predominantly of long-chain fatty acids, obtained from standard foods.

2.2.2 The medium-chain triglyceride (MCT) diet

In an effort to make the ketogenic diet more palatable, the MCT diet was introduced in the 1970s [22]. In its original form, the MCT diet is 60% fat by weight (roughly 75% fat by caloric intake), with fat sourced from MCT oils. Since medium-chain fatty acids yield more ketones per kilocalorie compared to long-chain fatty acids, the MCT diet allows for a lower overall fat intake, and a greater intake of protein and carbohydrate, compared to the CKD. A number of patients are prone to gastrointestinal side-effects on this diet, so a modified MCT diet was created in the 1980s, consisting of 30% medium-chain fatty acids plus 30% long-chain fatty acids by weight [23].

2.2.3 The modified Atkins diet (MAD)

In the early 2000s, the MAD was shown to be effective in treating epilepsy [24]. The MAD is approximately 50% fat by weight (65–70% fat by caloric intake),

Ketogenic diet	Macronutrient ratio (by weight)	Macronutrient ratio (by calorie intake)
CKD	Fat 80%	Fat 90%
	Protein 12%	Protein 6%
	Carbohydrate 8%	Carbohydrate 4%
MCT diet	Fat 60%	Fat 75%
	Protein 16%	Protein 10%
	Carbohydrate 24%	Carbohydrate 15%
MAD	Fat 50%	Fat 65–70%
	Protein 35%	Protein 25–30%
	Carbohydrate 15%	Carbohydrate 5%
LGIT diet	Fat 40%	Fat 60%
	Protein 45%	Protein 30%
	Carbohydrate 15%	Carbohydrate 10%

CKD = classic ketogenic diet; MCT = medium-chain triglyceride; MAD = modified Atkins diet; LGIT = low glycemic index treatment.

Table 2.
Conventional ketogenic diets supported by published evidence in treating epilepsy.

translating to a 1:1 ratio of fat to protein plus carbohydrate, although no set ratio is mandated; it may even approach a 4:1 ratio [2]. The MAD eases up on the protein and carbohydrate restrictions imposed by the CKD and MCT diet, and does not require food weighing.

2.2.4 The low glycemic index treatment (LGIT) diet

The LGIT, roughly 40% fat by weight (60% fat by caloric intake), was introduced in the early 2000s as a treatment for epilepsy [25]. The design of the LGIT was based on the hypothesis that stable glucose levels contribute to the seizure control conferred by ketogenic diets. The LGIT allows for relatively liberal levels of protein and carbohydrate intake, emphasizing carbohydrates with glycemic indices less than 50.

3. Ketogenic diet therapies in children with epilepsy

Unfortunately, many children throughout the world still lack access to a pediatric epilepsy center containing a specialized ketogenic service with both inpatient and outpatient management options [2]. Such a service should consist of a pediatric neurologist, nurse, dietitian, and ideally case managers, psychologists, social workers, and pharmacists [2, 26].

3.1 Selecting the right child for a ketogenic diet

Ketogenic diets in children are strongly indicated in drug-resistant epilepsy, two disorders of brain metabolism, and several other seizure disorders (**Table 3**) [2]. There is virtually no age restriction as to when the diet may be commenced; in fact, infants younger than 2 years may be an ideal age group [27].

3.1.1 Drug-resistant epilepsy in children

In 2010, the International League Against Epilepsy (ILAE) defined drug-resistant epilepsy as the failure of adequate trials of two appropriately chosen, tolerated, and used anti-epileptic drug schedules (whether as monotherapies or in combination) to achieve sustained seizure freedom [28]. The drugs must have been appropriate for the seizure type, tolerated at therapeutic doses, and given a reasonable period of time to work (at least 6 months) [29] before declaring drug resistance.

When drug-resistant epilepsy is declared, further anti-epileptic drug trials or epilepsy surgery may be helpful [30]. However, even after carefully excluding confounding factors and optimizing the drug approach, subsequent trials have only a slight (about 5%) chance of inducing seizure remission [31]. Surgery should always be considered in children with drug-resistant epilepsy, especially when a lesion concordant to the epilepsy is detected on imaging [30], but many children are not surgical candidates due to a generalized or multifocal epilepsy syndrome, or nonresectable location of ictal onset.

When drug trials and surgery are no longer feasible, a ketogenic diet is indicated [2]. Numerous studies have demonstrated the efficacy and safety of using ketogenic diets to treat drug-resistant epilepsy in children, but until the previous decade there were no randomized controlled trials. Since 2008, four published randomized controlled trials have compared the efficacy of a ketogenic diet with continued medications or a placebo arm in children with drug-resistant epilepsy [32–35].

General disorder	Specific disorder
Drug-resistant epilepsy	2010 ILAE definition
Disorders of brain metabolism	GLUT1 DS
	PDHD
Specific seizure disorders	Angelman syndrome
	Complex I mitochondrial disorders
	Doose syndrome
	Dravet syndrome
	FIRES
	Formula-fed
	Infantile spasms
	Ohtahara syndrome
	Super-refractory status epilepticus
	Tuberous sclerosis complex

ILAE = International League Against Epilepsy; GLUT1 DS = glucose transporter type 1 deficiency syndrome; PDHD = pyruvate dehydrogenase complex deficiency; FIRES = febrile infection-related epilepsy syndrome.

Table 3.
Epilepsy disorders in children for which a ketogenic diet may be strongly indicated.

The first randomized controlled trial compared the efficacy of a CKD versus no diet intervention in 145 children with drug-resistant epilepsy [32]. After 3 months, 28 children (38%) in the CKD group had a greater than 50% seizure reduction compared to four children (6%) in the control group. One weakness of the study was its unblinded design, with both patients and assessors aware of the group allocations.

The following year, a randomized controlled trial was published in 20 children with drug-resistant Lennox-Gastaut syndrome [33]. All patients were fasted 36 hours and then randomized to receive either a CKD plus a daily solution containing 60 g glucose per day or a solution containing saccharin (an artificial sweetener); the aim of the design was to ensure that both patients and assessors remained blinded to treatment. To the surprise of the investigators, both groups had positive blood BHB levels after 6 days, indicating that the glucose solution did not suppress physiological ketosis. Perhaps as a result of this, the study demonstrated only a borderline, non-statistically significant reduction in seizures in the saccharin arm.

The next randomized controlled trial compared the efficacy of a MAD versus no diet intervention in 102 children with drug-resistant epilepsy [34]. Surgical candidates were not excluded. After 3 months, 52% of children in the MAD group had a greater than 50% seizure reduction compared to 11.5% of those in the control group. A weakness of the study was its unblinded design, with both patients and assessors aware of the group allocations.

The most recent randomized controlled trial compared the efficacy of a ketogenic diet (CKD or MCT diet) versus no diet intervention in 57 children and adolescents with drug-resistant epilepsy [35]. None of the patients were eligible for surgery. After 4 months, 13 children (50%) in the ketogenic diet group had a greater than 50% seizure reduction compared to 4 children (18.2%) in the control group.

Pooling the results from these randomized controlled trials suggests that 40–50% of children experience a greater than 50% seizure reduction after 3–4 months on a ketogenic diet, compared to 10–15% of children receiving no dietary intervention. Given these encouraging results, many epilepsy specialists advocate that ketogenic diets be used earlier in the management of children with drug-resistant epilepsy [2].

3.1.2 Disorders of brain metabolism in children

Since ketogenic diets induce a shift away from glycolytic energy production towards mitochondrial oxidative phosphorylation, they are the treatment of choice in two childhood disorders of impaired brain glucose metabolism: glucose transporter type 1 deficiency syndrome (GLUT1 DS) and pyruvate dehydrogenase complex deficiency (PDHD) [2]. In both cases, the ketones produced by the diet bypass the metabolic defects, serving as an alternative energy source for the brain.

GLUT1 DS results from impaired glucose transport across the blood-brain barrier due to mutations in the SLC2A1 gene, which encodes the glucose transporter, GLUT1 [36]. Clinically, GLUT1 DS is characterized by cognitive impairment, mixed seizure types, and a complex movement disorder. The vast majority of children with GLUT1 DS achieve seizure freedom with a CKD, which should be introduced as early as possible and continued through to adulthood [36]. The CKD may be difficult to tolerate in older children and adolescents, in which case the MAD is also effective [2]. In GLUT1 DS, ketogenic diets may also enhance the child's alertness, and they frequently improve the movement disorder [36].

In PDHD, pyruvate is unable to be metabolized into acetyl-CoA, resulting in abnormal mitochondrial metabolism and lactic acidosis [37]. Clinically, PDHD is characterized by seizures, severe encephalopathy, and—usually—death during childhood. The CKD is effective and safe in PDHD, and appears to increase longevity and improve mental development [37]. However, severe forms of PDHD may not be appropriate for the diet if quality of life is not improved [2].

3.1.3 Specific seizure disorders in children

Ketogenic diets should be considered early in the management of children with seizure disorders that consistently demonstrate a 60–70% improvement in seizure control, well above the "usual" 40–50% improvement [2]. These disorders include Angelman syndrome, complex I mitochondrial disorders, Doose syndrome, Dravet syndrome, febrile infection-related epilepsy syndrome (FIRES), formula-fed infants or children, infantile spasms, Ohtahara syndrome, super-refractory status epilepticus, and tuberous sclerosis complex [2].

3.2 Preparing a child (and caregiver) for a ketogenic diet

Once the child is selected for a ketogenic diet, a medical and nutritional evaluation is both strongly advised (**Table 4**) [2, 26]. In addition to the caregiver (usually a parent), anyone else who will be helping institute the diet should attend.

3.2.1 Medical evaluation

A medical evaluation should be performed by a pediatric neurologist experienced in managing ketogenic diets in children, and include an assessment of the child's epilepsy, comorbidities, psychological and socioeconomic factors, medications, and investigations [2].

First, the pediatric neurologist must assess the child's baseline epilepsy state and any comorbidities that may complicate a ketogenic diet. Seizure symptomatology and frequency should be documented in sufficient detail so as to later gauge diet

Evaluation	Steps
Medical	Assess baseline epilepsy state and comorbidities
	Identify psycho-socioeconomic, cultural, and religious factors
	Review anti-epileptic drugs and medications
	Provide blood glucose and ketone monitor; show how to use
	Order investigations
Nutritional	Assess baseline physical parameters
	Select most appropriate conventional ketogenic diet
	Provide supplements
	Educate caregiver

Table 4.
Preparing a child (and caregiver) for a ketogenic diet.

efficacy on seizure control. Potential complicating comorbidities include gastrointestinal issues (such as gastroesophageal reflux and constipation), hypercholesterolemia, low weight gain, kidney stones, chronic metabolic acidosis, and cardiomyopathy [2]. Once identified, most comorbidities can be preventatively managed.

Second, it is critical to identify psychological, socioeconomic, cultural, and religious factors that may affect the child's diet [2]. Challenging behavior traits in the child or caregiver should be addressed early. Since many patients with epilepsy are of lower socioeconomic status, an appraisal of the family environment, including finances, is essential before deciding to proceed; even if deemed adequate, the caregiver must be made aware of the impact of a ketogenic diet on time and resources, including separate meal preparation from the rest of the family and increased costs [26]. It is also necessary to consider the family's cultural and religious background, which may result in some recipes being more suitable than others [2].

Third, the child's medications should be reviewed. Generally, blood levels of common anti-epileptic drugs are not significantly altered by a ketogenic diet, therefore dose adjustments are not required. However, it may be worth considering dose reductions in the case of valproate, zonisamide, and topiramate; although these drugs are generally safe alongside a ketogenic diet, there have been rare instances of hepatotoxicity and secondary carnitine deficiency with valproate, as well as chronic metabolic acidosis and a slight increase in kidney stones with zonisamide and topiramate [2]. All medications should be reviewed for carbohydrate content, which may necessitate a switch to lower carbohydrate preparations [26].

Fourth, the child and caregiver should be provided with a means of self-monitoring the diet, which critically provides feedback as to how effectively the child is achieving physiological ketosis [2]. Traditionally, this has been done using urine ketone dipstick testing, but it is now possible to prescribe a blood glucose and ketone monitor in many countries. The former is less expensive and avoids finger pricks, but the latter is easier, more specific, and more accurate [38]. Unless there is a compelling reason to measure urinary ketones, a blood glucose and ketone monitor should be prescribed and the caregiver instructed on its use.

Finally, investigations should be ordered before commencing a ketogenic diet in a child, primarily to rule out contraindications (a ketogenic diet is absolutely contraindicated in disorders of fat metabolism, including carnitine deficiency, carnitine palmitoyltransferase I and II deficiency, any of the short, medium, or long-chain acyl dehydrogenase deficiencies, and porphyria) [2]. Basic laboratory investigations include complete blood count, electrolytes, liver and kidney function tests, fasting lipid profile, calcium, vitamin D, serum acylcarnitine profile, and a urinalysis [2]. Baseline anti-epileptic drug levels can be measured, although few concerns for drug-diet interactions exist. A recent EEG and MRI brain should be obtained to identify potential surgical candidates. Further tests, such as ECG and renal ultrasound, may be ordered as clinically indicated.

3.2.2 Nutritional evaluation

A nutritional evaluation should be performed by a dietitian experienced in managing ketogenic diets in children, and include an assessment of baseline physical parameters, selection of the most suitable ketogenic diet, and education of the caregiver on what to expect with the diet.

Baseline weight, body-mass index, and height are routinely measured (in infants, head circumference is also measured) [2]. The child's recommended calorie and fluid intake should be calculated, as well as the desired fat to protein to carbohydrate ratio. Food aversions and allergies must be clearly documented.

When selecting a conventional ketogenic diet for a child, the most important factor to consider is the family environment, rather than perceived diet efficacy [2]. The CKD is highly effective for seizure control, but restrictive and time-consuming; depending on the family environment, it may be more feasible to implement the MCT diet, MAD, or LGIT diet. Regarding diet efficacy, the CKD appears to be superior to the MAD in infants under 2 years of age, whereas both are equally effective in older children [27]. For the transition to adolescence, the MAD and LGIT diet are less restrictive and more appropriate; the LGIT diet may not provide an adequate level of ketosis to treat GLUT1 DS and PDHD, although it is highly effective in Angelman syndrome [2, 39]. For infants and children on enteral feeds, ketogenic diets can be administered in liquid form, which may be more convenient and efficacious [2].

Given the limited fruit, vegetable, and calcium content in conventional ketogenic diets, supplementation with a carbohydrate-free multivitamin containing minerals, as well as supplementation with calcium and vitamin D, is considered mandatory in children [26]. No particular recommendations exist for supplementing a ketogenic diet with magnesium, selenium, carnitine, laxatives, probiotics, or exogenous ketones [2, 26].

Caregiver education is essential; the caregiver needs to understand exactly what is required of them to implement the diet. A classroom-based format, with several different caregivers present, can be advantageous [26]. The dietitian should demonstrate how to identify sources of fat, protein, and carbohydrate, how to count net carbohydrate (total carbohydrate minus fiber) for those on a MAD, how to identify foods with a low glycemic index for those on an LGIT diet, and how to navigate potential pitfalls [26]. Helpful additional resources should be provided [40, 41] and any expectations addressed.

3.3 Implementing a ketogenic diet in a child

Once the child and caregiver have been prepared, it is time to implement the diet (**Table 5**) [2]. The pediatric ketogenic service should take on a strong supportive role, aiding the caregiver as much as possible in troubleshooting problems.

3.3.1 Diet initiation

Currently, it is recommended that the CKD be initiated with the child in hospital [2]. The advantages of an inpatient admission include the ability to closely observe

Stage	Steps
Initiation	Decide whether to initiate as inpatient or outpatient
	If inpatient, decide on induction fast and diet introduction
	If outpatient, provide clear instructions to caregiver
Maintenance	Caregiver monitors seizure control and ketone levels
	Review at 1, 3, 6, 9, 12 months, and 6-monthly after
	Monitor for adverse effects
Cessation	Identify when diet should be ceased (if ever)
	If to be ceased, consider switching to another ketogenic diet
	If to be ceased, decide on rate of diet cessation

Table 5.
Implementing a ketogenic diet in a child with epilepsy.

the child, medically intervene if necessary, and provide more time to educate the caregiver on how to maintain the diet upon returning home.

Traditionally, a 12–24 hours fast has been used to commence the diet in an inpatient setting [2]. Fasting may lead to a quicker onset of seizure reduction, which may be useful in refractory status epilepticus [2]. However, induction fasts do not improve ketosis or seizure control at 3 months, and fasted children experience weight loss, hypoglycemia, and acidosis more frequently, which may increase the length of hospital stay [42]. Thus, although an induction fast should be considered, most pediatric ketogenic services no longer routinely fast children, and none recommend fasting infants under 2 years of age [2].

Regardless of whether an induction fast is utilized, several approaches may be used to introduce the CKD in hospital [2]. One approach involves starting the diet at one-third or one-half of the final calorie level, increasing the calories by one-third or one-half over several days until full calorie intake is achieved, keeping the fat to protein to carbohydrate ratio constant. Another approach is to start with full calorie intake, but increase the ratio of fat to protein plus carbohydrate daily, from 1:1 to 2:1 to 3:1 to 4:1, allowing the child to gradually adapt to the increasing fat intake. Yet another approach is to simply commence the CKD at full calories and a 4:1 ratio on the first day, which does not appear to prolong hospital stay, increase adverse effects, or decrease diet efficacy at 3 months.

In older children, the CKD may be initiated as an outpatient, the advantages of which include reduced family stress and fewer hospital-associated costs [2]. Most pediatric ketogenic services also routinely initiate the less-restrictive MAD and LGIT diet in the outpatient setting. If a graded introduction is required at home, clear instructions must be given to the caregiver on how to do so.

3.3.2 Diet maintenance

Once initiated, ketogenic diets tend to work rapidly and effectively, with 75% of children responding within 14 days [43]. Complete seizure freedom often occurs within several months of initiation, although it may take up to 18 months [44]. The caregiver should monitor the child's ketone levels (ideally, the blood BHB level) daily for the first several weeks, then two or three times a week once readings consistently show the child to be in physiological ketosis. Most pediatric ketogenic services recommend a blood BHB level of 4–6 mmol/L, although this is not based on clinical evidence [3]. If seizure control or ketone levels are not responding as expected, a 3-day food diary may be useful to discover potential oversights in diet implementation.

The pediatric neurologist and dietitian should be in frequent phone or email contact with the caregiver during the initial weeks of the diet, with additional follow-up visits occurring at 1, 3, 6, 9, and 12 months, and every 6 months thereafter [2]. The pediatric neurologist should document the child's seizure response, and regardless of any improvement, resist altering their anti-epileptic drugs unless necessary; alterations may make it difficult to gauge diet efficacy on seizure control. Recommended follow-up tests include complete blood count, electrolytes, liver and kidney function tests, fasting lipid profile, calcium, and vitamin D [2]. Since ketogenic diets and anti-epileptic drugs may predispose a child to osteopenia, some pediatric ketogenic services perform a bone density scan after 2 years on the diet [2]. The dietitian should monitor the child's physical parameters and nutritional intake at every visit. Ketogenic diets have a diuretic effect and fluid content in the food may be lessened, therefore fluid hydration must be monitored, and increased if necessary [26].

Both the caregiver and the pediatric ketogenic service must monitor the child for adverse effects. Gastrointestinal symptoms such as nausea, vomiting, abdominal pain, and constipation appear in up to 50% of children on the CKD, but are easily remedied by increasing fluid, salt, and fiber intake [2]. Hyperlipidemia is common, with raised triglyceride and low-density lipoprotein (LDL) levels seen in up to 60% of children on the CKD, but the increase is usually transient and normalizes within 1 year; if desired, the LDL can be lowered by altering the types of fats ingested (for example, by increasing olive oil and decreasing saturated fats) [2]. Moreover, ketogenic diets may slightly inhibit a child's growth; adjustments in calorie intake may compensate. Kidney stones may occur in 3–7% of children on the CKD, but can be prevented with oral citrates [2]. Ultimately, such common adverse effects are rarely sufficient reasons to discontinue the CKD, but rarer adverse effects such as cardiomyopathy, prolonged QT interval, and pancreatitis may provide sufficient reason to do so.

3.3.3 Diet cessation

Upon ceasing a ketogenic diet, the long-term benefits on seizure control often outlast the diet itself. In children who become seizure-free on a ketogenic diet, 80% will remain so after diet cessation [45], an effect that can persist for many years.

The child's ketogenic diet should be maintained for at least 3 months before passing judgment on its efficacy in seizure control [2]. The exception to this rule is if the seizures worsen for longer than 1–2 weeks after commencing the diet, or if a serious adverse effect occurs—in either case, it may be wise to discontinue the diet sooner.

If a child experiences the "usual" greater than 50% seizure reduction, the ketogenic diet is usually discontinued after 2 years [2]. In new-onset infantile spasms, the diet can be ceased at 6 months [46]. In drug-resistant epilepsy in which seizure control is virtually complete (over 90% seizure reduction) and GLUT1 DS, the diet can be carried into adulthood [2]. Older children may start to see their diet as overly restrictive; if it effectively controls the seizures, it may be switched over to another type of ketogenic diet (for example, from a CKD or MCT diet to a MAD or LGIT diet).

A child's ketogenic diet should be ceased gradually (over several months) [2]. In the case of the CKD, the ratio can be reduced by decreasing the ratio of fat to protein plus carbohydrate monthly, from 4:1 to 3:1 to 2:1 to 1:1, allowing the child to gradually adapt to the decreasing fat intake, followed by the reintroduction of regular foods. However, it is usually still possible to cease the diet more rapidly (over several weeks) without negative consequences, although some children may experience a higher risk of increased seizures during the tapering-down period. If medically necessary, ketogenic diets can be stopped abruptly; this is best done in hospital.

4. Ketogenic diet therapies in adults with epilepsy

Few epilepsy centers in the world offer a dedicated adult ketogenic service [3]. Such a service should consist of a neurologist, nurse, dietitian, and ideally a psychologist and social worker [3, 47].

4.1 Selecting the right adult for a ketogenic diet

Ketogenic diets in adults are indicated in drug-resistant epilepsy and certain seizure disorders (**Table 6**); they may be used in adults of all ages [47].

4.1.1 Drug-resistant epilepsy in adults

In 2010, the ILAE defined drug-resistant epilepsy as the failure of adequate trials of two appropriately chosen, tolerated, and used anti-epileptic drug schedules (whether as monotherapies or in combination) to achieve sustained seizure freedom [28]. Since adults may suffer from drug-resistant epilepsy for decades, many adult patients have already failed multiple trials of anti-epileptic drugs over their lifetime.

Further anti-epileptic drug trials and epilepsy surgery may be feasible options in adults with drug-resistant epilepsy [30]. However, subsequent drug trials confer only a slight (about 5%) chance of inducing seizure remission [31]. Surgery should always be considered, but some eligible adults may not be ready to pursue surgery [48], and many others will not be eligible due to a generalized or multifocal epilepsy syndrome, or nonresectable lesion of ictal onset.

When drug trials and surgery are not feasible, a ketogenic diet may be indicated [48]. Many single-arm studies have demonstrated the efficacy and safety of ketogenic diets in treating drug-resistant epilepsy in adults, but to date there are no randomized controlled trials of a ketogenic diet in adults with drug-resistant epilepsy.

Surprisingly, a 1930 study remains the largest retrospective case series to examine a ketogenic diet in adults with epilepsy [49]. In this study, 100 adolescents and adults with epilepsy were treated with a CKD. After 1–46 months, 56% of patients had a greater than 50% seizure reduction.

General disorder	Specific disorder
Drug-resistant epilepsy	2010 ILAE definition
Disorders of brain metabolism	GLUT1 DS
	PDHD
Specific seizure disorders	JME
	Lennox-Gastaut syndrome
	Rett syndrome

ILAE = International League Against Epilepsy; GLUT1 DS = GLUT1 deficiency syndrome; PDHD = pyruvate dehydrogenase complex deficiency; JME = juvenile myoclonic epilepsy.

Table 6.
Epilepsy disorders in adults for which a ketogenic diet may be indicated; this list is not comprehensive.

In 2014, a review of all subsequently published ketogenic diet studies in adults with drug-resistant epilepsy was published [50]. Five studies examined the use of a CKD to treat a combined total of 47 adults with drug-resistant epilepsy. After 3–26 months, 15 patients (32%) had a greater than 50% seizure reduction, with 24 patients (51%) stopping the diet before study completion. Another five studies examined the use of a MAD to treat a combined total of 85 adults with drug-resistant epilepsy. After 3–12 months, 24 patients (28%) had a greater than 50% seizure reduction, with 36 patients (42%) stopping the diet before completion. For both diets, most patients withdrew due to culinary and social restrictions.

In 2016, the largest observational study of a ketogenic diet in adults with drug-resistant epilepsy was published, in which 106 patients were treated with a MAD [48]. After 3 months, 38 patients (36%) had a greater than 50% seizure reduction, with 47 patients (44%) not completing the study, largely due to diet restrictiveness.

Pooling the results from these single-arm studies suggests that 30–40% of adults with drug-resistant epilepsy experience a greater than 50% seizure reduction after 3 or more months on a ketogenic diet. While these results are encouraging, they emanate from single-arm studies; moreover, 40–50% of adults stopped their diet before study completion. Clearly, randomized controlled trials involving less restrictive ketogenic diets are needed in adults with drug-resistant epilepsy.

4.1.2 Specific seizure disorders in adults

Ketogenic diets remain standard treatments for disorders of impaired brain glucose metabolism in adults [47]. In GLUT1 DS, ketogenic diets have been shown to confer seizure freedom in up to 90% of patients, including adults [47]. The prognosis in more severe forms of PDHD may be poor, but less severely affected individuals may benefit from a ketogenic diet as they transition to adulthood.

In addition to GLUT1 DS and PDHD, ketogenic diet therapy may be warranted in several seizure disorders often seen in adults, including juvenile myoclonic epilepsy (JME), Lennox-Gastaut syndrome, and Rett syndrome [48]. JME is particularly common, representing 5–10% of all epilepsy cases, and typically manifests in adolescence or early adulthood with a combination of myoclonic jerks or seizures, absence seizures, and generalized tonic-clonic seizures. In two separate case series, 60–70% of adolescents and adults with JME experienced a 50% seizure reduction after 3 months of MAD therapy [51, 52].

4.2 Preparing an adult (and partner) for a ketogenic diet

Once the adult has been selected for the diet, a medical and nutritional evaluation is advised (**Table 7**) [3, 47]. If possible, a cohabiting partner (spouse or family member) should accompany the adult to the evaluations, and ideally participate in the diet alongside them.

4.2.1 Medical evaluation

A brief medical evaluation should be performed by a neurologist with experience managing ketogenic diets in adults, and should include a history of the epilepsy, comorbidities, psychological and socioeconomic factors, level of commitment to the diet, medications, and investigations [47].

First, the neurologist must ascertain the adult's baseline epilepsy state and any comorbidities that may complicate their ketogenic diet. The symptomatology and frequency of the various types of seizures should be documented in sufficient detail so as to later gauge diet efficacy on seizure control. Potentially complicating

Evaluation	Steps
Medical	Assess baseline epilepsy state and comorbidities
	Identify psycho-socioeconomic, cultural, and religious factors
	Elucidate level of commitment
	Review anti-epileptic drugs and medications
	Provide blood glucose and ketone monitor; show how to use
	Order investigations
Nutritional	Assess baseline physical parameters
	Select most appropriate conventional ketogenic diet
	If none appropriate, offer a non-conventional ketogenic diet
	Provide list of foods for social settings
	Provide supplements
	Educate patient

Table 7.
Preparing an adult (and partner) for a ketogenic diet.

comorbidities include hypercholesterolemia, underweight body-mass index, kidney stones, osteopenia or osteoporosis, gastrointestinal issues (such as gastroesophageal reflux and constipation), cardiomyopathy, and diabetes [3]. Adults with type 1 diabetes can safely pursue a ketogenic diet, but must be closely monitored as their insulin requirements often decline, putting them at risk of hypoglycemia if they do not adjust their insulin doses accordingly [53]. Adults with type 2 diabetes may also start a ketogenic diet [3]; in fact, such adults may be ideal candidates.

Second, it is critical to identify psychological, socioeconomic, cultural, and religious factors with the potential to disrupt the adult's ketogenic diet [3]. Diet adherence in adults may be endangered by any number of factors, including personality traits, alcohol habits, income, cultural influences, and religious preferences; each must be realistically appraised before the adult and ketogenic service commit to the diet.

Third, the adult's level of commitment to ketogenic diet therapy must be elucidated. Diet modification often involves a major change in lifestyle, therefore anything less than a full commitment is likely to fail. If the adult holds any reservations about commencing the diet, these should be explored; if unsolvable, the adult may not yet be ready for the diet. The neurologist should counsel the adult on how to deal with inevitable "mixed messages" regarding the purported negative aspects of high-fat diets from friends, family, and even other medical professionals. Lastly, it can be helpful to emphasize the additional positive aspects of a ketogenic diet, such as beneficial effects on cognition, energy, and mood [47].

Fourth, the adult's medications should be reviewed. In general, anti-epileptic drug blood levels are not altered by a ketogenic diet, therefore dose adjustments are not usually required. However, for the same reasons as in children, exceptions might be made in the case of valproate, zonisamide, or topiramate [2]. All medications should be reviewed for carbohydrate content, which may necessitate a switch to lower carbohydrate preparations [47].

Fifth, the adult should be provided with a means of self-monitoring their diet, which critically provides feedback as to how effectively they are achieving physiological ketosis. In adults, it is best to prescribe a blood glucose and ketone monitor given that this method is easier, more specific, and more accurate than urine dipstick testing [38]. The adult should be shown how to use the monitor.

Finally, investigations should be ordered to rule out contraindications to a ketogenic diet (as a rule, it is not necessary to screen for disorders of fat metabolism in adults, unless the history suggests otherwise) [47]. Laboratory investigations include complete blood count, electrolytes, liver and kidney function tests, fasting lipid profile, calcium, vitamin D, and a urinalysis [3]. Given that the effects of a ketogenic diet on pregnancy are not known [3], pregnancy testing may be indicated in women of childbearing age. Baseline anti-epileptic drug levels can be measured, although few concerns for drug-diet interactions exist. A recent EEG and MRI brain should be obtained to identify potential surgical candidates. Given that ketogenic diets and anti-epileptic drugs may predispose adults to osteopenia, a baseline bone density scan may be wise. Further tests, such as ECG and renal ultrasound, are ordered as clinically indicated.

4.2.2 Nutritional evaluation

A nutritional evaluation should be performed by a dietitian experienced in managing ketogenic diets in adults, and ought to include an assessment of baseline physical status, a decision as to which is the most appropriate ketogenic diet option for that adult, and education about their chosen ketogenic diet.

Baseline weight and body-mass index should be measured and recommended calorie and fluid intake calculated, including the desired ratio of fat to protein to carbohydrate [48]. Food aversions and allergies must be clearly documented.

When selecting which conventional ketogenic diet to use, the most important factors to consider in adults are culinary and social restrictions [48, 50]. Since the CKD is the most restrictive of the four, it is rarely a viable long-term option in adults (unless given as a formula). The MCT diet is slightly less restrictive, but still not viable in most adults due to the copious quantities of MCT oil and resulting gastrointestinal side-effects. The MAD and LGIT are less restrictive conventional options in adults, but both are still associated with considerable dropout rates [54]. Thus, although conventional ketogenic diets should be offered, the adult may not be motivated to pursue any of them; this will negatively impact diet implementation.

If conventional ketogenic diets do not appeal to the adult, a fifth option, that of a non-conventional ketogenic diet, can be considered. Such a diet might consist of dietitian-verified recipes obtained from trusted ketogenic diet books and websites, a major advantage of which is that it can be specifically tailored towards the adult's food preferences, reducing the perception that their diet is restrictive. It is now possible to prepare a variety of ketogenic diets, including vegetarian and culturally-tailored ketogenic diets (theoretically, as long as a ketogenic diet sustains physiological ketosis, it is "ketogenic"). Given that each conventional ketogenic diet is decades old (nearly a century old in the case of the CKD), a newer, less restrictive, patient-tailored ketogenic diet is appealing to many adults, although it must be emphasized that evidence for such a diet in epilepsy may be lacking.

Since many adults with epilepsy are of lower socioeconomic status, the dietitian must strive to minimize any socioeconomic impediments that may disrupt their ketogenic diet. Social activities are to be encouraged, but they can also jeopardize the diet; it is extremely helpful if the dietitian provides a list of appropriate food options relevant to most restaurants and social gatherings that will inform the adult as to what they can and cannot eat, so as not to disrupt the diet. For meals made at home, the dietitian should recommend foods that are both within the adult's budget range as well as readily available at their local food markets.

Given the limited fruit, vegetable, and calcium content in many ketogenic diets, adults should be commenced on a carbohydrate-free multivitamin [3, 47]. Some ketogenic services also supplement adults with calcium, vitamin D, and magnesium [3, 47].

Lastly, education is essential; the adult needs to understand exactly what is required of them to implement their diet. A classroom-based format, with multiple adult patients present, can be advantageous [26]. The dietitian should demonstrate how to identify sources of fat, protein, and carbohydrate, how to count net carbohydrate (total carbohydrate minus fiber) for those on a MAD or non-conventional ketogenic diet, how to identify foods with a low glycemic index for those on an LGIT diet, and how to navigate potential pitfalls [26]. Helpful additional resources should be provided [55] and any expectations addressed.

4.3 Implementing a ketogenic diet in an adult

Once the adult has been prepared, their chosen diet can be implemented (**Table 8**) [47]. The ketogenic service should provide as much support as the adult needs, but also encourage them to develop a sense of "ownership" over their diet, thus conferring a feeling of empowerment over their epilepsy.

4.3.1 Diet initiation

In younger and disabled adults, it may be more appropriate to initiate a ketogenic diet as an inpatient [48]. The advantages of an admission include the ability to observe the patient and medically intervene if needed, and provide more time to educate the caregiver on how to maintain the diet upon returning home. In general, fasting is not employed in adults, although an induction fast might be useful if a quicker response is required (for example, if the adult is having multiple daily seizures, an induction fast might lessen the interference of the epilepsy on the initiation of the diet) [48]. The same graded approach used to introduce the diet in children may also be used in adults [48].

In most cases, adults with epilepsy can initiate their ketogenic diet as an outpatient, especially if they have selected the MAD, LGIT diet, or a non-conventional ketogenic diet. In most adults, it is not necessary to employ a graded approach when initiating a ketogenic diet at home, but if required then clear instructions should be provided on how to do so.

Stage	Steps
Initiation	Decide whether to initiate as inpatient or outpatient
	If inpatient, decide on induction fast and diet introduction
	If outpatient, provide clear instructions to caregiver
Maintenance	Adult self-monitors seizure control and ketone levels
	Review at 3 and 6 months, and 6-monthly after
	Monitor for adverse effects
	Document beneficial effects
Cessation	Identify when diet should be ceased (if ever)
	If to be ceased, consider switching to another ketogenic diet
	If to be ceased, decide on rate of diet cessation
	If relevant, consider diet cessation and driving

Table 8.
Implementing a ketogenic diet in an adult with epilepsy.

4.3.2 Diet maintenance

Ketogenic diets often work rapidly, within days [43]. The adult should regularly monitor their blood BHB level daily for the first several weeks, then two or three times a week once readings indicate that constant physiological ketosis has been achieved. There are no firm recommendations regarding optimal blood BHB levels in adults [3], although aiming for at least 2 mmol/L at all times seems reasonable. If seizure control or ketone levels are not responding as expected, a 3-day food diary may be useful to discover potential oversights in diet implementation.

The neurologist or dietitian should be in regular phone or email contact during the initial weeks of the diet, with multidisciplinary follow-up visits at 3 and 6 months, and every 6 months thereafter [3]. The neurologist should document the adult's seizure response to the diet; regardless of any improvement, anti-epileptic drugs should not be altered unless necessary, as alterations may make it difficult to gauge diet efficacy on seizure control. Recommended follow-up tests include complete blood count, electrolytes, liver and kidney function tests, fasting lipid profile, calcium, and vitamin D [47]. If osteopenia is a concern, a bone density scan may be warranted every 5 years or less [47], and bone protection therapy prescribed as needed. The dietitian should monitor weight, nutritional intake, and fluid hydration at every visit, and alter each as required.

Adverse effects may occur in adults on a ketogenic diet, but are generally transient, and rarely serious enough to necessitate stopping the diet [47]. The two most common adverse effects in adults are hyperlipidemia and weight loss [48]. Raised LDL levels are seen in least one-quarter of adults with epilepsy [48]. However, triglyceride levels often decline, and HDL levels usually increase [47]. Moreover, among healthy adults following a low-carbohydrate diet, the LDL increase is due to increased LDL particle size rather than particle number, which may be associated with a lower risk of atherosclerosis [56]. Furthermore, LDL and total cholesterol levels typically normalize within a year of commencing the diet [57], and return to baseline within 3 months of stopping it [50]. Weight loss is also common on a ketogenic diet, seen in at least one-fifth of adult with epilepsy [48], but since many such adults are overweight or obese, this adverse effect is often desired and beneficial [47]. Other adverse effects, such as kidney stones and osteopenia or osteoporosis, are rare in adults [47].

Benefits other than seizure control may also occur with a ketogenic diet, including improved arousal, alertness, concentration, energy, and mood [3, 47]. Moreover, adults on a ketogenic diet often report increased quality of life scores [58]. Given that many adults with epilepsy suffer from impaired quality of life, these additional benefits may be significant and should be documented.

4.3.3 Diet cessation

Unlike children, the long-term benefits on seizure control in adults with epilepsy may not outlast dietary therapy [59]. Further studies are needed to determine if this is the case for all adults.

It is customary to maintain a ketogenic diet for at least 3 months before passing judgment on its efficacy in seizure control [3]. The exception to this rule is if the seizures worsen for longer than 1–2 weeks after commencing the diet, or if a serious adverse effect occurs—in either case, it may be wise to discontinue the diet sooner.

If the adult experiences a greater than 50% seizure reduction and no serious adverse effects, their ketogenic diet can be maintained indefinitely [3]. If the adult starts to perceive their diet as overly restrictive, yet it remains effective at controlling seizures, it can be switched over to another type of ketogenic diet.

Most ketogenic diets in adults are ceased slowly, over weeks or months on an individual basis [3], although many can be ceased abruptly without negative consequences. The sole exception may be the CKD, which can be ceased gradually by decreasing the ratio of fat to protein plus carbohydrate weekly or monthly, from 4:1 to 3:1 to 2:1 to 1:1, followed by the reintroduction of regular foods.

An important consideration during diet cessation is the effect on driving restrictions. If a ketogenic diet has conferred complete seizure freedom for a long enough period of time such that the adult has returned to driving, stopping the diet applies the same driving restrictions as when anti-epileptic drugs are altered or modified [3].

5. Conclusions

Historically, ketogenic diets have been utilized as "end of the line" therapeutic options in children and adults with epilepsy. However, given recent advances in the possible mechanisms through which these diets improve seizure control and the growing evidence base supporting their use in epilepsy, this is changing. Significant challenges to the more widespread use of ketogenic diets in children and adults with epilepsy remain, most conspicuously a lack of access to ketogenic services in many regions of the world. Moreover, the culinary and social restrictions associated with conventional ketogenic diets are barriers to their use in adults. If these issues can be addressed, there may come a day when ketogenic diet therapies are utilized more widely, as first-line options alongside drugs and surgery, in the management of children and adults with epilepsy.

Acknowledgements

The author is grateful for the support of Waikato Hospital, Hamilton, New Zealand.

Conflict of interest

The author declares no conflict of interest.

Author details

Matthew Charles Lee Phillips
Waikato Hospital, Hamilton, New Zealand

*Address all correspondence to: matthew.phillips@waikatodhb.health.nz

References

[1] Granata T, Marchi N, Carlton E, et al. Management of the patient with medically refractory epilepsy. Expert Review of Neurotherapeutics. 2009; **9**(12):1791-1802. DOI: 10.1586/ern.09.114

[2] Kossoff EH, Zupec-Kania BA, Auvin S, et al. Optimal clinical management of children receiving dietary therapies for epilepsy: Updated recommendations of the International Ketogenic Diet Study Group. Epilepsia Open. 2018;**3**(2): 175-192. DOI: 10.1002/epi4.12225

[3] Schoeler NE, Cross JH. Ketogenic dietary therapies in adults with epilepsy: A practical guide. Practical Neurology. 2016;**16**:208-214. DOI: 10.1136/practneurol-2015-001288

[4] Wilder RM. The effect on ketonemia on the course of epilepsy. Mayo Clinic Bulletin. 1921;**2**:307-318. DOI: 10.1001/jama.1927.02680470024012

[5] Kim JM. Ketogenic diet: Old treatment, new beginning. Clinical Neurophysiology Practice. 2017;**2**: 161-162. DOI: 10.1016/j.cnp.2017.07.001

[6] Stewart WK, Fleming LW. Features of a successful therapeutic fast of 382 days' duration. Postgraduate Medical Journal. 1973;**49**(569):203-209

[7] Rho J. How does the ketogenic diet induce anti-seizure effects? Neuroscience Letters. 2017;**637**:4-10. DOI: 10.1016/j.neulet.2015.07.034

[8] Lutas A, Yellen G. The ketogenic diet: Metabolic influences on brain excitability and epilepsy. Trends in Neurosciences. 2013;**36**(1):32-40. DOI: 10.1016/j.tins.2012.11.005

[9] Puchalska P, Crawford PA. Multi-dimensional roles of ketone bodies in fuel metabolism, signaling, and therapeutics. Cell Metabolism. 2017; **25**(2):262-284. DOI: 10.1016/j.cmet.2016.12.022

[10] Paoli A. Ketogenic diet for obesity: Friend or foe? International Journal of Environmental Research and Public Health. 2014;**11**(2):2092-2107. DOI: 10.3390/ijerph110202092

[11] Simeone TA, Simeone KA, Stafstrom CE, et al. Do ketone bodies mediate the anti-seizure effects of the ketogenic diet? Neuropharmacology. 2018;**133**:233-241. DOI: 10.1016/j.neuropharm.2018.01.011

[12] Politi K, Shemer-Meiri L, Shuper A, et al. The Ketogenic diet 2011: How it works. Epilepsy Research and Treatment. 2011;**2011**:1-4. DOI: 10.1155/2011/963637

[13] Ma W, Berg J, Yellen G. Ketogenic diet metabolites reduce firing in central neurons by opening K(ATP) channels. The Journal of Neuroscience. 2007;**27**: 3618-3625. DOI: 10.1523/JNEUROSCI.0132-07.2007

[14] Juge N, Gray JA, Omote H, et al. Metabolic control of vesicular glutamate transport and release. 2010;**68**(1): 99-112. DOI: 10.1016/j.neuron.2010.09.002

[15] Keith HM. Factors influencing experimentally produced convulsions. Archives of Neurology & Psychiatry. 1933;**29**(1):148-154. DOI: 10.1001/archneurpsyc.1933.02240070154009

[16] Keith HM, Stavraky GW. Experimental convulsions induced by administration of thujone. Archives of Neurology and Psychiatry. 1935;**34**(5): 1022-1040. DOI: 10.1001/archneurpsyc.1935.02250230094008

[17] Shimazu T, Hirschey MD, Newman J, et al. Suppression of oxidative stress

by β-hydroxybutyrate, an endogenous histone deacetylase inhibitor. Science. 2013;**339**(6116):211-214. DOI: 10.1126/science.1227166

[18] Youm YH, Nguyen KY, Grant RW, et al. The ketone metabolite β-hydroxybutyrate blocks NLRP3 inflammasome-mediated inflammatory disease. Nature Medicine. 2015;**21**:263-269. DOI: 10.1038/nm.3804

[19] Augustin K, Khabbush A, Williams S, et al. Mechanisms of action for the medium-chain triglycerideketogenic diet in neurological and metabolic disorders. Lancet Neurology. 2018;**17**: 84-93. DOI: 10.1016/S1474-4422(17) 30408-8.

[20] Masino SA, Li T, Theofilas P, Sandau US, et al. A ketogenic diet suppresses seizures in mice through adenosine A(1) receptors. The Journal of Clinical Investigation. 2011;**121**(7): 26792683. DOI: 10.1172/JCI57813.

[21] Chang P, Augustin K, Boddum K, et al. Seizure control by decanoic acid through direct AMPA receptor inhibition. Brain. 2016;**139**(2):431-443. DOI: 10.1093/brain/awv325

[22] Huttenlocher PR, Wilbourn AJ, Signore JM. Medium-chain triglycerides as a therapy for intractable childhood epilepsy. Neurology. 1971;**21**:1097-1103. DOI: 10.1212/WNL.21.11.1097

[23] Schwartz RH, Eaton J, Bower BD, et al. Ketogenic diets in the treatment of epilepsy: Short-term clinical effects. Developmental Medicine and Child Neurology. 1989;**1**:145-151. DOI: 10.1111/j.1469-8749.1989.tb03972.x

[24] Kossoff EH, McGrogan JR, Bluml RM, et al. A modified Atkins diet is effective for the treatment of intractable pediatric epilepsy. Epilepsia. 2006;**47**: 421-424. DOI: 10.1111/j.1528-1167.2006.00438.x

[25] Pfeifer HH, Thiele EA. Low-glycemic-index treatment: A liberalized ketogenic diet for treatment of intractable epilepsy. Neurology. 2005; **65**:1810-1812. DOI: 10.1212/01.wnl.0000187071.24292.9e

[26] Roehl K, Sewak SL. Practice paper of the academy of nutrition and dietetics: Classic and modified ketogenic diets for treatment of epilepsy. Journal of the Academy of Nutrition and Dietetics. 2017;**117**:1279-1292. DOI: 10.1016/j.jand.2017.06.006

[27] Kim JA, Yoon JR, Lee EJ, et al. Efficacy of the classic ketogenic and the modified Atkins diets in refractory childhood epilepsy. Epilepsia. 2016;**57**: 51-58. DOI: 10.1111/epi.13256

[28] Kwan P, Arzimanoglou A, Berg AT, et al. Definition of drug resistant epilepsy: Consensus proposal by the ad hoc task force of the ILAE commission on therapeutic strategies. Epilepsia. 2010;**51**(6):1069-1077. DOI: 10.1111/j.1528-1167.2009.02397.x

[29] Kwan P, Schachter SC, Brodie MJ. Drug-resistant epilepsy. The New England Journal of Medicine. 2011; **365**(10):919-926. DOI: 10.1056/NEJMra1004418

[30] Dalic L, Cook MJ. Managing drug-resistant epilepsy: Challenges and solutions. Neuropsychiatric Disease and Treatment. 2016;**2016**:2605-2616. DOI: 10.2147/NDT.S84852

[31] Callaghan B, Schlesinger M, Rodemer W, et al. Remission and relapse in a drug-resistant epilepsy population followed prospectively. Epilepsia. 2011;**52**(3): 619-626. DOI: 10.1111/j.1528-1167.2010.02929.x

[32] Neal EG, Chaffe HM, Schwartz RH, et al. The ketogenic diet in the treatment of epilepsy in children: A randomised, controlled trial. Lancet Neurology.

2008;7:500-506. DOI: 10.1016/S1474-4422(08)70092-9

[33] Freeman JM, Vining EP, Kossoff EH, et al. A blinded, crossover study of the efficacy of the ketogenic diet. Epilepsia. 2009;**50**:322-325. DOI: 10.1111/j.1528-1167.2008.01740.x

[34] Sharma S, Sankhyan N, Gulati S, et al. Use of the modified Atkins diet for treatment of refractory childhood epilepsy: A randomized controlled trial. Epilepsia. 2013;**54**:481-486. DOI: 10.1111/epi.12069

[35] Lambrechts DA, de Kinderen RJ, Vles JS, et al. A randomized controlled trial of the ketogenic diet in refractory childhood epilepsy. Acta Neurologica Scandinavica. 2017;**135**:231-239. DOI: 10.1111/ane.12592

[36] De Giorgis V, Veggiotti P. GLUT1 deficiency syndrome 2013: Current state of the art. Seizure. 2013;**22**(10):803-811. DOI: 10.1016/j.seizure.2013.07.003

[37] Sofou K, Dahlin M, Hallböök T, et al. Ketogenic diet in pyruvate dehydrogenase complex deficiency: Short- and long-term outcomes. Journal of Inherited Metabolic Disease. 2017;**40**: 237-245. DOI: 10.1007/s10545-016-0011-5

[38] Arora S, Henderson SO, Long T, et al. Diagnostic accuracy of point-of-care testing for diabetic ketoacidosis at emergency-department triage: {Beta}-hydroxybutyrate versus the urine dipstick. Diabetes Care. 2011;**34**: 852-854. DOI: 10.2337/dc10-1844

[39] Grocott OR, Herrington KS, Pfeifer HH, et al. Low glycemic index treatment for seizure control in Angelman syndrome: A case series from the Center for Dietary Therapy of Epilepsy at the Massachusetts General Hospital. Epilepsy & Behavior. 2017;**68**:45-50. DOI: 10.1016/j.yebeh.2016.12.018

[40] Whitmer E, Riether JL. Fighting Back with Fat: A parent's Guide to Battling Epilepsy through the Ketogenic Diet and Modified Atkins Diet. New York: Demos Health; 2013. 136 p

[41] Martenz DM, Cramp L. The Keto Cookbook: Innovative Delicious Meals for Staying on the Ketogenic Diet. New York: Demos Health; 2012. 160 p

[42] Bergqvist AG, Schall JI, Gallagher PR, et al. Fasting versus gradual initiation of the ketogenic diet: A prospective, randomized clinical trial of efficacy. Epilepsia. 2005;**46**:1810-1819. DOI: 10.1111/j.1528-1167.2005.00282.x

[43] Kossoff EH, Laux LC, Blackford R, et al. When do seizures improve with the ketogenic diet? Epilepsia. 2008;**49**: 329-333. DOI: 10.1111/j.1528-1167.2007.01417.x

[44] Taub KS, Kessler SK, Bergqvist AG. Risk of seizure recurrence after achieving initial seizure freedom on the ketogenic diet. Epilepsia. 2014;**55**: 579-583. DOI: 10.1111/epi.12583

[45] Martinez CC, Pyzik PL, Kossoff EH. Discontinuing the ketogenic diet in seizure-free children: Recurrence and risk factors. Epilepsia. 2007;**48**:187-190. DOI: 10.1111/j.1528-1167.2006.00911.x

[46] Hong AM, Turner Z, Hamdy RF, et al. Infantile spasms treated with the ketogenic diet: Prospective single-center experience in 104 consecutive infants. Epilepsia. 2010;**51**:1403-1407. DOI: 10.1111/j.1528-1167.2010.02586.x

[47] Williams TJ, Cervenka MC. The role for ketogenic diets in epilepsy and status epilepticus in adults. Clinical Neurophysiology Practice. 2017;**2**: 154-160. DOI: 10.1016/j.cnp.2017.06.001

[48] Cervenka MC, Henry BJ, Felton EA, et al. Establishing an adult epilepsy diet center: Experience, efficacy and

challenges. Epilepsy & Behavior. 2016; **58**:61-68. DOI: 10.1016/j.yebeh.2016.02.038

[49] Barborka CJ. Epilepsy in adults: Results of treatment by ketogenic diet in one hundred cases. Archives of Neurology and Psychiatry. 1930;**23**: 904-914. DOI: 10.1001/archneurpsyc.1930.02220110066004

[50] Klein P, Tyrlikova I, Mathews GC. Dietary treatment in adults with refractory epilepsy: A review. Neurology. 2014;**83**(21):1978-1985. DOI: 10.1212/WNL.0000000000001004

[51] Kossoff EH, Henry BJ, Cervenka MC. Efficacy of dietary therapy for juvenile myoclonic epilepsy. Epilepsy & Behavior. 2013;**26**:162-164. DOI: 10.1016/j.yebeh.2012.11.007

[52] Kverneland M, Selmer KK, Nakken KO, et al. A prospective study of the modified Atkins diet for adults with idiopathic generalized epilepsy. Epilepsy & Behavior. 2015;**53**:197-201. DOI: 10.1016/j.yebeh.2015.10.021

[53] Phillips MCL, Murtagh DKJ, Gilbertson LJ, et al. Low-fat versus Ketogenic diet in Parkinson's disease: A pilot randomized controlled trial. Movement Disorders. 2018;**33**(8): 1306-1314. DOI: 10.1002/mds.27390

[54] Payne NE, Cross JH, Sander JW, et al. The ketogenic and related diets in adolescents and adults—A review. Epilepsia. 2011;**52**(11):1941-1948. DOI: 10.1111/j.1528-1167.2011.03287.x

[55] Diet Doctor [Internet]. 2018. Available from: http://www.dietdoctor.com [Accessed: Dec 11, 2018]

[56] Song TJ, Cho HJ, Chang Y, et al. Low-density lipoprotein particle size predicts a poor outcome in patients with atherothrombotic stroke. Journal of Clinical Neurology. 2015;**11**(1):80-96. DOI: 10.3988/jcn.2015.11.1.80

[57] Cervenka MC, Patton K, Eloyan A, et al. The impact of the modified Atkins diet on lipid profiles in adults with epilepsy. Nutritional Neuroscience. 2014;**19**(3):131-137. DOI: 10.1179/1476830514Y.0000000162

[58] Lambrechts DAJE, Wielders LHP, Aldenkamp AP, et al. The ketogenic diet as a treatment option in adults with chronic refractory epilepsy: Efficacy and tolerability in clinical practice. Epilepsy & Behavior. 2012;**23**:310-314. DOI: 10.1016/j.yebeh.2012.01.002

[59] Klein P, Janousek J, Barber A, et al. Ketogenic diet treatment in adults with refractory epilepsy. Epilepsy & Behavior. 2010;**19**:575-579. DOI: 10.1016/j.yebeh.2010.09.016

Section 6

Recent Advances in Epilepsy

Chapter 10

Ion Channels in Epilepsy: Blasting Fuse for Neuronal Hyperexcitability

Shuzhang Zhang, Yudan Zhu, Jiwei Cheng and Jie Tao

Abstract

Voltage-gated ion channels (VGICs), extensively distributed in the central nervous system (CNS), are responsible for the generation as well as modulation of neuroexcitability and considered as vital players in the pathogenesis of human epilepsy, with regulating the shape and duration of action potentials (APs). For instance, genetic alterations or abnormal expression of voltage-gated sodium channels (VGSCs), Kv channels, and voltage-gated calcium channels (VGCCs) are proved to be associated with epileptogenesis. This chapter aims to highlight recent discoveries on the mutations in VGIC genes and dysfunction of VGICs in epilepsy, especially focusing on the pathophysiological and pharmacological properties. Understanding the role of epilepsy-associated VGICs might not only contribute to clarify the mechanism of epileptogenesis and genetic modifiers but also provide potential targets for the precise treatment of epilepsy.

Keywords: ion channels, VGSCs, Kv channels, Cav channels, TRPs, mutation, epilepsy

1. Introduction

Epilepsy is one of the chronic brain disorders characterized by recurrent seizures due to abnormal excessive electrical discharges of cerebral neurons [1]. It is believed that genetic factors play a crucial role in the etiopathogenesis of epilepsy. So far ~1000 genes have been proved to be associated with epilepsy, among which genes encoding VGIC predominate [2].

VGICs are pore-forming membrane proteins. Their functions include establishing APs and maintaining homeostasis by gating the ionic flow traversing the cell membrane, managing the ionic flow across cells and regulating Ca^{2+} signal transduction, which are essential to the neuroexcitability, so VGICs are potentially involved in epileptogenesis [2]. The association of VGIC genes and epilepsy might provide insights into the etiopathogenesis underlying epilepsy. Pathophysiological studies illuminated that two key defects are (i) a neuronal disinhibition induced by loss-of-function of VGIC gene expressed specifically in inhibitory interneurons (for example, Nav1.1 and P/Q VGCCs) or (ii) dysfunction of axon initial segments, the neuronal structure in which APs are generated and many VGICs (such as Nav1.2 and Kv7) are mainly localized (**Figure 1**). Moreover, clinically originated studies identified novel genes, defined their neuronal functions, and sometimes established novel physiological principles [2].

IntechOpen

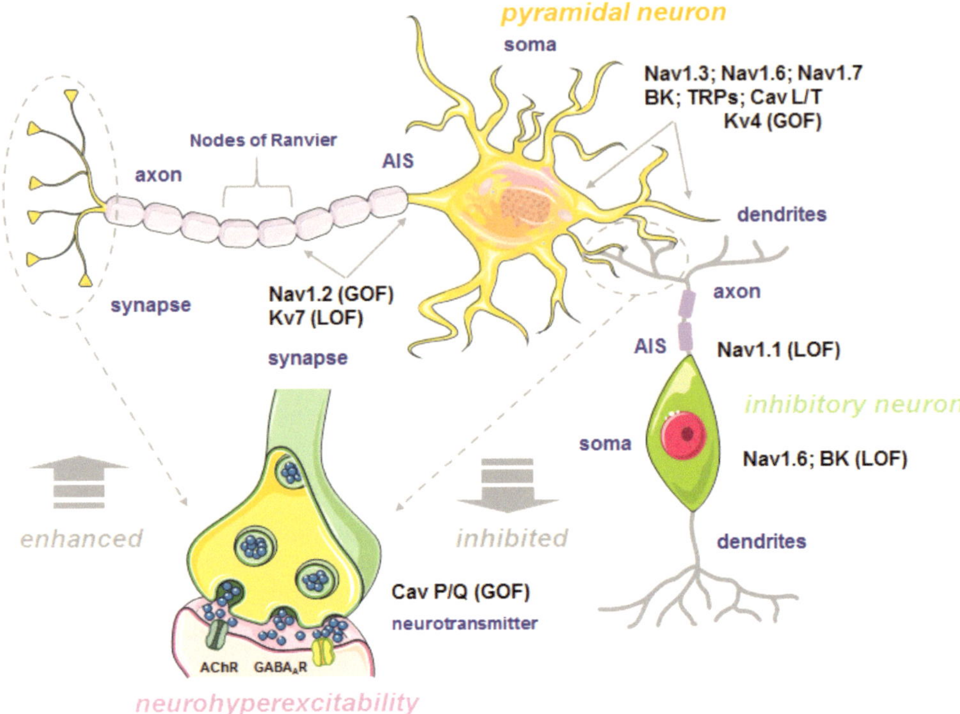

Figure 1.
Neuronal localization of some relevant voltage-gated ion channels. A schematic view of an excitatory pyramidal (orange), an inhibitory (green) neuron, and their synaptic connections is shown. Distinctive intracellular compartments are targeted by different populations of VGICs. Examples of which as mentioned in this chapter are shown here: in the somatodendritic compartment, Nav, Cav (L- and T-type), TRP, BK, and Kv channels; at axon initial segments (AIS) and nodes of Ranvier in pyramidal neurons, Nav1.2, Kv7 channels; at AIS of inhibitory neurons, Nav1.1; in the somatodendritic compartment of inhibitory neurons, BK and Nav1.6; in the presynaptic terminals, Cav P/Q type. GOF represents the gain-of-function mutation of VGICs-induced human epilepsy. LOF represents the loss-of-function mutation of VGICs.

In this chapter, we summarize the epilepsy-associated VGIC genes, the mutations, corresponding phenotypes, and functional changes, aiming to provide clues for evaluating the relationship between VGIC genes and epileptogenesis.

2. Voltage-gated sodium channels

VGSCs play a critical role in the generation and propagation of APs in neurons, genetic alterations in VGSC genes are considered to be associated with epileptogenesis. Mammalian VGSC is composed of a large pseudotetrameric pore-forming α subunit with a molecular weight of 260 KDa, and one or more auxiliary β subunits (30–40 KDa) [3–5] (**Figure 2**). Nine subtypes of VGSC α subunits have been found in humans, including Nav1.1-Nav1.9, encoded by the genes SCN1A-SCN5A, SCN8A-SCN11A, respectively.

2.1 Nav1.1

Nav1.1 is mainly distributed in the inhibitory GABAergic neurons of cerebellum and hippocampus. The Nav1.1 gene SCN1A is the clinically most relevant SCN gene for epilepsy. More than 1200 mutants have been identified to be associated with epilepsy; most of them are febrile seizures [6]. M145T mutation, a well-conserved amino acid in the first transmembrane segment of domain I of the

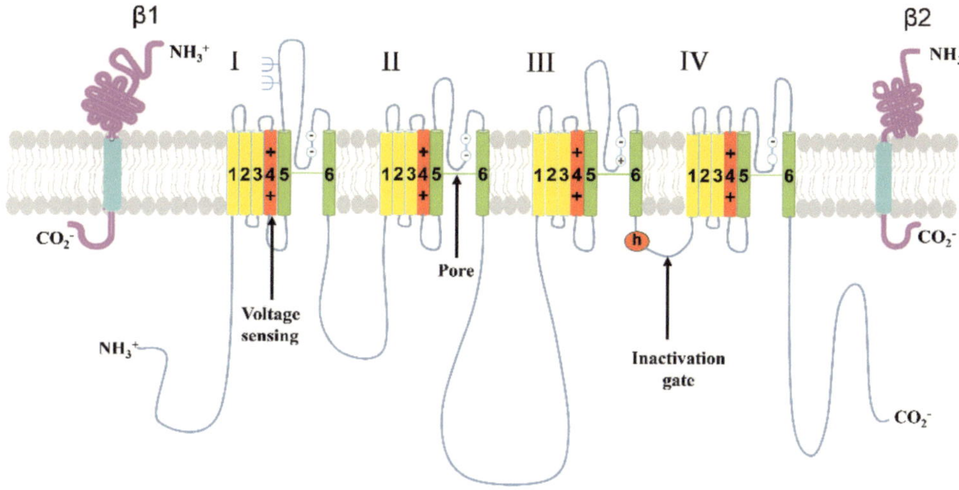

Figure 2.
Structure of voltage-gated sodium channels. Schematic representation of VGSC subunits. The α subunit of the VGSC is illustrated together with β1 and β2 subunits; extracellular domains of the β subunits are shown as immunoglobulin-like folds, interacting with the loops in α subunits. Roman numerals indicate the domains of the α subunit; segments 5 and 6 (shown in green) are the pore-lining segments, and S4 helices (red) make up the voltage sensors. The red circle in the intracellular loop of domains III and IV indicates the inactivation gate IFM motif; Ψ, probable N-linked glycosylation site. The circles in reentrant loops in each domain represent the residues that form the ion selectivity filter.

Nav1.1 α-subunit, caused a reduction in peak sodium currents and a positive shift in the voltage dependence of activation [7], which provided the first evidence that the mild loss-of-function mutations in Nav1.1 may cause a significant portion of febrile seizures. Complete loss-of-function mutations in Nav1.1 cause severe myoclonic epilepsy of infancy (SMEI or Dravet's syndrome), which includes severe, intractable epilepsy and comorbidities of ataxia and cognitive impairment. Besides, homozygous null Nav1.1$^{-/-}$ mice developed ataxia and died on half a month of postnatal and did not change the voltage-dependent activity of VGSCs in hippocampal neurons. However, heterozygous Nav1.1$^{+/-}$ mice exhibited spontaneous seizures and sporadic deaths after 3 weeks, and the sodium current density was substantially reduced in inhibitory interneurons, except in excitatory pyramidal neurons [8]. So loss-of-function mutations in Nav1.1 can severely impair sodium currents and AP firing in hippocampal GABAergic inhibitory neurons. The functional downregulation in inhibitory neurons might cause the hyperexcitability of dentate granule or pyramidal neurons, which could lead to epilepsy in patients with SMEI. Experiments in mice have demonstrated that haploinsufficiency of Nav1.1 channels is sufficient to allow induction of seizures by elevated body temperature, supporting that haploinsufficiency of SCN1A is pathogenic in human SMEI which has striking temperature and age dependence of onset and progression of epilepsy [9]. What is more, SCN1A mutations were mostly missense mutations in GEFS+ patients, which are typically well controlled by treatment with antiepileptic drugs and no cognitive impairment is observed. The R1648H channels showed the reduced function in both excitatory and inhibitory neurons although the biophysical mechanisms were different, reducing peak sodium currents and enhancing slow inactivation in inhibitory neurons versus negatively shifted voltage dependence of fast inactivation in excitatory neurons [10]. The similar conclusion had been drawn when the R1648H mutation has been inserted into the mouse genome under the native promoter [11]. In light of these results, GEFS+ and SMEI may be caused by a continuum of mutational effects that selectively impair firing of GABAergic inhibitory neurons, which lead to increase in the excitability of the neural network [12].

2.2 Nav1.2

The mutation of the Nav1.2 gene SCN2A is associated with various epilepsies, such as benign familial neonatal seizures (BFNIS), hereditary epilepsy with febrile seizures plus (GEFS+), Dravet's syndrome (DS), and other stubborn childhood epilepsy encephalopathy. Nav1.2 subunit is mainly distributed in the axon-initiating segment (AIS) and node of Ranvier. SCN2A mutations cause changes in VGSC function and expression and result in abnormal neuronal discharge. Because Nav1.2 plays an important role in the AIS area during the development, it is more common for infants to show SCN2A mutant-induced epilepsy encephalopathy [13]. BFNIS is the most common phenotype caused by gain-of-function missense mutations in SCN2A [14]. Up to now, at least 10 SCN2A mutations associated with BFNIS have been identified. SCN2A mutations are also found to result in the reduced expression of Nav1.2 on the surface of neurons [15]. Therefore, SCN2A mutants will lead to the decrease of sodium current density at node of Ranvier and AIS, seriously affecting the excitability of neurons [16]. For missense mutation of SCN2A, p.Tyr1589Cys causes a depolarizing shift of steady-state inactivation, increased persistent Na^+ current, a slowing of fast inactivation, and an acceleration of its recovery, which contribute to neuronal hyperexcitability and familial epilepsy [17]. Due to the SCN2A mutation, early infantile epileptic encephalopathy (EIEE) patients with burst suppression and tonic-clonic migrating partial seizures showed a specific dose-dependent efficacy of VGSC blockers [18]. It is mainly caused by the dysfunction of VGSC [19]. By replacing neonatal Nav1.2 with adult Nav1.2 in mice, it has been suggested that neonatal Nav1.2 reduced neuronal excitability and had a significant impact on seizure susceptibility and behavior.

2.3 Nav1.3

The SCN3A gene, clustered on human chromosome 2q24, encodes the Nav1.3 subtype [20], which is usually located in the soma of neurons. It is important in the integration of synaptic signals, determination of the depolarization threshold, and AP transmission [21]. In contrast to the rodent gene which is transiently expressed during development, human SCN3A is widely expressed in adult brain [22]. The first epilepsy-associated mutation (K354Q) in SCN3A was found in 2008. K354Q mutation decreased inactivation rate and increased I_{NaP} [23]. The mutation is not sensitive to antiepilepsy drug carbamazepine or oxcarbazepine. K354Q mutation causes neuronal abnormal spontaneous discharge and membrane potential paroxysmal depolarization [24]. In 2014, four more missense variants were identified in SCN3A, which are R357Q, D766N, E1111K, and M1323V [25]. Compared to wild-type channels, R357Q caused smaller currents, slower activation, and depolarized voltage dependences of activation and inactivation. The E1111K mutation evoked a significantly greater level of persistent sodium current. All four mutants increase current activation in response to depolarizing voltage ramps. These findings support for a contribution of Nav 1.3 to childhood epilepsy. Recently, a novel SCN3A variant (L247P) was identified by whole exome sequencing of a child with focal epilepsy, developmental delay, and autonomic nervous system dysfunction. Voltage clamp analysis showed no detectable sodium currents in a heterologous expression system. To further test the possible clinical consequences of reduced SCN3A activity, they investigated the effect of a hypomorphic Scn3a allele (Scn3a Hyp) on seizure susceptibility and behavior using a gene trap mouse line. Heterozygous SCN3A mutant mice ($SCN3A^{+/Hyp}$) neither exhibit spontaneous seizures nor hyperthermia-induced seizures, but they displayed increased susceptibility to electroconvulsive- and chemiconvulsive-induced seizures, which provide evidence that loss-of-function of SCN3A may contribute to increased seizure susceptibility [26].

2.4 Nav1.6

Nav1.6, mainly distributed to the soma and synaptic origin, is important for APs generation and propagation [27]. In the development process, Nav1.2 is gradually replaced by Nav1.6 in the mature node of Ranvier [28]. The first heterozygous missense mutation (p.Asn1768Asp) in the Nav1.6 gene SCN8A was identified in 2012 by whole-genome sequencing (WGS) in a patient with severe epileptic encephalopathy who exhibited early-onset seizures, autistic features, intellectual disability, ataxia, and sudden unexpected death in epilepsy (SUDEP) [29]. Since this initial discovery, more than 100 pathogenic SCN8A variants have been identified in patients with epilepsy [30]. Most of the SCN8A variants have been detected in individuals with EIEE.

Different mutations in the SCN8A gene encoding Nav1.6 have different effects on epilepsy. For the missense mutation V929F, an evolutionarily conserved residue in the pore loop of domain II of Nav1.6, it was found that heterozygous mutations produced well-defined spike-wave discharges and are associated to absence epilepsy in mice [31]. However, missense mutations in $Scn8a^{med-jo}$ were able to improve the epilepsy symptoms of $SCN1A^{+/-}$ heterozygotes. The mechanism might be the decrease in Nav1.6 expression of excitatory neurons compensating for the loss of Nav1.1 in inhibitory neurons [32]. Recently, more and more de novo and inherited SCN8A epilepsy mutations were detected by gene panel analysis [33]. For example, loss-of-function mutants [34], underlying the complex seizure phenotype, were identified using specific mouse line. It was suggested that decreasing Scn8a expression in cortical excitatory neurons could reduce seizures. On the contrary, the decreasing expression of SCN8A in the thalamic reticular nucleus (RT) leads to absence seizures. Loss of Scn8a will impair tonic firing mode behavior and impair desynchronizing recurrent RT-RT synaptic inhibition in the thalamic reticular nucleus, which suggested that Scn8a-mediated hypofunction in cortical circuits, conferring convulsive seizure resistance, while hypofunction in the thalamus is sufficient to generate absence seizures.

2.5 Nav1.7

The SCN9A gene encodes the Nav1.7 subtype, which was initially identified in the peripheral nervous system, sympathetic ganglion, and olfactory sensory neurons [35–38]. Nav1.7 is also found expressed in the central nervous system such as in the cerebral cortex and hippocampus [39]. A missense mutation of SCN9A (N641Y), at a conserved amino acid residue located at the intracellular loop between domain I and II, is associated with a family of febrile seizures (FS, N641Y). Mice carrying N641Y mutations were more susceptible to electrical stimulation-induced clonic and tonic seizures [40]. However, it is still unclear how SCN9A gene mutation caused epilepsy in the CNS.

3. Potassium channels

K^+ channels control the resting membrane potential and enable rapid repolarization of the AP by producing outward K^+ currents, thus limiting neuronal excitability. K^+ channels are composed of four pore forming a subunits and modulatory b subunits. Kv channels are the largest ion channel group (Kv1–Kv12) that are expressed substantially in the CNS. Dysfunction of Kv channels including Ca^{2+}-activated K^+ channels, are associated with epilepsy [2].

3.1 Large conductance calciumactivated potassium channel

Large conductance calcium-activated potassium (BK) channels, consisting of functional α subunit and the tissue-specific regulatory subunits (β1–4 and γ1–4), are widely distributed in the CNS. BK channels are usually considered as vital players in the development of epilepsy (**Figure 3**), with the evidence including the K^+ derangement and regulating AP shape and duration [41, 42].

Gain-of-function mutation of BK, promoting the high-frequency neuron firing, is associated with spontaneous epileptic seizures paradoxically in both humans and rodents [43]. In fact, patients suffering from generalized epilepsy were detected a site mutation D434G at the RCK1 domain of BK α subunit. D434G increased the opening time of BK, through the enhancement of Ca^{2+} sensitivity [43]. In terms of functionality, the enhanced membrane excitability is associated with the increased BK activity and fAHP consequent [43, 44]. The augment seems to be induced by an increased recovery rate, underlying fast currents of VGSCs with a APs' reduced refractory period and/or through disinhibiting thalamocortical circuits by blocking brain GABAergic interneurons [43, 45, 46].

The knockout mice of BK channel β4 subunit exhibit temporal lobe epilepsy (TLE) seizure associated with a gain-of-function phenotype of BK, which not only sharpens APs but also induces a higher neuronal firing frequency in hippocampus DG granule cells [47].It is worth mentioned that epileptic seizures themselves also could induce a gain-of-function effect to BK. Picrotoxin and pentylenetetrazol (PTZ) caused generalized tonic-clonic epileptic seizures, with giving rise to a gain-of-function effect on BK channels, presenting increased BK currents and neuron firing in the neocortex [48]. It is of interest that BK-specific inhibitors attenuated generalized tonic-clonic epileptic seizures in picrotoxin or PTZ-induced epilepsy models, which suppressed the increase of neuron firing [48, 49].

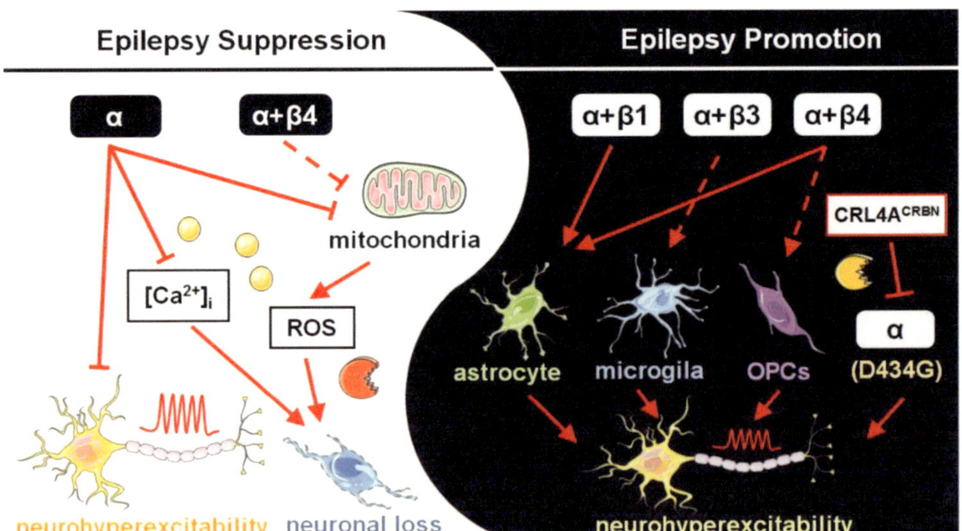

Figure 3.
Yin and Yang of BK channels in epilepsy. For epilepsy suppression, BK (α) channels act as negative feedback regulators on calcium rise and transmitter release in most synapses. Activation of mitoBK channel subtypes (α or α+β4) may contribute to suppressing seizure as well as conferring neuroprotection via the inhibition of ROS synthesis [54]. For epilepsy promotion, astrocyte and OPCs BK channel subtypes (α+β1 or α+β4) may induce elevate $[K^+]_o$, causing membrane depolarization as well as neuronal hyperexcitation. Microglial BK channels (α+β3) may involve in the neuroinflammation during status epilepsy. Mutation D434G of α causes the neurohyperexcitation in hereditary epilepsy. However, ubiquitin ligase $CRL4A^{CRBN}$ could inhibit the overactivation of BK channels.

Loss-of-function phenotype of BK might also contribute to the pathological process of clinical TLE. It was reported that two siblings suffered from the severe cerebellar atrophy and developmental delay, who adopted the exome analysis that identified a homozygous frameshift duplication in BK gene *KCNMA1* (c.2026dupT; p.(Tyr676 Leufs*7)) in children from a consanguineous family with epilepsy [50].

KCNMB3, encoding the auxiliary BK β3, mapping the human chromosome 3 (3q26.3-q27) [51], is duplicated in the dup (3q) syndrome, which is characterized by neurological abnormalities, especially epileptic seizures [51]. Because of the dup (3q) syndrome having early onset during developmental process, the *KCNMB3* duplication implies that β3 subunits overexpression might contribute to the etiology of epilepsy. Similarly, site mutations might also contribute to both neurohyperexcitation by a single nucleotide deletion at *KCNMB3* exon 4 (delA750), which is associated with the generalized epilepsy, especially in the form of the typical absence epilepsy [52]. BK coexpressed with β3 variant of β3b-V4 (delA750) shows fast inactivation properties [53], which suggest that BK currents were reduced and the repolarization of cell membrane was attenuated during an action potential, eventually leading to neurohyperexcitation.

3.2 Voltage-gated potassium channel subfamily KQT (KCNQ)

Kv7 is its seventh member of Kv channel family (Kv1–Kv12). The Kv7.1 mutation mediates type 1 long QT syndrome (long-QT syndrome type 1, LQT1) and is therefore named KCNQ1 (K, potassium; CN, channel; Q, LQT). KCNQ has five subtypes of KCNQ1–KCNQ5, which play crucial roles in physiological functions. Dysfunction of KCNQ is associated with many diseases.

KCNQ1 is mainly distributed in the heart, which mediates cardiac delayed-rectifier K^+ current and maintains the normal repolarization process of cardiomyocytes [55]. KCNQ2–KCNQ5 are mainly distributed in central and peripheral neuronal tissues, of which KCNQ2 and KCNQ3 are distributed in brain regions [56]. KCNQ2 and KCNQ3 form functional heterotetramers, which are the main molecular bases for the formation of M currents that can be inhibited by acetylcholine M1 receptor activation [57]. Abundant KCNQ2 and KCNQ3 mutations could induce abnormal M currents, causing similarities in neonatal seizures and other nervous system diseases.

Benign familial neonatal seizure (BFNS) is an autosomal dominant idiopathic epilepsy syndrome that occurs on the 2nd to 8th day after birth and stops spontaneously after a few weeks. Whereas 15% of patients in later life may have recurrence of epilepsy [58]. With the study of pathogenic genes in epilepsy, 60–70% of patients with BFNS were found to be associated with KCNQ2 and KCNQ3 mutations. More than 80 different mutations have been reported on KCNQ2, and multiple mutations on KCNQ3 are associated with BFNS. Soldovieri et al. [58] studied the genes of 17 BFNS clinical patients. Sixteen different heterozygous mutations were found in KCNQ2, including 10 substitutions, 3 insertions/deletions, and 3 large deletions. One substitution was found in KCNQ3. Most of these mutations were novel, except for four KCNQ2 substitutions that were shown to be recurrent. Electrophysiological studies in mammalian cells revealed that homomeric or heteromeric KCNQ2 and/or KCNQ3 channels carrying mutant subunits with newly found substitutions displayed reduced current densities. Borgatti studied a BFNS family with four affected members: two of them exhibit BFNS only, while the other two, in addition to BFNS, present either with a severe epileptic encephalopathy or with focal seizures and mental retardation. All affected members of this family carry a novel missense mutation in the KCNQ2 gene (K526N), disrupting the tridimensional conformation of a C-terminal region of the channel subunit involved in accessory protein binding. When heterologously expressed in CHO cells, potassium channels containing mutant subunits in homomeric or heteromeric configuration with wild-type KCNQ2 and KCNQ3 subunits exhibit an altered voltage-dependence of activation, without changes in intracellular trafficking and plasma membrane expression. The KCNQ2 K526N mutation might affect M-channel function by disrupting the complex biochemical signaling involving KCNQ2 C-terminus [59, 60]. KCNQ2 or KCNQ3 mutations cause M current to be downregulated, and the frequency of neuronal firing increases, leading to epilepsy.

3.3 G protein-coupled Kir channel

Inward-rectifier potassium channels (Kir, IRK) are a specific subset of potassium channels. To date, seven subfamilies have been identified, which are associated with a variety of diseases [61]. The G-protein-coupled Kir (GIRK) channels belong to the subfamily of Kir3 (GIRKs) which are activated by ligand-stimulated G protein-coupled receptors (GPCRs). GPCRs, interacting with GIRK channels, facilitate their activation, resulting in hyperpolarization of the cell membrane [61].

GIRK channels have four identified subunits (GIRK1–4, encoded by KCNJ3, KCNJ6, KCNJ9, and KCNJ5, respectively) in mammals, existing in vivo both as homotetramers and heterotetramers with unique biophysical properties, regulation, and distribution [61, 62]. GIRK 1, 2, 3, and 4 subunits are expressed in the brain, localized in certain axons, postsynaptic, and presynaptic regions [63]. GIRK channels may be involved not only in slow inhibitory postsynaptic potentials but also in the presynaptic modulation of neuronal activity [61].

GIRK in the CNS is a heterotetramer composed of GIRK1 and GIRK2 subunits [63], which is responsible for maintaining the resting membrane potential and excitability of the neuron [64]. GIRK1 and GIRK2 subunits are found in the dendritic areas of neurons highly [63] correlate with the large concentration of $GABA_B$ receptors. Once the $GABA_B$ receptors are activated by their ligands, they can in turn activate IRK, mediating a significant part of the GABA postsynaptic inhibition [63].

Alterations in GIRK function have been associated with pathophysiology of severe brain disorders, including epilepsy. In this regard, a GIRK2 knockout mouse model resulted to be more susceptible to develop both spontaneous and induced seizures in respect to wild-type mice [65]. In particular, mice carrying a p Gly156Ser mutation displayed an epileptic phenotype [66]. Indeed, this mutation has been found to alter the putative ion-permeable, pore-forming domain of the channel, inducing Ca^{2+} overload in cells and reducing channel availability, leading thus to neurodegeneration and seizure susceptibility [67].

An increased expression of GIRK was observed in rat brain after an electroconvulsive shock, probably altering the excitability of granule cells and the functions of neurotransmitter receptors which are coupled to these channels [68]. Another evidence in support of a role of GIRK in epilepsy was provided by the demonstration that ML297, a potent and selective activator of GIRK, showed epileptogenic properties in mice [69]. On the other hand, the inhibition of GIRK activity by drugs causes seizures [70]. All these considerations imply that changes in Kir3 channel activity may alter the susceptibility to seizures.

4. Calcium channels

As an important second messenger, Ca^{2+} plays a vital role in normal brain function and in the pathophysiological process of different neurodegenerative diseases. Ca^{2+} entry via VGCCs conveys the electric signals to intracellular transduction cascades in a wide variety of cells [71]. VGCCs were first identified by Fatt and Katz [72] and shown to consist of several subunits [73, 74]. VGCCs were divided into low-voltage-activated (LVA) and high-voltage-activated (HVA), based on electrophysiological and pharmacological properties. HVA channels, composed of α_1, β, $\alpha_2\delta$, γ subunit, are further divided into L, N, P, and Q types, which have an activation threshold at membrane voltage positive to −20 mV [75]. LVA channels, also called T type, consist only of the α_1 subunit, activated at a membrane voltage positive to −70 mV. It is composed of transmembrane topology with four homologous transmembrane domains, each containing six transmembrane segments and a pore region between segments S5 and S6.

4.1 L-type Cav

The L-type VGCC family has four members, Cav1.1–1.4, of which α subunits present tissue-specific expression, such as the α_1D subunit in the brain. The L-type VGCC family shapes neuronal firing and activates Ca^{2+}-dependent pathways involved in regulation of gene expression [76]. Cav1.2 channels appear to contribute critically to the generation of febrile seizures, which was proved by testing the excitability of hippocampal pyramidal cells in rat brain slices [77]. The Wistar Albino Glaxo/Rij (WAG/Rij) model experiments suggest that L-type calcium channels play a positive role in the frequency and duration of epileptic spikes [78]. Verapamil, an L-type VGCC blocker, could significantly reduce TLE seizure, enhancing the expression of the α subunit of γ-$GABA_AR$ [79].

4.2 P/Q-, N-, and R-type Cav

P/Q-, N-, and R-type are corresponding to Cav2.1, Cav2.2, and Cav2.3, respectively, which initiate rapid synaptic transmission, regulated primarily by direct interaction with G proteins and SNARE (soluble N-ethylmaleimide-sensitive factor attachment protein receptor) and secondarily by protein phosphorylation. The loss function of P/Q VGCC could lead to epileptic spikes, paroxysmal dystonia and ataxia. If P/Q VGCCs were blocked, it could disrupt the triggering synaptic neurotransmitter release [80]. Spikes of Cacna1aNtsr$^{-/-}$ mice are increased in layer VI corticothalamic neurons compared with control group, suggesting that Cav P/Q deletion generates absence epilepsy [81]. Cacna1a LOF from parvalbumin (PV)(+) and somatostatin (SST)(+) interneurons results in severe generalized epilepsy. It might be the mechanism for severe generalized epilepsy that the loss of Cav2.1 channel function from cortical PV(+) interneurons inhibits GABA release from these cells, which impairs their ability to constrain cortical pyramidal cell excitability [82]. When knocking out the cerebellar Cav2.1 channel in mice, cortical function is changeable, which caused movement disorders and epilepsy [83]. In two families with idiopathic epilepsy, the loss of function mutation in γ4 subunits, auxiliary subunit of Cav2.1 channels, could also cause seizures, and maybe aggravate seizures [84]. Downregulation of $\alpha 2\delta 2$ subunits in rats will generate 5–7 Hz epileptic wave accompanied by ataxia [85]. N-type calcium channels are mainly distributed in the nucleus of different neurons and glial cells. In the pilocarpine model, Cav2.2 expression decreased in the granule layer of the dentate gyrus and the pyramidal cells of the CA3 region during the acute phase of seizure. However, the expression of N-type calcium channels increased in the subsequent chronic phase, which demonstrated that the increase of N-type calcium channels might be associated with recurrent status epilepticus [86]. R-type calcium channel, Cav2.3, is mainly distributed in the presynaptic membrane, such as hippocampal mossy fibers, globus pallidus, and neuromuscular junctions. Knocking out R-type calcium channels could increase the susceptibility of seizures, with altering the seizure form [87]. The lack of Cav2.3 resulted in a marked decrease in the sensitivity of the animal to γ-butyrolactone-induced absence epilepsy and change thalamocortical network oscillations [88]. Administration of kainic acid revealed alteration in behavioral seizure architecture, dramatic resistance to limbic seizures and excitotoxic effects in Cav2.3$^{-/-}$ mice compared with controls. It indicated that the Cav2.3 plays a crucial role in both hippocampal ictogenesis and seizure generalization and is of central importance in neuronal degeneration after excitotoxic events [89].

4.3 T-type Cav

T-type channels, widely distributed in the thalamus, are important for the repetitive firing of APs in rhythmically firing cells, which could be activated and inactivated more rapidly at more negative membrane potentials than other VGCCs [90]. Three subtypes of T-type channels have been identified, designated as Cav3.1, Cav3.2, and Cav3.3; they correspond to complexes containing the pore-forming α1 subunits, α1G, α1H, and α1I, respectively [91]. It has long been suggested that generalized absence seizures are accompanied by hyperexcitable oscillatory activities in the thalamocortical network [92]. The evidence that succinimide and related anticonvulsants could block thalamic T-type channels make researchers speculate that T-type Ca2+ channels might be related to the pathogenesis of spike-and-wave discharges (SWDs) in generalized absence seizures [93]. In the kainate epilepsy model, Cav3.1$^{-/-}$ mice display significantly reduced duration of seizures compared to wild type, but the frequency of seizures increased slightly [94]. In the WAG/Rij model, the expression of Cav3.1 may be related to age, and blocking Cav3.1 can reduce the onset of epilepsy [94, 95] which suggested that decrease in Cav3.1 channel expression and Ca^{2+} current component that they carry in thalamocortical relay neurons serves as a protective measure against early onset of SWD and absence seizures [96]. Notably, Cav3.1$^{-/-}$ mice are resistant to SWD seizures specifically induced by γ-$GABA_BR$ agonists. Simultaneously, the γ-$GABA_BR$ agonists induced only very weak and intermittent SWDs in Cav3.1$^{-/-}$ mice [97]. Cav3.2 single nucleotide mutation has been reported in patients with childhood absence epilepsy and other types of idiopathic generalized epilepsies [98, 99]. Gain-of-function mutations (C456S) in Cav3.2 channels increase seizure susceptibility by directly altering neuronal electrical properties and indirectly by changing gene expression [100].

5. Transient receptor potential channels

Transient receptor potential (TRP) channels, which could induce a transient voltage changes to continuous light mutations of *Drosophila melanogaster*, are expressed in photoreceptors carrying trp gene. The first homologous human gene was reported in 1995. There are 30 trp genes, and more than 100 TRP channels have been identified so far, and TRP channels were divided into 7 subfamilies, including TRPC, TRPV, TRPM, TRPA, TRPP, TRPML, and TRPN. Focus on TRPs, one family of Ca^{2+} channels, plays a role in neuronal excitability. It is obviously known that Ca^{2+} is an important second messenger, which is related to the etiology of epilepsy [101]. Therefore, TRP channels are thought to be partially responsible for epileptic seizures, especially for TPRC and TRPV1 channels.

5.1 Canonical transient receptor potential (TRPC)

TRPC channels are the closet homolog to Drosophila TRP channels. Based on the functional comparisons and sequence alignments, four subsets of mammalian TRPCs (TRPC1, TRPC2, TRPC3/6/7, and TRPC4/5) have been generated [101]. These channels form receptor-modulated currents in the mammalian brain and important to SE-induced neuronal cell death. These channels could play a critical role in the generation of spontaneous seizures. TRPC1 and TRPC4 are expressed in CA1 pyramidal neurons. The amplitude of the plateau and the number of spikes were significantly reduced in mice without TRPC1 and TRPC4 [102]. TRPC3 channels are found to be responsible for pilocarpine-induced status epilepticus (SE) in mice. The reduction on SE in TRPC3 KO mice is caused by a selective attenuation of pilocarpine-induced theta wave activity [103]. TRPC7 can be detected in CA3 pyramidal neurons largely. The spontaneous seizures in CA3 pyramidal neurons and the pilocarpine-induced increase in gamma wave activities during the latent period could be significantly reduced by ablating the gene TRPC7 [104].

5.2 Transient receptor potential vanilloid 1 (TRPV1)

TRPV1 is one subfamily of TRP channels, expressing in most neurons. The expression of TRPV1 protein in epileptic brain areas was increased [105], but the epileptic activity in hippocampal slices was decreased by iodoresiniferatoxin (IRTX), a selective TRPV1 channel antagonist [106]. It is well known that glutamate could be released when the TRPV1 channel was activated [107], and the glutamate neurotransmitters are related to the etiology of epilepsy. Thus, focusing the TRPV1 channels activity may be important for the modulating neuronal excitability in epilepsy [106]. Recent studies showed that the high expression of TRPV1 channels could induce the temporal lobe epilepsy [105]. Cytosolic calcium elevation through activation of TRPV1 channels plays a physiologically relevant role in the regulation of epileptic seizures [108], decreasing the calcium accumulation by inhibiting the TRPV1 channels, could play a neuronal protective role against epilepsy-induced Ca^{2+} entry in hippocampal neurons. As mentioned above, the TRPV1 could be activated by hyperthermia; the hyperthermia-induced TRPV1 might be an effective candidate therapeutic target in heat-induced hyperexcitation [109, 110]. The activation of TRPV1 promotes glutamate release by increasing the excitability of neurons and synaptic terminals [111]. Whereas the activities would be reduced in hippocampus slices of rats after given the CPZ and ITRX, which were the TRPV1 channel blockers.

6. Antiepileptic therapy and beyond

At present, the treatment of epilepsy is still dominated by drugs. More than 35% of marketed antiepileptic drugs target VGICs, such as phenytoin, carbamazepine, oxcarbazepine, and ethosuximide. Phenytoin and carbamazepine are broad-spectrum antiepileptic drugs blocking VGSCs as their primary mechanism of action. For example, phenytoin is a more effective inhibitor of SCN8A-I1327V than other drugs [112], which could be used in treating patients with gain-of-function mutations of SCN8A. Different types of VGCCs play different roles in the pathological process of epilepsy. Decreased expression of P/Q type could induce epilepsy, whereas increased expression of N-type and T-type calcium channels could lead to epilepsy. Calcium blockers including ethosuximide have been widely accepted for the treatment of absence epilepsy [71]. Gain-of-function BK channels contribute to epileptogenesis and seizure generation. BK-blocking agents, like paxilline [49], might be used as potential therapeutic drugs.

In the future, novel techniques might contribute to develop reasonable therapies for treating inherited or acquired epileptic syndromes. For instance, induced pluripotent stem cells (IPS) and genetically engineering animal models could be used for accurate treatments of epilepsy. Single-nucleotide polymorphisms (SNPs) of VGIC genes from hereditary epilepsy patients could be detected by *de novo* genomic sequencing. VGICs of IPS cells could be mutated by CRISPR-Cas9 according to the information of these SNPs [113]. Through inducing IPS cells differentiated into neurons, phenotype of VGIC gene SNPs could be well investigated. It is also a well-detection platform for selecting antiepileptic drugs that would be sensitive to mutated VGICs *in vitro* [112]. For *in vivo* tests, besides transgenic mice, construction of nematode or zebrafish epileptic models may be creating a shortcut for choosing suitable and personalized antiepileptic drugs [114, 115]. In addition to drug control, optogenetics and ultrasonic control are hopeful to suppress the epileptic seizures induced by VGIC dysfunction [116, 117].

7. Conclusion

We systemically summarized the mutations and phenotype information of 21 epilepsy-associated VGIC genes. The dysfunctional VGICs are like the blasting fuse for neuronal hyperexcitability. We have good reason to believe that epilepsy-associated mutations of VGICs could be considered as a biomarker, which is possible to be one of the molecular bases underlying the classification of epilepsy syndromes identified by modern medicine. VGICs are the important targets for many antiepileptic drugs. Novel VGIC modulators are potentially effective strategy for the development of novel antiepileptic drugs. Individualized precise treatment using matching VGIC drugs will provide novel research directions and antiepileptic strategies.

Acknowledgements

This work was supported by National Science Foundation of China (Nos. 81603410 and 31771191), Innovation Fund of Putuo District Health System (No. 17-PT-10), Shanghai Municipal Commission of Health and Family Planning Fund (Nos. 20184Y0086, 2016JP007, and 2018JQ003), Project within budget of Shanghai University of Traditional Chinese Medicine (No. 18TS086), the Key Speciality Program (No. 2016102A) and Research Project (No. 2016208A) of Putuo Hospital, Shanghai University of Traditional Chinese Medicine.

Conflict of interest

The authors confirm that this article content has no conflict of interest.

Author details

Shuzhang Zhang[1,2], Yudan Zhu[1], Jiwei Cheng[1] and Jie Tao[1*]

1 Department of Central Laboratory and Neurology, Putuo Hospital, Shanghai University of Traditional Chinese Medicine, Shanghai, China

2 Laboratory of Neuropharmacology and Neurotoxicology, Shanghai University, Shanghai, China

*Address all correspondence to: jietao_putuo@foxmail.com

References

[1] Chang BS, Lowenstein DH. Epilepsy. The New England Journal of Medicine. 2003;**349**(13):1257-1266. DOI: 10.1056/NEJMra022308

[2] Wei F, Yan LM, Su T, et al. Ion channel genes and epilepsy: Functional alteration, pathogenic potential, and mechanism of epilepsy. Neuroscience Bulletin. 2017;**33**(4):455-477. DOI: 10.1007/s12264-017-0134-1

[3] Catterall WA. From ionic currents to molecular mechanisms: The structure and function of voltage-gated sodium channels. Neuron. 2000;**26**(1):13-25. DOI: 10.1016/S0896-6273(00)81133-2

[4] Fozzard HA, Hanck DA. Structure and function of voltage-dependent sodium channels: Comparison of brain II and cardiac isoforms. Physiological Reviews. 1996;**76**(3):887-926. DOI: 10.1152/physrev.1996.76.3.887

[5] Goldin AL, Barchi RL, Caldwell JH, et al. Nomenclature of voltage-gated sodium channels. Neuron. 2000;**28**(2):365-368. DOI: 10.1016/S0896-6273(00)00116-1

[6] Meng H, Xu HQ, Yu L, et al. The SCN1A mutation database: Updating information and analysis of the relationships among genotype, functional alteration, and phenotype. Human Mutation. 2015;**36**(6):573-580. DOI: 10.1002/humu.22782

[7] Mantegazza M, Gambardella A, Rusconi R, et al. Identification of an Nav1.1 sodium channel (SCN1A) loss-of-function mutation associated with familial simple febrile seizures. Proceedings of the National Academy of Sciences of the United States of America. 2005;**102**(50):18177-18182. DOI: 10.1073/pnas.0506818102

[8] Yu FH, Mantegazza M, Westenbroek RE, et al. Reduced sodium current in GABAergic interneurons in a mouse model of severe myoclonic epilepsy in infancy. Nature Neuroscience. 2006;**9**(9):1142-1149. DOI: 10.1038/nn1754

[9] Oakley JC, Kalume F, Yu FH, et al. Temperature- and age-dependent seizures in a mouse model of severe myoclonic epilepsy in infancy. Proceedings of the National Academy of Sciences of the United States of America. 2009;**106**(10):3994-3999. DOI: 10.1073/pnas.0813330106

[10] Tang B, Dutt K, Papale L, et al. A BAC transgenic mouse model reveals neuron subtype-specific effects of a generalized epilepsy with febrile seizures plus (GEFS+) mutation. Neurobiology of Disease. 2009;**35**(1):91-102. DOI: 10.1016/j.nbd.2009.04.007

[11] Martin MS, Dutt K, Papale LA, et al. Altered function of the SCN1A voltage-gated sodium channel leads to gamma-aminobutyric acid-ergic (GABAergic) interneuron abnormalities. The Journal of Biological Chemistry. 2010;**285**(13):9823-9834. DOI: 10.1074/jbc.M109.078568

[12] Catterall WA, Kalume F, Oakley JC. NaV1.1 channels and epilepsy. The Journal of Physiology. 2010;**588**(Pt 11):1849-1859. DOI: 10.1113/jphysiol.2010.187484

[13] Liao Y, Deprez L, Maljevic S, et al. Molecular correlates of age-dependent seizures in an inherited neonatal-infantile epilepsy. Brain. 2010;**133**(Pt 5):1403-1414. DOI: 10.1093/brain/awq057

[14] Heron SE, Crossland KM, Andermann E, et al. Sodium-channel defects in benign familial neonatal-infantile seizures. Lancet. 2002;**360**(9336):851-852. DOI: 10.1016/s0140-6736(02)09968-3

[15] Misra SN, Kahlig KM, George AL Jr. Impaired NaV1.2 function and reduced cell surface expression in benign familial neonatal-infantile seizures. Epilepsia. 2008;**49**(9):1535-1545. DOI: 10.1111/j.1528-1167.2008.01619.x

[16] Boiko T, Van Wart A, Caldwell JH, et al. Functional specialization of the axon initial segment by isoform-specific sodium channel targeting. The Journal of Neuroscience. 2003;**23**(6):2306-2313. DOI: 10.1523/JNEUROSCI.23-06-02306.2003

[17] Lauxmann S, Boutry-Kryza N, Rivier C, et al. An SCN2A mutation in a family with infantile seizures from Madagascar reveals an increased subthreshold Na(+) current. Epilepsia. 2013;**54**(9):e117-e121. DOI: 10.1111/epi.12241

[18] Dilena R, Striano P, Gennaro E, et al. Efficacy of sodium channel blockers in SCN2A early infantile epileptic encephalopathy. Brain & Development. 2017;**39**(4):345-348. DOI: 10.1016/j.braindev.2016.10.015

[19] Gazina EV, Leaw BT, Richards KL, et al. 'Neonatal' Nav1.2 reduces neuronal excitability and affects seizure susceptibility and behaviour. Human Molecular Genetics. 2015;**24**(5): 1457-1468. DOI: 10.1093/hmg/ddu562

[20] Catterall WA, Goldin AL, Waxman SG. International Union of Pharmacology. XLVII. Nomenclature and structure-function relationships of voltage-gated sodium channels. Pharmacological Reviews. 2005;**57**(4):397-409. DOI: 10.1124/pr.57.4.4

[21] Yu FH, Catterall WA. Overview of the voltage-gated sodium channel family. Genome Biology. 2003;**4**(3):207. DOI: 10.1186/gb-2003-4-3-207

[22] Whitaker WR, Faull RL, Waldvogel HJ, et al. Comparative distribution of voltage-gated sodium channel proteins in human brain. Brain Research. Molecular Brain Research. 2001;**88**(1-2):37-53. DOI: 10.1016/s0169-328x(00)00289-8

[23] Holland KD, Kearney JA, Glauser TA, et al. Mutation of sodium channel SCN3A in a patient with cryptogenic pediatric partial epilepsy. Neuroscience Letters. 2008;**433**(1):65-70. DOI: 10.1016/j.neulet.2007.12.064

[24] Estacion M, Gasser A, Dib-Hajj SD, et al. A sodium channel mutation linked to epilepsy increases ramp and persistent current of Nav1.3 and induces hyperexcitability in hippocampal neurons. Experimental Neurology. 2010;**224**(2):362-368. DOI: 10.1016/j.expneurol.2010.04.012

[25] Vanoye CG, Gurnett CA, Holland KD, et al. Novel SCN3A variants associated with focal epilepsy in children. Neurobiology of Disease. 2014;**62**:313-322. DOI: 10.1016/j.nbd.2013.10.015

[26] Lamar T, Vanoye CG, Calhoun J, et al. SCN3A deficiency associated with increased seizure susceptibility. Neurobiology of Disease. 2017;**102**: 38-48. DOI: 10.1016/j.nbd.2017.02.006

[27] Blumenfeld H, Lampert A, Klein JP, et al. Role of hippocampal sodium channel Nav1.6 in kindling epileptogenesis. Epilepsia. 2009;**50**(1):44-55. DOI: 10.1111/j.1528-1167.2008.01710.x

[28] Boiko T, Rasband MN, Levinson SR, et al. Compact myelin dictates the differential targeting of two sodium channel isoforms in the same axon. Neuron. 2001;**30**(1):91-104. DOI: 10.1016/s0896-6273(01)00265-3

[29] Veeramah KR, O'Brien JE, Meisler MH, et al. De novo pathogenic SCN8A mutation identified by whole-genome sequencing of a family quartet affected by infantile epileptic encephalopathy

and SUDEP. American Journal of Human Genetics. 2012;**90**(3):502-510. DOI: 10.1016/j.ajhg.2012.01.006

[30] Meisler MH, Helman G, Hammer MF, et al. SCN8A encephalopathy: Research progress and prospects. Epilepsia. 2016;**57**(7):1027-1035. DOI: 10.1111/epi.13422

[31] Papale LA, Beyer B, Jones JM, et al. Heterozygous mutations of the voltage-gated sodium channel SCN8A are associated with spike-wave discharges and absence epilepsy in mice. Human Molecular Genetics. 2009;**18**(9):1633-1641. DOI: 10.1093/hmg/ddp081

[32] Martin MS, Tang B, Papale LA, et al. The voltage-gated sodium channel Scn8a is a genetic modifier of severe myoclonic epilepsy of infancy. Human Molecular Genetics. 2007;**16**(23):2892-2899. DOI: 10.1093/hmg/ddm248

[33] Butler KM, da Silva C, Shafir Y, et al. De novo and inherited SCN8A epilepsy mutations detected by gene panel analysis. Epilepsy Research. 2017;**129**:17-25. DOI: 10.1016/j.eplepsyres.2016.11.002

[34] Makinson CD, Tanaka BS, Sorokin JM, et al. Regulation of thalamic and cortical network synchrony by Scn8a. Neuron. 2017;**93**(5):1165-1179. e6. DOI: 10.1016/j.neuron.2017.01.031

[35] Toledo-Aral JJ, Moss BL, He ZJ, et al. Identification of PN1, a predominant voltage-dependent sodium channel expressed principally in peripheral neurons. Proceedings of the National Academy of Sciences of the United States of America. 1997;**94**(4):1527-1532. DOI: 10.1073/pnas.94.4.1527

[36] Rush AM, Dib-Hajj SD, Liu S, et al. A single sodium channel mutation produces hyper- or hypoexcitability in different types of neurons. Proceedings of the National Academy of Sciences of the United States of America. 2006;**103**(21):8245-8250. DOI: 10.1073/pnas.0602813103

[37] Ahn HS, Black JA, Zhao P, et al. Nav1.7 is the predominant sodium channel in rodent olfactory sensory neurons. Molecular Pain. 2011;7:32. DOI: 10.1186/1744-8069-7-32

[38] Weiss J, Pyrski M, Jacobi E, et al. Loss-of-function mutations in sodium channel Nav1.7 cause anosmia. Nature. 2011;**472**(7342):186-190. DOI: 10.1038/nature09975

[39] Mechaly I, Scamps F, Chabbert C, et al. Molecular diversity of voltage-gated sodium channel alpha subunits expressed in neuronal and non-neuronal excitable cells. Neuroscience. 2005;**130**(2):389-396. DOI: 10.1016/j.neuroscience.2004.09.034

[40] Singh NA, Pappas C, Dahle EJ, et al. A role of SCN9A in human epilepsies, as a cause of febrile seizures and as a potential modifier of Dravet syndrome. PLoS Genetics. 2009;**5**(9):e1000649. DOI: 10.1371/journal.pgen.1000649

[41] Latorre R, Castillo K, Carrasquel-Ursulaez W, et al. Molecular determinants of BK channel functional diversity and functioning. Physiological Reviews. 2017;**97**(1):39-87. DOI: 10.1152/physrev.00001.2016

[42] Tao J, Lan Z, Wang Y, et al. Large-conductance calcium-activated potassium channels in glomerulus: From cell signal integration to disease. Frontiers in Physiology. 2016;**7**:248. DOI: 10.3389/fphys.2016.00248

[43] Du W, Bautista JF, Yang H, et al. Calcium-sensitive potassium channelopathy in human epilepsy and paroxysmal movement disorder. Nature Genetics. 2005;**37**(7):733-738. DOI: 10.1038/ng1585

[44] Yang J, Krishnamoorthy G, Saxena A, et al. An epilepsy/

dyskinesia-associated mutation enhances BK channel activation by potentiating Ca^{2+} sensing. Neuron. 2010;**66**(6):871-883. DOI: 10.1016/j.neuron.2010.05.009

[45] Gu N, Vervaeke K, Storm JF. BK potassium channels facilitate high-frequency firing and cause early spike frequency adaptation in rat CA1 hippocampal pyramidal cells. The Journal of Physiology. 2007;**580**(Pt. 3):859-882. DOI: 10.1113/jphysiol.2006.126367

[46] Martire M, Barrese V, D'Amico M, et al. Pre-synaptic BK channels selectively control glutamate versus GABA release from cortical and hippocampal nerve terminals. Journal of Neurochemistry. 2010;**115**(2):411-422. DOI: 10.1111/j.1471-4159.2010.06938.x

[47] Brenner R, Chen QH, Vilaythong A, et al. BK channel beta4 subunit reduces dentate gyrus excitability and protects against temporal lobe seizures. Nature Neuroscience. 2005;**8**(12):1752-1759. DOI: 10.1038/nn1573

[48] Shruti S, Clem RL, Barth AL. A seizure-induced gain-of-function in BK channels is associated with elevated firing activity in neocortical pyramidal neurons. Neurobiology of Disease. 2008;**30**(3):323-330. DOI: 10.1016/j.nbd.2008.02.002

[49] Sheehan JJ, Benedetti BL, Barth AL. Anticonvulsant effects of the BK-channel antagonist paxilline. Epilepsia. 2009;**50**(4):711-720. DOI: 10.1111/j.1528-1167.2008.01888.x

[50] Tabarki B, AlMajhad N, AlHashem A, et al. Homozygous KCNMA1 mutation as a cause of cerebellar atrophy, developmental delay and seizures. Human Genetics. 2016;**135**(11):1295-1298. DOI: 10.1007/s00439-016-1726-y

[51] Riazi MA, Brinkman-Mills P, Johnson A, et al. Identification of a putative regulatory subunit of a calcium-activated potassium channel in the dup (3q) syndrome region and a related sequence on 22q11.2. Genomics. 1999;**62**(1):90-94. DOI: 10.1006/geno.1999.5975

[52] Lorenz S, Heils A, Kasper JM, et al. Allelic association of a truncation mutation of the KCNMB3 gene with idiopathic generalized epilepsy. American Journal of Medical Genetics. Part B, Neuropsychiatric Genetics. 2007;**144B**(1):10-13. DOI: 10.1002/ajmg.b.30369

[53] Uebele VN, Lagrutta A, Wade T, et al. Cloning and functional expression of two families of beta-subunits of the large conductance calcium-activated K+ channel. The Journal of Biological Chemistry. 2000;**275**(30):23211-23218. DOI: 10.1074/jbc.M910187199

[54] Zhu Y, Zhang S, Feng Y, et al. The yin and Yang of BK channels in epilepsy. CNS & Neurological Disorders Drug Targets. 2018. DOI: 10.2174/1871527317666180213142403

[55] Abbott GW. KCNE1 and KCNE3: The yin and yang of voltage-gated K(+) channel regulation. Gene. 2016;**576**:(1 Pt 1):1-13. DOI: 10.1016/j.gene.2015.09.059

[56] Yang WP, Levesque PC, Little WA, et al. Functional expression of two KvLQT1-related potassium channels responsible for an inherited idiopathic epilepsy. The Journal of Biological Chemistry. 1998;**273**(31):19419-19423. DOI: 10.1074/jbc.273.31.19419

[57] Grigorov AO, Moskalyuk AA, Fedulova SA, et al. Differentiation of potassium currents in cultured inhibitory interneurons of the rat hippocampus (identification of the potassium M-type current). Neurophysiology. 2006;**38**(3):163-168

[58] Soldovieri MV, Boutry-Kryza N, Milh M, et al. Novel KCNQ2 and KCNQ3 mutations in a large cohort of families with benign neonatal epilepsy: First evidence for an altered channel regulation by syntaxin-1A. Human Mutation. 2014;**35**(3):356-367. DOI: 10.1002/humu.22500

[59] Miceli F, Striano P, Soldovieri MV, et al. A novel KCNQ3 mutation in familial epilepsy with focal seizures and intellectual disability. Epilepsia. 2015;**56**(2):e15-e20. DOI: 10.1111/epi.12887

[60] Borgatti R, Zucca C, Cavallini A, et al. A novel mutation in KCNQ2 associated with BFNC, drug resistant epilepsy, and mental retardation. Neurology. 2004;**63**(1):57-65. DOI: 10.1212/01.WNL.0000132979.08394.6D

[61] Hibino H, Inanobe A, Furutani K, et al. Inwardly rectifying potassium channels: Their structure, function, and physiological roles. Physiological Reviews. 2010;**90**(1):291-366. DOI: 10.1152/physrev.00021.2009

[62] Luscher C, Slesinger PA. Emerging roles for G protein-gated inwardly rectifying potassium (GIRK) channels in health and disease. Nature Reviews. Neuroscience. 2010;**11**(5):301-315. DOI: 10.1038/nrn2834

[63] Koyrakh L, Lujan R, Colon J, et al. Molecular and cellular diversity of neuronal G-protein-gated potassium channels. The Journal of Neuroscience. 2005;**25**(49):11468-11478. DOI: 10.1523/jneurosci.3484-05.2005

[64] Mark MD, Herlitze S. G-protein mediated gating of inward-rectifier K+ channels. European Journal of Biochemistry. 2000;**267**(19):5830-5836. DOI: 10.1046/j.1432-1327.2000.01670.x

[65] Signorini S, Liao YJ, Duncan SA, et al. Normal cerebellar development but susceptibility to seizures in mice lacking G protein-coupled, inwardly rectifying K+ channel GIRK2. Proceedings of the National Academy of Sciences of the United States of America. 1997;**94**(3):923-927. DOI: 10.1073/pnas.94.3.923

[66] Patil N, Cox DR, Bhat D, et al. A potassium channel mutation in weaver mice implicates membrane excitability in granule cell differentiation. Nature Genetics. 1995;**11**(2):126-129. DOI: 10.1038/ng1095-126

[67] Slesinger PA, Patil N, Liao YJ, et al. Functional effects of the mouse weaver mutation on G protein-gated inwardly rectifying K+ channels. Neuron. 1996;**16**(2):321-331. DOI: 10.1016/S0896-6273(00)80050-1

[68] Pei Q, Lewis L, Grahame-Smith DG, et al. Alteration in expression of G-protein-activated inward rectifier K+−channel subunits GIRK1 and GIRK2 in the rat brain following electroconvulsive shock. Neuroscience. 1999;**90**(2):621-627. DOI: 10.1016/S0306-4522(98)00453-9

[69] Kaufmann K, Romaine I, Days E, et al. ML297 (VU0456810), the first potent and selective activator of the GIRK potassium channel, displays antiepileptic properties in mice. ACS Chemical Neuroscience. 2013;**4**(9): 1278-1286. DOI: 10.1021/cn400062a

[70] Mazarati A, Lundstrom L, Sollenberg U, et al. Regulation of kindling epileptogenesis by hippocampal galanin type 1 and type 2 receptors: The effects of subtype-selective agonists and the role of G-protein-mediated signaling. The Journal of Pharmacology and Experimental Therapeutics. 2006;**318**(2):700-708. DOI: 10.1124/jpet.106.104703

[71] Catterall WA. Voltage-gated calcium channels. Cold Spring Harbor Perspectives in Biology.

2011;**3**(8):a003947. DOI: 10.1101/cshperspect.a003947

[72] Fatt P, Katz B. The electrical properties of crustacean muscle fibres. The Journal of Physiology. 1953;**120**(1-2):171-204. DOI: 10.1113/jphysiol.1953.sp004884

[73] Borsotto M, Barhanin J, Fosset M, et al. The 1,4-dihydropyridine receptor associated with the skeletal muscle voltage-dependent Ca^{2+} channel. Purification and subunit composition. The Journal of Biological Chemistry. 1985;**260**(26):14255-14263

[74] Takahashi M, Seagar MJ, Jones JF, et al. Subunit structure of dihydropyridine-sensitive calcium channels from skeletal muscle. Proceedings of the National Academy of Sciences of the United States of America. 1987;**84**(15):5478-5482. DOI: 10.1073/pnas.84.15.5478

[75] Furukawa T. Types of voltage-gated calcium channels: Molecular and electrophysiological views. Current Hypertension Reviews. 2013;**9**(3):170-181. DOI: 10.2174/1573402110666140131155912

[76] Ma H, Cohen S, Li B, et al. Exploring the dominant role of Cav1 channels in signalling to the nucleus. Bioscience Reports. 2012;**33**(1):97-101. DOI: 10.1042/bsr20120099

[77] Radzicki D, Yau HJ, Pollema-Mays SL, et al. Temperature-sensitive Cav1.2 calcium channels support intrinsic firing of pyramidal neurons and provide a target for the treatment of febrile seizures. The Journal of Neuroscience. 2013;**33**(24):9920-9931. DOI: 10.1523/jneurosci.5482-12.2013

[78] Durmus N, Kaya T, Gulturk S, et al. The effects of L type calcium channels on the electroencephalogram recordings in WAG/RIJ rat model of absence epilepsy. European Review for Medical and Pharmacological Sciences. 2013;**17**(9):1149-1154

[79] Han DY, Guan BJ, Wang YJ, et al. L-type calcium channel blockers enhance trafficking and function of epilepsy-associated alpha1(D219N) subunits of GABA(a) receptors. ACS Chemical Biology. 2015;**10**(9):2135-2148. DOI: 10.1021/acschembio.5b00479

[80] Qian J, Noebels JL. Presynaptic Ca^{2+} channels and neurotransmitter release at the terminal of a mouse cortical neuron. The Journal of Neuroscience. 2001;**21**(11):3721-3728. DOI: 10.1523/JNEUROSCI.21-11-03721.2001

[81] Bomben VC, Aiba I, Qian J, et al. Isolated P/Q calcium channel deletion in layer VI corticothalamic neurons generates absence epilepsy. The Journal of Neuroscience. 2016;**36**(2):405-418. DOI: 10.1523/jneurosci.2555-15.2016

[82] Rossignol E, Kruglikov I, van den Maagdenberg AM, et al. CaV 2.1 ablation in cortical interneurons selectively impairs fast-spiking basket cells and causes generalized seizures. Annals of Neurology. 2013;**74**(2):209-222. DOI: 10.1002/ana.23913

[83] Maejima T, Wollenweber P, Teusner LU, et al. Postnatal loss of P/Q-type channels confined to rhombic-lip-derived neurons alters synaptic transmission at the parallel fiber to purkinje cell synapse and replicates genomic Cacna1a mutation phenotype of ataxia and seizures in mice. The Journal of Neuroscience. 2013;**33**(12):5162-5174. DOI: 10.1523/jneurosci.5442-12.2013

[84] Letts VA, Mahaffey CL, Beyer B, et al. A targeted mutation in Cacng4 exacerbates spike-wave seizures in stargazer (Cacng2) mice. Proceedings of the National Academy of Sciences of the United States of America. 2005;**102**(6):2123-2128. DOI: 10.1073/pnas.0409527102

[85] Barclay J, Balaguero N, Mione M, et al. Ducky mouse phenotype of epilepsy and ataxia is associated with mutations in the Cacna2d2 gene and decreased calcium channel current in cerebellar Purkinje cells. The Journal of Neuroscience. 2001;**21**(16):6095-6104. DOI: 10.1523/JNEUROSCI.21-16-06095.2001

[86] Xu JH, Long L, Wang J, et al. Nuclear localization of Ca(v)2.2 and its distribution in the mouse central nervous system, and changes in the hippocampus during and after pilocarpine-induced status epilepticus. Neuropathology and Applied Neurobiology. 2010;**36**(1):71-85. DOI: 10.1111/j.1365-2990.2009.01044.x

[87] Weiergraber M, Henry M, Ho MS, et al. Altered thalamocortical rhythmicity in Ca(v)2.3-deficient mice. Molecular and Cellular Neurosciences. 2008;**39**(4):605-618. DOI: 10.1016/j.mcn.2008.08.007

[88] Zaman T, Lee K, Park C, et al. Cav2.3 channels are critical for oscillatory burst discharges in the reticular thalamus and absence epilepsy. Neuron. 2011;**70**(1):95-108. DOI: 10.1016/j.neuron.2011.02.042

[89] Weiergraber M, Henry M, Radhakrishnan K, et al. Hippocampal seizure resistance and reduced neuronal excitotoxicity in mice lacking the Cav2.3 E/R-type voltage-gated calcium channel. Journal of Neurophysiology. 2007;**97**(5):3660-3669. DOI: 10.1152/jn.01193.2006

[90] Catterall WA. Structure and regulation of voltage-gated Ca^{2+} channels. Annual Review of Cell and Developmental Biology. 2000;**16**:521-555. DOI: 10.1146/annurev.cellbio.16.1.521

[91] Catterall WA, Perez-Reyes E, Snutch TP, et al. International Union of Pharmacology. XLVIII. Nomenclature and structure-function relationships of voltage-gated calcium channels. Pharmacological Reviews. 2005;**57**(4):411-425. DOI: 10.1124/pr.57.4.5

[92] Shin HS, Cheong EJ, Choi S, et al. T-type Ca^{2+} channels as therapeutic targets in the nervous system. Current Opinion in Pharmacology. 2008;**8**(1):33-41. DOI: 10.1016/j.coph.2007.12.003

[93] Huguenard JR. Neuronal circuitry of thalamocortical epilepsy and mechanisms of antiabsence drug action. Advances in Neurology. 1999;**79**:991-999

[94] Talley EM, Solorzano G, Depaulis A, et al. Low-voltage-activated calcium channel subunit expression in a genetic model of absence epilepsy in the rat. Brain Research. Molecular Brain Research. 2000;**75**(1):159-165. DOI: 10.1016/S0169-328X(99)00307-1

[95] Rimoli MG, Russo E, Cataldi M, et al. T-type channel blocking properties and antiabsence activity of two imidazo[1,2-b]pyridazine derivatives structurally related to indomethacin. Neuropharmacology. 2009;**56**(3):637-646. DOI: 10.1016/j.neuropharm.2008.11.003

[96] Sharop BR, Boldyriev OI, Batiuk MY, et al. Compensatory reduction of Cav3.1 expression in thalamocortical neurons of juvenile rats of WAG/Rij model of absence epilepsy. Epilepsy Research. 2016;**119**:10-12. DOI: 10.1016/j.eplepsyres.2015.11.008

[97] Kim D, Song I, Keum S, et al. Lack of the burst firing of thalamocortical relay neurons and resistance to absence seizures in mice lacking alpha(1G) T-type Ca(2+) channels. Neuron. 2001;**31**(1):35-45. DOI: 10.1016/S0896-6273(01)00343-9

[98] Khosravani H, Bladen C, Parker DB, et al. Effects of Cav3.2 channel

mutations linked to idiopathic generalized epilepsy. Annals of Neurology. 2005;**57**(5):745-749. DOI: 10.1002/ana.20458

[99] Chen Y, Lu J, Pan H, et al. Association between genetic variation of CACNA1H and childhood absence epilepsy. Annals of Neurology. 2003;**54**(2):239-243. DOI: 10.1002/ana.10607

[100] Eckle VS, Shcheglovitov A, Vitko I, et al. Mechanisms by which a CACNA1H mutation in epilepsy patients increases seizure susceptibility. The Journal of Physiology. 2014;**592**(4):795-809. DOI: 10.1113/jphysiol.2013.264176

[101] Venkatachalam K, Montell C. TRP channels. Annual Review of Biochemistry. 2007;**76**:387-417. DOI: 10.1146/annurev.biochem.75.103004.142819

[102] Phelan KD, Shwe UT, Abramowitz J, et al. Canonical transient receptor channel 5 (TRPC5) and TRPC1/4 contribute to seizure and excitotoxicity by distinct cellular mechanisms. Molecular Pharmacology. 2013;**83**(2):429-438. DOI: 10.1124/mol.112.082271

[103] Phelan KD, Shwe UT, Cozart MA, et al. TRPC3 channels play a critical role in the theta component of pilocarpine-induced status epilepticus in mice. Epilepsia. 2017;**58**(2):247-254. DOI: 10.1111/epi.13648

[104] Nagamine K, Kudoh J, Minoshima S, et al. Molecular cloning of a novel putative Ca^{2+} channel protein (TRPC7) highly expressed in brain. Genomics. 1998;**54**(1):124-131. DOI: 10.1006/geno.1998.5551

[105] Bhaskaran MD, Smith BN. Effects of TRPV1 activation on synaptic excitation in the dentate gyrus of a mouse model of temporal lobe epilepsy. Experimental Neurology. 2010;**223**(2):529-536. DOI: 10.1016/j.expneurol.2010.01.021

[106] Iannotti FA, Hill CL, Leo A, et al. Nonpsychotropic plant cannabinoids, cannabidivarin (CBDV) and cannabidiol (CBD), activate and desensitize transient receptor potential vanilloid 1 (TRPV1) channels in vitro: Potential for the treatment of neuronal hyperexcitability. ACS Chemical Neuroscience. 2014;**5**(11):1131-1141. DOI: 10.1021/cn5000524

[107] Fawley JA, Hofmann ME, Andresen MC. Cannabinoid 1 and transient receptor potential vanilloid 1 receptors discretely modulate evoked glutamate separately from spontaneous glutamate transmission. The Journal of Neuroscience. 2014;**34**(24):8324-8332. DOI: 10.1523/JNEUROSCI.0315-14.2014

[108] Naziroglu M, Ovey IS. Involvement of apoptosis and calcium accumulation through TRPV1 channels in neurobiology of epilepsy. Neuroscience. 2015;**293**:55-66. DOI: 10.1016/j.neuroscience.2015.02.041

[109] Ghazizadeh V, Naziroglu M. Electromagnetic radiation (Wi-fi) and epilepsy induce calcium entry and apoptosis through activation of TRPV1 channel in hippocampus and dorsal root ganglion of rats. Metabolic Brain Disease. 2014;**29**(3):787-799. DOI: 10.1007/s11011-014-9549-9

[110] Naziroglu M, Ozkan FF, Hapil SR, et al. Epilepsy but not mobile phone frequency (900 MHz) induces apoptosis and calcium entry in hippocampus of epileptic rat: Involvement of TRPV1 channels. The Journal of Membrane Biology. 2015;**248**(1):83-91. DOI: 10.1007/s00232-014-9744-y

[111] Edwards JG, Gibson HE, Jensen T, et al. A novel non-CB1/TRPV1 endocannabinoid-mediated mechanism depresses excitatory synapses on hippocampal CA1 interneurons.

Hippocampus. 2012;**22**(2):209-221. DOI: 10.1002/hipo.20884

[112] Barker BS, Ottolini M, Wagnon JL, et al. The SCN8A encephalopathy mutation p.Ile1327Val displays elevated sensitivity to the anticonvulsant phenytoin. Epilepsia. 2016;**57**(9): 1458-1466. DOI: 10.1111/epi.13461

[113] Liu J, Gao C, Chen W, et al. CRISPR/Cas9 facilitates investigation of neural circuit disease using human iPSCs: Mechanism of epilepsy caused by an SCN1A loss-of-function mutation. Translational Psychiatry. 2016;**6**:e703. DOI: 10.1038/tp.2015.203

[114] Jiang Q , Li K, Lu WJ, et al. Identification of small-molecule ion channel modulators in *C. elegans* channelopathy models. Nature Communications. 2018;**9**(1):3941. DOI: 10.1038/s41467-018-06514-5

[115] Sourbron J, Smolders I, de Witte P, et al. Pharmacological analysis of the anti-epileptic mechanisms of fenfluramine in scn1a mutant zebrafish. Frontiers in Pharmacology. 2017;**8**:191. DOI: 10.3389/fphar.2017.00191

[116] Ye J, Tang S, Meng L, et al. Ultrasonic control of neural activity through activation of the mechanosensitive channel MscL. Nano Letters. 2018;**18**(7):4148-4155. DOI: 10.1021/acs.nanolett.8b00935

[117] Tonnesen J, Kokaia M. Epilepsy and optogenetics: Can seizures be controlled by light? Clinical Science (London, England). 2017;**131**(14):1605-1616. DOI: 10.1042/CS20160492

Chapter 11

Components of Soft Computing for Epileptic Seizure Prediction and Detection

B. Suguna Nanthini

Abstract

Components of soft computing include machine learning, fuzzy logic, evolutionary computation, and probabilistic theory. These components have the cognitive ability to learn effectively. They deal with imprecision and good tolerance of uncertainty. Components of soft computing are needed for developing automated expert systems. These systems reduce human interventions so as to complete a task essentially. Automated expert systems are developed in order to perform difficult jobs. The systems have been trained and tested using soft computing techniques. These systems are required in all kinds of fields and are especially very useful in medical diagnosis. This chapter describes the components of soft computing and review of some analyses regarding EEG signal classification. From those analyses, this chapter concludes that a number of features extracted are very important and relevant features for classifier can give better accuracy of classification. The classifier with a suitable learning method can perform well for automated epileptic seizure detection systems. Further, the decomposition of EEG signal at level 4 is sufficient for seizure detection.

Keywords: soft computing, intelligence, EEG signals, epilepsy, seizure, classification, accuracy, detection, prediction

1. Introduction

The human brain contains billions of neurons which vibrate and generate oscillatory activity. This neural activity of nervous system is studied through brainwaves. These waves are highly complex and can be recorded using the method called electroencephalography (EEG). An epileptic seizure is a symptom due to abnormal and irregular excessive neuronal activity in the brain. The neuronal activity can be recorded by medical tests. Various methods are available for diagnosing brain diseases. Among those methods, the electroencephalogram test is mainly used for diagnosing epilepsy. EEG includes different types of waveforms with different frequency, amplitude, and spatial distribution. The electrical activity of the brain differs due to different stimuli and physiological variables. An EEG test can provide detailed information about the electrical activity of the brain at the testing time. The neurologist recognizes the brain pattern from the EEG test results to diagnose epilepsy. EEG recordings by visual scanning will take time and are inaccurate for detecting epilepsy [1]. Nowadays, the technology of computer-aided diagnosis (CAD) has been used in hospitals; it cannot replace the doctor, but it can assist the professionals to diagnose the disease accurately. The main aim of the CAD systems is to identify the disease in early stages of its development. The CAD supportive tool is developed by using highly complex recognition techniques and machine learning algorithms. The CAD systems are approved by US Food and Drug Administration. They can reduce the false negative rate of recognition of diseases. Recent research studies have identified that the performance of CAD is better in the clinical environment. Establishing CAD systems in medical practice contains some risk and complexity. Sometimes, the interpretation of given data may not yield 100% accurate result. It provides only secondary opinion to the physicians. Especially in epileptic seizure detection, machine learning is very difficult because of understanding the brainwaves. The patterns of brainwaves are completely unique to individuals. Since 1998, CAD tools have been useful for diagnosing disease. It does not mean that they are meant for diagnostic purposes, but the approved CAD system can provide accurate results. Early diagnosis of disease is very important for saving life. Different information can be extracted by using medical image and signal technologies such as X-ray, computed tomography (CT), positron emission tomography (PET), single positron emission computed tomography (SPECT), magnetic resonance imaging (MRI), ultrasound, EEG, electrocardiography (ECG), electromyography (EMG), etc. for diagnosing diseases like cancer and coronary artery, cardiovascular, and neurological disorders. CAD supports accurate diagnosis in early stages of a chronic disease. Soft computing techniques are used in computer-aided diagnosis and computer-aided detection. In the earlier stage of computational approaches, the problem-solving methods were carried out using conventional mathematics and specific analytical models [2].

The traditional way of computing would be less efficient for problem-solving. In the growth of computational science, researchers focus on soft computing in order to overcome the drawbacks of hard computing. Just like artificial

Hard computing	Soft computing
There are different types of conventional methods such as Boolean logic, crisp analysis, numerical analysis, deterministic search, analytical model, and binary logic. These conventional methods are also called hard computing techniques	To make something better to handle uncertainty, imprecision, robustness, low solution cost, partial truth, and approximation, the soft computing techniques are introduced
These techniques commonly use arithmetic, science, and computing	It imitates the model from nature
Since conventional methods are used from the beginning of computational science, these traditional ways of approach require a lot of computation time	It mimics biological procedures and plays a greater role in the development of computational science and acts efficiently
The hard computing techniques are inaccurate, inadequate, and unreliable	The soft computing methods can be approached in different ways for finding solution
The programs that are written by using these techniques are deterministic	The soft computing techniques are developed mainly to get better results for any NP (nondeterministic polynomial)-complete problems
It involves precise input data and sequential procedures	Unlike hard computing, the inputs are adjusted to optimize the result
It can produce exact but not an approximate answer	For any given information, the process can give the best result by maximizing the desired benefit and minimizing the undesired one at low solution cost

Table 1.
Comparison of hard and soft computing.

intelligence (AI), soft computing method works similar to the human brain. A comparison of hard computing and soft computing is given in **Table 1**. Soft computing techniques can be applicable in various fields such as signal and image processing, system integration, decision support process and system control, pattern recognition, fault diagnosis, data mining, forecasting applications, robotics, virtual reality, etc. Machine learning, fuzzy logic, evolutionary computation, Bayesian network, and chaos theory techniques are the main components of soft computing. These methods are very useful for automation and necessary for technology development [2]. The following sections of this chapter explain the merits and demerits of soft computing and the procedure for automated epileptic seizure prediction and detection.

2. Components of soft computing

Machine learning, fuzzy logic, evolutionary computation, and probabilistic ideas are the main components of soft computing. The following sections give detailed descriptions of each component.

2.1 Machine learning

Problem-solving is a challenging task for intelligent entities. It has been proved that "a machine can learn new things." It can adapt to new situations and has an ability to learn from the storage information. Machine learning techniques include artificial neural networks (ANNs), perceptron, and support vector machine (SVM) whereas evolutionary computations include evolutionary algorithms, meta-heuristic and swam intelligence. Just like human brain, a machine is capable of acquiring knowledge from data. It is developed from the field of AI. In order to build intelligent machines, we need machine learning techniques. These techniques deal with huge data in minimum time. There are different types of machine learning methods. They are as follows:

- supervised learning;
- unsupervised learning; and
- reinforcement learning.

Supervised learning technique is used in majority of analyses. In this technique, the system learns from training examples, whereas in unsupervised learning, the system is challenged to discover some patterns directly from the given data. Classification and regression are two different supervised learning problems. The next section gives detailed description about classification using EEG signals for epileptic seizure detection. Regression gives the statistical relationship between two or more variables. An association rule learning problem and clustering problem are major examples explaining unsupervised learning problems. Association rule learning is based on rule-based machine learning method and used to discover the interesting relationship between variables in a huge database whereas clustering method discovers the patterns from the groupings of given data. Reinforcement learning is the third type of machine learning which learns how to behave in an environment merely by interaction. It is a dynamic way of learning. It learns directly and controls the data (no supervisor). Machine learning algorithms have the ability of learning from data and make predictions and classifications for a model based on the sample inputs. ANN is a technique composed of artificial neurons (processing units or elements) and mimics the function of the human brain, whereas SVM is based on associate learning method and performs data classification. It separates the data into corresponding groups using hyperplanes. Perceptron and support vector are very similar linear classifiers. A network with no hidden layers is called a single layer perceptron. Back propagation algorithm and perceptron are second-generation neural networks. Back propagation is a technique used to train the neural network in order to minimize the objective function. It can learn from mistakes. It looks for the minimum value of the error function in weight space. The weight that minimizes the error function is then considered to be a solution for the learning problem. "It is a supervised learning method, and is a generalization of the delta rule or gradient descent" [2].Neural networks can be classified as follows:

- single-layer neural network;
- multi-layer neural network; and
- competitive neural network.

The back propagation algorithm works as follows: each neuron has an activation function in the neural network with respect to weights w_{ij} defined as:

$$A_j(\overline{x},\overline{w}) = \sum_{i=0}^{n} x_i w_{ji} \quad (1)$$

The sigmoid function with respect to output function is defined as:

$$O_j(\overline{x},\overline{w}) = \frac{1}{1+e^{A(\overline{x},\overline{w})}} \quad (2)$$

Therefore, the error functions of each neuron in the output are defined as:

$$E_j(\overline{x},\overline{w},d) = \left(O_j(\overline{x},\overline{w}) - d_j\right)^2 \quad (3)$$

where d_j denotes the jth element of the desired response vector and the sum of the errors in the output layer from all the neurons is defined as:

$$E_j(\overline{x},\overline{w},d) = \Sigma_j \left(O_j(\overline{x},\overline{w}) - d_j\right)^2 \quad (4)$$

Since $\Delta w \,\alpha - \frac{\partial E}{\partial w}$, the overall error is reduced by using the *gradient descendent* method. The partial derivative of errors with respect to weight using the delta rule is defined as:

$$w_{ji} = -\eta \frac{\partial E}{\partial w_{ji}} \quad (5)$$

where η denotes the learning rate parameter. Eqs. (1) and (2) provide the dependency with respect to output as:

$$\frac{\partial E}{\partial O_j} = 2(O_j - d_j) \quad (6)$$

$$\text{Also, } \frac{\partial O_j}{\partial w_{ji}} = \frac{\partial O_j}{\partial A_j}\frac{\partial A_j}{\partial w_{ji}} = O_j(1 - O_j)x_i \quad (7)$$

From (6) and (7)

$$\frac{\partial E}{\partial w_{ji}} = \frac{\partial E}{\partial O_j}\frac{\partial O_j}{\partial w_{ji}} = 2(O_j - d_j)\,O_j(1 - O_j)\,x_i \quad (8)$$

Therefore, the weight adjustment of each neuron (from (5) and (8)) is:

$$\Delta w_{ji} = -2\eta(O_j - d_j)\,O_j(1 - O_j)\,x_i \quad (9)$$

Feed forwarding the inputs, calculating the error, and propagating it back to the previous layers are the main steps of an ANN classifier. The error is identified as the difference between the desired response and actual response of the network. Each classifier is based on some learning method. There are different types of learning methods such as error correction learning, memory-based learning, associative learning, neural net learning, genetic learning, etc. SVM is based on the associative learning method. There are many advantages in SVM. The performance of SVM is very competitive with other methods. A drawback is the problem complexity for large sample sizes. Special optimizers are used for optimization. Basically, SVM is a linear classifier that classifies the two different classes (normal and seizure) efficiently. The features of the two classes are categorized by the labels "−1" and "+1." The features that are extracted from the signal are defined as:

$$S = \left\{ (x_i, y_i)_{i=1}^{n} \right\} \quad (10)$$

where y_i denotes the label related to the pattern x_i and n refers to the number of samples. Dot product or the scalar product of linear classifier is defined as:

$$W^T(x) = \sum_i w_i x_i \quad (11)$$

This Eq. (11) in the function form is:

$$f(x) = W^T(x) + b \quad (12)$$

where w_i denotes the weight vector and b refers to the bias. For the case b = 0, the set of vectors in $W^T(x) = 0$ produce a hyperplane through the origin, which divides the features into two classes. The kernel is an algorithm that can produce non-linear decision boundaries. Replacing the normal SVM (linear kernel) dot product with a kernel function defines a Gaussian radial basis function classifier which is expressed as

$$k(x_i x_j) = e^{-\|x_i - x_j\|^2/2\sigma^2} \quad (13)$$

The variables x_i and x_j represent the two sample data from the dataset. The default sigma value is one that has been associated with all the attributes in the dataset. The features are separated into two different classes with respect to their feature label. ANN and SVM are supervised learning methods. Both have different working patterns. SVM with kernels is highly suitable for non-linear mapping functions. The classification process is important because a machine has to learn how to classify the data into groups [3].

2.2 Fuzzy logic

Machine learning, fuzzy logic, and evolutionary computations can be applicable for any decision-making problems. Unlike Boolean logic, fuzzy logic is an approach that deals with a problem by the level of truth values which lie between 0 and 1. Fuzzy refers to vagueness. The Boolean logic results in true or false for the question (**Figure 1**) "Is it raining?" but fuzzy logic gives a number in the range from 0 to 1. Here 1.0 represents absolute truth and 0.0 represents absolute false.

This is a logic used for fuzziness. It was introduced in 1965 by Lofti A.Zadeh. Fuzzy classifier is a classifier (algorithm) that uses fuzzy logic for classification and prediction problems. It is based on fuzzy sets (membership functions). The data-driven and trial and error (heuristic) approaches are two different approaches of fuzzy logic. An automated system can be designed using these approaches. Among these approaches, data-driven is most essential for the model to learn and update continuously. Fuzzy logic uses trial and error approach in tuning process for obtaining a satisfactory result. It is a technique that can handle imprecise data and especially analyze crisp/standard data. The data-driven approach is similar to event-driven approach and it is well structured. In classification processes, appropriate features are required to train and test the system. The performance of the system depends on selecting the apt features from the data for modeling the detection system. The heuristic method is not an optimal approach for problem-solving. It gives satisfactory solution. Heuristics, hyper-heuristics, and meta-heuristics are commonly used with machine learning and optimization techniques. Mostly, machine learning techniques are heuristic. Genetic algorithm or any optimization technique can be used to get optimal solution for the given problem. Fuzzy if then rule is the simple form of fuzzy rule based classifier. Fuzzy if-then rule statements are the form of fuzzy logic. Any classifier that uses fuzzy logic is fuzzy rule based classifier. These classifiers are well suited for linear model of classification whereas ANN can predict better on test data. Recently, deep learning has been the popular tool for prediction and detection processes. Fuzzy logic gives multi-value answers, whereas in machine learning, the system learns from data especially with the control or supervisor [2].

2.3 Evolutionary computation

Evolutionary computation (EC) is a subdiscipline of AI and soft computing. In computational intelligence, evolutionary algorithms are inspired by biological systems and give optimal solution for problems. Meta-heuristic and swarm intelligence may also yield enough good solutions for any optimization problem. EC is a computational intelligence method involved in a lot of optimization techniques for problem-solving methods. It is a subfield of AI. The algorithms of EC are inspired by biological evolution. These algorithms can give highly optimum solutions for any kind of problems. Ant colony optimization, genetic algorithm (GA), genetic programming, self-organization maps, competitive learning, and swarm intelligence are some examples of EC techniques. Genetic algorithm is a technique used for optimization in problem-solving of various fields. It is derived from the natural genetic systems. It gives accurate results, exhibits robustness, and produces optimal solution for the problem.

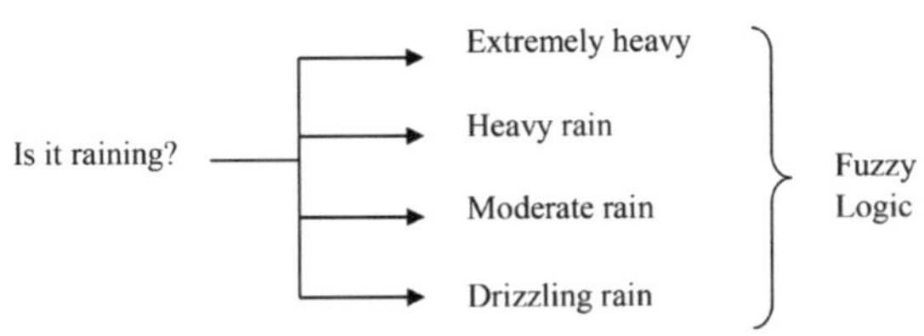

Figure 1.
Example for fuzzy logic.

In computational intelligence, the application program differs among various problems in various fields. GA starts with the production of the initial chromosome in the population. Chromosomes are binary digits representing the control parameters in the coding of the given problem. Like natural reproduction systems, crossover and mutation processes take place for generating a new population. Fitness calculation is evaluated in successive iterations called generations. After several generations, GA selects the best chromosome using probabilistic transition rules and obtains the optimal or closest optimal solution to the problem. In the automated epileptic seizure detection problem, genetic algorithm is used for feature selection. Selecting relevant features is important for the performance of the system [2].

2.4 Probabilistic ideas

Both probabilistic ideas and logic are used in probabilistic reasoning in order to handle uncertainty situations. Most of the problems use probability and statistics. "Clean data is greater than more data." Machine learns from data. Quality of data is important rather than quantity of data. Bayesian analysis is one of the most important approaches for probabilistic reasoning. Unknown information or imperfectness is the situation of uncertainty. Bayesian inference is a statistical inference based on Bayes theorem that can be used for accurate prediction. It is very useful when the available data are insufficient for solving the problem. Data analysis is a procedure of evaluating data that are gathered from various sources. The soft computing techniques play a challenging part in data analysis. For example, data mining techniques are especially used for discovering new information from a huge database, whereas soft computing techniques mimic the process of human brain in order to find effective solutions for any NP-complete problem.

3. Epileptic seizure prediction and detection

There is a link between data analysis and soft computing. Data may be qualitative or quantitative. Quantitative data can give exact solution for the problem. The data are pre-processed once they have been collected. The raw data are transformed effectively for the purpose of analysis in the pre-processing stage. Any type of data has to be initially pre-processed for analysis. The main principle of data pre-processing is to eliminate the irrelevant and redundant data (noise data) in order to get better detection accuracy of the system. In signal processing, the error is referred to as an artifact or noise. Unwanted information can be removed from the raw data using noise reduction. Different types of algorithms are available for data pre-processing. For example, in the case of EEG signal processing for epileptic seizure detection, artifacts can occur from physiological or mechanical sources. Respiratory, cardiac/pulse, eye movement, and electromyography signals are biological artifacts [4]. These artifacts should be recognized and eliminated for proper diagnosis. More than one variety of artifacts can appear in the recorded EEG. Preprocessing is the first step in classification and diagnostics where the artifacts have to be removed. After pre-processing, the signals are filtered and free from noise. These filtered signals are used for feature extraction process in the next step.

3.1 Feature extraction/selection and classification

The process that converts the huge samples to a set of features is called feature extraction and feature selection is the process that filters the redundant or irrelevant features. These methods are used to reduce the actual dimension of the given data.

Data are important to build a machine learning model. The performance of the classifier depends on the given data. The noise must be removed from data. Classifier cannot separate the noise from data. Pre-processing is the process that is most important for removing noise. Analysis of EEG signals is important to diagnose epilepsy in clinical practice [3]. Fourier transform-based analysis is suitable for stationary signals. Studies have proved that EEG signals change over time and frequency components. Several time-frequency domain-based methods such as short time Fourier transform, discrete wavelet transform (DWT), and multiwavelet transform can be used to decompose the EEG signals [5]. Removing artifacts from the signal especially in biomedical applications is a challenging task, because it creates some signals and disturbs the epilepsy diagnosis. Pre-processing is the process to remove artifacts, and they can be extracted well by a method called independent component analysis (ICA) [6]. In order to reduce the dimension of the raw data and to find optimal solution, feature extraction process with kernel trick is frequently used [7]. **Figure 2** explains the EEG signal classification.

In earlier days, reading and interpretations of the EEG signals were very difficult for a neurophysiologist. This drawback has been overcome in the latest computer technology. EEG is a non-stationary signal and is very difficult to understand by an ordinary person. For EEG signal analysis, features are extracted from the EEG vectors and appropriate features are selected for classification. Feature selection is a subset of feature extraction. The irrelevant and redundant features are eliminated for better performance of the system. Feature selection algorithms can be used to select

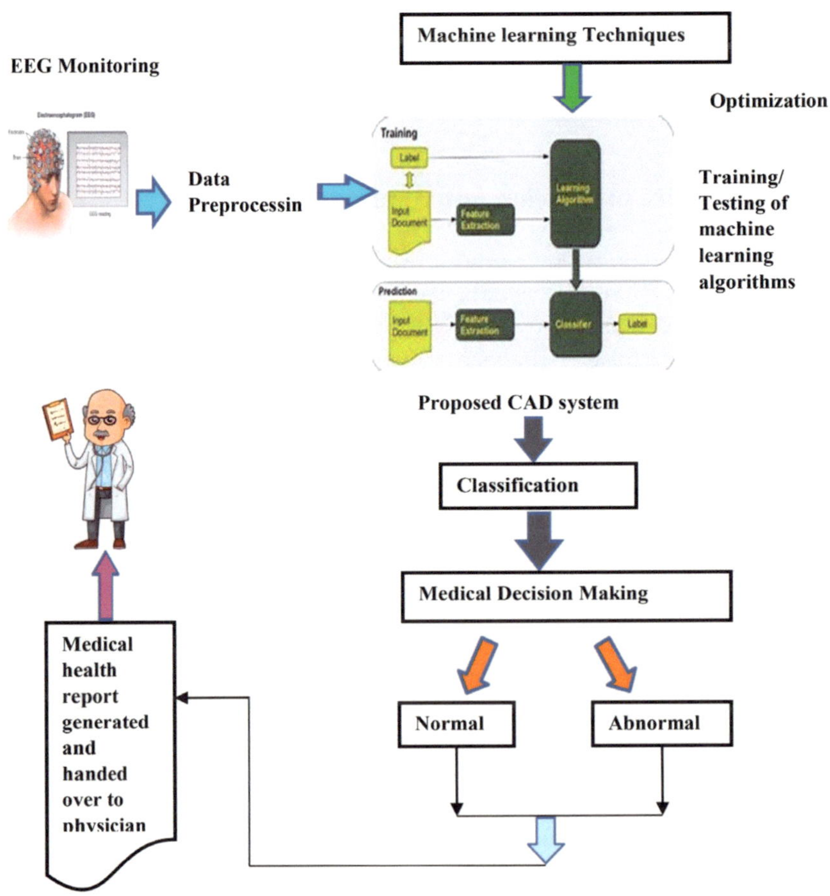

Figure 2.
EEG signal classification.

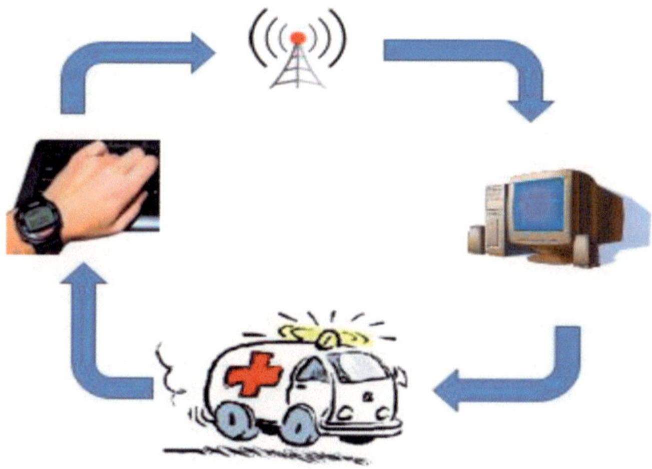

Figure 3.
Warning system in epilepsy.

appropriate features. Genetic algorithm is an exact tool for feature selection. It can reduce the computing time and space required to run the algorithms. Filter method, Pearson's correlation co-efficient, mutual information, wrapper methods, and greedy forward search are some of the methods used to select features for classification. In machine learning, classification is the process of categorizing the data by training the machine with the class label. For example, labels like "Seizure" or "Normal" are used in the case of supervised learning. The clustering technique also known as grouping technique is based on inherence in unsupervised learning and can handle unlabeled data. An algorithm that maps the data into a particular group is called a classifier.

3.2 Warning system in epilepsy

ECG and EEG data are used in seizure detection. Several electronic mobile applications are developed to track seizure information from the patient electronically. The information includes type of seizure, frequency, and duration. The application provides useful data for the epileptologist to treat epilepsy accurately. Already, many applications have been developed and are available on the market. **Figure 3** represents the closed-loop warning system for epilepsy.

A new high tech bracelet developed by Netherlands scientists can detect 85% of all severe night time epilepsy seizures. Automated seizure detection methods can overcome some of the difficulties that occur from data collection, patient monitoring, and prediction modeling. Closed-loop system monitors the seizures and can detect, anticipate, and even respond to the real-time information from the patients. These systems have been used in emergency and intensive care settings of medical diagnosis [8].

4. Review of EEG signal analyses

B. Suguna Nanthini [3] had carried out six different analyses for detecting seizures using EEG signals under supervised learning method. The performance of the system in all the analyses is measured by the confusion matrix method. Online available EEG database (Bonn University Database) and real-time data from the EEG center, Coimbatore, India, are used for EEG signal classification analysis. EEG tests taken from 10 normal and seizure subjects for epileptic seizure detection are used in second database. These signals are examined and used for binary classification as well as for validation. Set A (perfectly normal) and Set E (merely seizure) have been chosen from online database. The first three analyses were carried out in the spatial domain and next three analyses were carried out in the frequency (wavelet) domain. In the first analysis [9], gray-level co-occurrence matrix (GLCM) features namely contrast, correlation, energy, and homogeneity are extracted from the EEG vectors. The system is well trained to identify the exact group and tested for classification of data using ANN classifier. The performance of the system is measured by the confusion matrix. The system achieves 85% accuracy. The same problem is examined with an SVM classifier in the second analysis [10]. The classifier achieves 90% accuracy for EEG signal classification. The computational complexity of analyses 1 and 2 are calculated and shown in the following **Table 2**.

When the analyses use ANN and SVM classifiers, the space complexity depends on the number of training samples used in the classification process. In the third analysis [11], eight statistical features are added with GLCM features. The EEG signals are segmented and combinations of normal and seizure signals are used for classification process. In extraction process, eight statistical features and four GLCM features are extracted from each of the segmented signal. An SVM classifier with different kernels is used for seizure detection. The computation complexity of analysis 3 is calculated and presented in the following **Table 3**. The complexity of the model depends on k-fold cross-validation method. The system executes the same learning algorithm k times. It takes different training sets of size (k−1)/k times the size of the original data. In the execution step, each sample is evaluated (k−1) times. The space complexity of the analysis for RBF kernel is (Number of samples) ^2*(Number of features) and for linear kernel is (Number of samples) * (Number of features). ANN with back propagation algorithm [9] and SVM with linear kernel have achieved almost similar results.

EEG signals are non-stationery and can be analyzed better through wavelet transform. Different types of wavelets are available to decompose the signal. The challenging part is to select a suitable wavelet and the level of decomposition of the signal. In the fourth analysis [12], statistical features namely mean, median, mode, standard deviation, skewness and kurtosis and four GLCM features are extracted

Analysis	Training time (seconds)	Testing time (seconds)	Precision (%)	Miss classification rate (%)
GLCM with ANN	105	0.05	100	24
GLCM with SVM	64	0.02	90	10

Table 2.
Computational complexity of analyses 1 and 2.

Analysis	Training time (seconds)	Testing time (seconds)
GLCM and statistical features with SVM linear kernel	275	245
GLCM and statistical features with SVM RBF kernel	127	182
GLCM and statistical features with SVM-tuned RBF kernel	220	129

Table 3.
Computation complexity of analysis 3.

from the EEG signal. The performance of the system is measured to select a suitable classifier for seizure detection. ANN and SVM are two classifiers used in the fourth analysis. The wavelets namely db1, db2, and haar are used for signal decomposition. The signal is decomposed up to level 3.

4.1 Significance of the analysis

1. Statistical and GLCM features are used to examine the EEG signals separately and further they are combined together as an input to the classifier.

2. Raw EEG data (0–60 Hz) as its subbands (30–60 Hz (cD1), 15–30 Hz (cD2), 8–15 Hz (cD3), and 0–8 Hz (cA3)) are verified and analyzed using all those features.

3. On comparison of features (statistical, GLCM, and their combination), wavelets (db1,db2, and haar), and classifiers (ANN and SVM), the analysis concluded that the combination of statistical and GLCM features using SVM classifier gives the best outcome.

To extract maximum information from the EEG signal, entropy features are used in the fifth analysis [13]. There are different types of entropies. In this analysis, Shannon, Renyi, and Tsallis entropies are extracted from the EEG signals. On comparison of entropy features, the analysis concluded that Renyi entropy can achieve successful result. Instead of using only statistical features over the wavelet coefficient, this analysis examines the EEG signals through entropy values obtained from different degrees of orders for classification. When comparing with the existing work, this research uses the extended version of Shannon, namely Renyi and Tsallis to extract the maximum information from each EEG signal vector in terms of probability events. In the sixth analysis [14], EEG signals are examined by combining all the features from the previous analysis. Altogether, 16 features from the methods namely GLCM, statistical, and Renyi entropy features are extracted from the raw EEG and its subbands. DWT (db2) is used for decomposition of the signal at level 4.The approximation and detail co-efficient are analyzed individually with 16 and 8 features, respectively. Genetic algorithm is used for selecting 8 appropriate features. The SVM is used as a classifier. Classification is carried out for seizure detection. Accuracies from 16 and 8 dimension features are compared and it is concluded that relevant features can give better accuracy. Moreover, level 4 is enough for decomposing the signal because the lower frequencies namely delta and theta can be obtained at level 4 of decomposition. Mostly, seizures are identified at lower frequencies; so, level 4 is sufficient for decomposition of the EEG signal. Further, the time to execute the algorithm is reduced and it occupies less memory space for the storage of data parameters. The complexity of this EEG signal analysis is calculated and presented in the following **Table 4**.

Summary and time complexity of the analyses are shown in **Tables 5** and **6**, respectively. All analyses are carried out in MATLAB environment. From the

Analysis	Training time (seconds)	Testing time (seconds)
16 Dimension features with SVM	0.76	10.0013
8 Dimension features with SVM classifier	0.72	0.0011

Table 4.
Computational complexity of analysis 6.

calculations, the analyses prove that the performance of SVM with significant features is good when compared with ANN using large number of features as the input. The major contributions of these analyses in view of the existing work are as follows:

1. Two different machine learning algorithms (ANN and SVM) that are based on two different learning methods (error correcting and associative learning) have been examined for seizure detection.

2. Unique set of features are extracted from the EEG signals for classification.

3. For optimization, genetic algorithm is used for feature selection and proved that the classifier can perform well with relevant features.

4. Accuracies are calculated for raw EEG signal and for all decomposed signals

EEG analysis #:	Domain	Feature extraction	Classifier	Conclusion
1	Spatial domain	GLCM features	ANN	85% Accuracy
2	Spatial domain	GLCM features	SVM	90% Accuracy
3	Spatial domain (EEG segments)	(GLCM and statistical)	SVM (Linear and RBF kernel)	Linear kernel (99.95% accuracy)
4	Frequency domain DWT (db1,db2)	GLCM, statistical, and hybrid features	ANN and SVM	Db2 wavelet and hybrid features to SVM classifier are the best outcomes (92.16% accuracy)
5	Frequency domain db2 at level 4	Entropy estimation (Shannon, Renyi, and Tsallis)	SVM	Renyi entropy gives better accuracy (99.9 accuracy)
6	Db2 at level 4	8 statistical features, 4 GLCM features, 4 Renyi entropy estimation (Genetic algorithm for feature selection)	SVM	Relevant features give successful result with 90% performance accuracy in system validation

Table 5.
Summary of EEG analyses.

Analysis	Database	LoD	Number of features	Number of features significant	Classifier	Tr time (seconds)	Test Time (seconds)
1	Bonn University	3	10	6	ANN	243	0.123
2	Bonn University	3	10	6	SVM	64	0.023
3	Bonn University	4	6	6	ANN	184	0.2
4	Bonn University	4	6	6	SVM	61	0.02
5	Real-time data	4	16	12	SVM	63	0.0013
6	Real-time data	4	8	4	SVM	62	0.0011
7	Validation	4	8	4	SVM	—	0.017
		4	12	12	SVM	—	0.09

LoD, Level of decomposition; Tr, Training.

Table 6.
Time complexity of EEG analyses.

5. Conclusion

An epileptic seizure is a symptom due to abnormal and excessive irregular neuronal activity in the brain. EEG test is mainly used for diagnosing epilepsy. EEG includes different types of waveforms with different frequency, amplitude, and spatial distribution. Traditional ways of computations would be less efficient for problem-solving. But, soft computing methods can work in an efficient way for discovering solutions from the given data. Components of soft computing are essential for developing automated expert systems. Early diagnosis of disease can save the life of a person. The approved CAD system is able to provide accurate results. Problem-solving is a challenging task for intelligent entities. It has been proved that "a machine can learn new things." It can adapt to new situations and has an ability to learn from the storage information. Supervised learning technique is used in majority of analyses. Fuzzy logic gives multi-value answers, whereas in machine learning, the system learns from data especially with the control or supervisor. In computational intelligence, evolutionary algorithms are inspired by biological systems and give optimal solution for the problem. "Clean data are greater than more data." Machine learns from data. Quality of data is important rather than quantity of data. This chapter gave an introduction about the components of soft computing and classification in machine learning. From the review of analyses, this chapter concludes that relevant features and less number of features can make the classifier perform well. Accuracies are compared in all decomposed signals and proved that level 4 of decomposition is enough for EEG signal classification. At level 4, the lower frequencies (delta and theta) can be analyzed perfectly because seizures occur mostly at lower frequencies. Also, from the analyses, it has been proved that the time required and memory space for data parameters are less.

Conflict of interest

There are no conflicts of interest.

Author details

B. Suguna Nanthini
SAAI Centre for research, Thanjavur, Tamilnadu, India

*Address all correspondence to: bs.nanthini@gmail.com

References

[1] Meier R, Dittrich H, Schulze-Bonhage A, Aertsen AD. Detecting epileptic seizures in long-term human EEG: A new approach to automatic online and real-time detection and classification of polymorphic seizure patterns. Journal of Clinical Neurophysiology. 2008;**25**(3)

[2] Padhy NP, Simon SP. Soft Computing with MATLAB Programming. New Delhi, India: Oxford University Press; 2015

[3] Suguna Nanthini B. EEG signal analysis for automated epileptic seizure detection using soft computing techniques [thesis]. Thanjavur: SASTRA University; 2017

[4] Misra UK, Kalita J. Clinical Electroencephalography. New Delhi, India: Reed Elsevier India Private Limited; 2005

[5] Bajaj V, Pachori RB. Classification of seizure and non seizure EEG signals using empirical mode decomposition. IEEE Transactions on information in Biomedicine. 2012;**16**(6)

[6] Mommone N, Morabito FC. Enhanced automatic artifact detection based on independent component analysis and Renyi's entropy. Neural Networks. 2008;**21**:1029-1040

[7] Han L, Embrechts MJ, Szymanski B. Sigma tuning of Gaussian Kernels: Detection of ischemia from magneto cardiograms. In: Computational Modeling and Simulation of Intellect: Current State and Future Perspective. IGI Global; 2011. pp. 206-223

[8] Ramgopal S, Souza ST, Jackson M, Kadish NE, Fernandez IS, Klehm J, et al. Seizure detection, seizure prediction and closed loop warning system in epilepsy. Epilepsy & Behavior. 2014;**37**:291-302

[9] Nanthini BS, Santhi B. Qualitative diagnostic criteria into objective quantitative signal feature classification. Journal of Theoretical and Applied Information Technolody. 2012;**42**:94-99

[10] Nanthini BS, Santhi B. Seizure detection using SVM classifier on EEG signal. Journal of Applied Sciences. 2014;**14**:1658-1661

[11] Nanthini BS, Santhi B. EEG signal classification and segmentation for automated epileptic seizure detection using SVM classifier. Research Journal of Pharmaceutical, Biological and Chemical Sciences. 2016;**7**:1231-1238

[12] Nanthini BS, Santhi B. Different approaches of analysing EEG signals for seizure detection. International Journal of signal and Imaging systems Engineering. 2015;**8**:28-38

[13] Nanthini BS, Santhi B. EEG signal classification through entropy measurements for seizure detection using soft computing techniques. International Journal of Pharmacy & Technology. 2016;**8**(4):21847-21858

[14] Nanthini BS, Santhi B. Electroencephalogram signal classification for automated epileptic seizure detection using genetic algorithm. Journal of Natural Science, Biology and Medicine. 2017;**8**:159-166